Contemporary Internal Medicine

Clinical Case Studies

Volume 3

Contemporary Internal Medicine

Clinical Case Studies

A collection of cases from The Ohio State University Hospitals discussed by faculty of the Department of Internal Medicine

Volume 3

Edited by

Juan M. Bowen, M.D., and Ernest L. Mazzaferri, M.D.

The Ohio State University
Columbus, Ohio

PLENUM MEDICAL BOOK COMPANY
NEW YORK AND LONDON

The Library of Congress cataloged the first volume of this series as follows:

Contemporary internal medicine.

Includes bibliographies and index.
1. Internal medicine—Case studies. I. Bowen, Juan. II. Mazzaferri, Ernest L.,
1936 –   . [DNLM: 1. Internal Medicine—case studies. WB 115 C761]
RC66.C66   1988   616.09   88-22379

ISBN 0-306-43684-1

© 1991 Plenum Publishing Corporation
233 Spring Street, New York, N.Y. 10013

Plenum Medical Book Company is an imprint of Plenum Publishing Corporation

Printed in the United States of America

This volume is dedicated to our patients,
who continue to enrich our lives with questions,
as well as with answers.

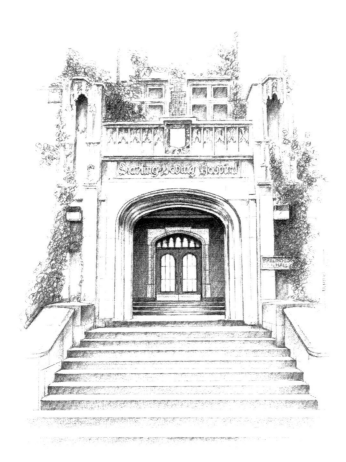

Starling-Loving Hall
By Robert L. Hummel

Contributors

JAMES BACON, MD, Clinical Assistant Professor of Medicine, The Ohio State University, Columbus, Ohio

LORRAINE M. BIRSKOVICH, MD, Assistant Professor of Clinical Medicine, The Ohio State University, Columbus, Ohio

HARISIOS BOUDOULAS, MD, Professor of Medicine, The Ohio State University, Columbus, Ohio

DAN CARUSO, MD, Assistant Professor of Clinical Medicine, The Ohio State University, Columbus, Ohio

SAMUEL CATALAND, MD, Professor of Medicine, The Ohio State University, Columbus, Ohio

DARYL A. COTTRELL, MD, Assistant Professor of Clinical Medicine, The Ohio State University, Columbus, Ohio

LORETTA S. DAVIS, MD, Assistant Professor of Clinical Medicine, The Ohio State University, Columbus, Ohio

JOHN J. FROMKES, MD, Associate Professor of Medicine, Director of Gastroenterology, The Ohio State University, Columbus, Ohio

JOHN S. HEINTZ, MD, Assistant Professor of Clinical Medicine, The Ohio State University, Columbus, Ohio

N. PAUL HUDSON, MD, Associate Professor of Clinical Medicine, The Ohio State University, Columbus, Ohio

SETH M. KANTOR, MD, Associate Professor of Clinical Medicine, The Ohio State University, Columbus, Ohio

GARY C. KINDT, MD, Assistant Professor of Medicine, The Ohio State University, Columbus, Ohio

CYNTHIA G. KREGER, MD, Assistant Professor of Clinical Medicine, The Ohio State University, Columbus, Ohio

ANDREW LIBERTIN, MD, Assistant Professor of Clinical Medicine, The Ohio State University, Columbus, Ohio

CHARLES LOVE, MD, Assistant Professor of Clinical Medicine, The Ohio State University, Columbus, Ohio

ERNEST L. MAZZAFERRI, MD, FACP, Chairman, Department of Internal Medicine, Professor of Medicine and Physiology, The Ohio State University, Columbus, Ohio

EARL N. METZ, MD, FACP, Vice Chairman, Department of Internal Medicine, Charles A. Doan Professor of Medicine, The Ohio State University, Columbus, Ohio

SCOTT MILLER, MD, Assistant Professor of Clinical Medicine, The Ohio State University, Columbus, Ohio

DOUGLAS MYERS, MD, Assistant Professor of Clinical Medicine, The Ohio State University, Columbus, Ohio

THOMAS M. O'DORISIO, MD, Professor of Medicine, Director of Endocrinology, The Ohio State University, Columbus, Ohio

KWAME OSEI, MD Associate Professor of Medicine, The Ohio State University, Columbus, Ohio

BHASKAR RAO, MD, FACP, Associate Professor of Clinical Medicine, The Ohio State University, Columbus, Ohio

JAMES M. RYAN, MD, FACP, Assistant Professor of Medicine, Director of Nuclear Cardiology, The Ohio State University, Columbus, Ohio

EDITH DE LOS SANTOS, MD, Assistant Professor of Clinical Medicine, The Ohio State University, Columbus, Ohio

DAVID B. THOMAS, MD, Assistant Professor of Clinical Medicine, The Ohio State University, Columbus, Ohio

FRED THOMAS, MD, Professor of Medicine, The Ohio State University, Columbus, Ohio

DONALD E. THORNTON, MD, Assistant Professor of Clinical Medicine, The Ohio State University, Columbus, Ohio

JEFFREY E. WEILAND, MD, Associate Professor of Clinical Medicine, The Ohio State University, Columbus, Ohio

JONATHAN K. WILKIN, MD, FACP, FAAD, Professor of Medicine, Director of Dermatology, The Ohio State University, Columbus, Ohio

CHARLES F. WOOLEY, MD, Professor of Medicine, The Ohio State University, Columbus, Ohio

JEFFREY P. YORK, MD, Assistant Professor of Surgery, The Ohio State University, Columbus, Ohio

Preface to Volume 1

Read with two objectives: first, to acquaint yourself with the current knowledge of a subject and the steps by which it has been reached; and secondly, and more important, read to understand and analyze your cases.

William Osler, The Student Life

What follows is a collection of cases — or more aptly, the stories of our patients and friends who have been seen at The Ohio State University Hospitals where our faculty have provided their care and about whom this volume is written. Today many fear that our patients are being moved from center stage while we are being distracted by the technology of medicine. This volume was written with patients in mind. The idea is that the most intriguing questions and the most rewarding answers begin and end at the bedside. This is a story of our patients, told by expert clinicians and spiced with commentary along the way. This volume in no way attempts to be comprehensive. Instead, it is like the practice of medicine, scattered, somewhat disjointed, while at the same time intensely personal and focused upon whatever problem the patient brings to us. The discussions are not so much about disease entities as they are about patients with problems. The two are uniquely different. For instance, when the physician suspects hepatitis, not every imaginable cause can be actively investigated. Instead, tests and procedures are discriminately chosen, a part of medicine that is still more art than science. The cases presented in this book are discussed in a format that shows the art of medicine in a framework of science. In all, 25 cases, both the common and the unusual, are presented. Each is summarized with the author's comments, which emphasize the important historical features and salient physical diagnostic points. This is followed by a discussion of the contemporary issues, including pathophysiology, diagnosis, treatment, and prognosis, as they relate to the patient's case. References selected are those which the author considers best or most important recent citations on the subject. This is the first in a series of volumes that will present our most interesting and challenging patients in a case study format. We hope the practicing clinician will find this book useful.

Juan M. Bowen, MD
Ernest L. Mazzaferri, MD, FACP

Preface

In the previous two volumes of this series, we presented classic problems in internal medicine as illustrated by actual cases cared for in our institution. It has been gratifying for us to see the interest that these volumes have generated with students and trainees. We remain committed to the case method of instruction, and believe that there is no better method to learn medicine than to have an individual patient problem as the basis for study of pathophysiology, natural history, diagnosis and management. We hope that our readers find this third volume as enjoyable and instructive as the editors found it.

Juan M. Bowen, MD
Ernest L. Mazzaferri, MD, FACP

Acknowledgement

The editors are grateful to Jeff Smith and Jenny Riegler for their unflagging professionalism and patience.

Contents

This case reviews the extensive differential diagnosis and appropriate management of an important cardiovascular problem.

Recent advances in the understanding of the pathophysiology and treatment of asthma are illustrated in the base discussion of the case.

The special significance of hypertension in the diabetic is presented by two workers in the field of diabetes.

Hypothyroidism — an extremely common problem, hypothyroidism remains a challenge to both primary physicians and consultants.

Patients with leukemia who develop skin lesions provide a diagnostic challenge which is often of an urgent nature.

Thyrotoxicosis, one of the classic problems in internal medicine, still presents diagnostic and management dilemmas.

An expert presents the differential diagnosis and management strategy of flushing disorders.

Recent technological and pharmacologic advances are reviewed by an expert in cardiac rhythm disorders.

One of the classic diseases of the elderly is discussed by an expert.

Diagnostic strategies for the evaluation of chest pain and the management of postinfarction patients are reviewed.

The distinction between Crohn's disease and ulcerative colitis is emphasized with an illustrative case.

Current understanding and pathophysiology, diagnosis and management of this common but treacherous disease are presented.

Case 1

Mitral Regurgitation – Chronic Versus Acute: Implications for Timing of Surgery

Harisios Boudoulas, MD and Charles F. Wooley, MD

Normal mitral valve closure is a complex mechanism resulting from a combination of atrial and ventricular events. Effective systolic sealing of the mitral valve depends on proper function, size, position, motion, and integrity of the mitral leaflets, chordae tendineae, papillary muscles, and mitral valve annulus in the presence of a normal left atrium (LA) and a normal left ventricle (LV). Mitral regurgitation (MR) occurs when mitral valve closure is ineffective.

Etiology

Acute or chronic abnormalities of the mitral valve apparatus may lead to MR. In the past rheumatic heart disease was reported to be the most common cause of chronic MR. More recently mitral valve prolapse (MVP) resulting from a floppy mitral valve has become the most frequent cause of MR necessitating surgery in the Western world.[1,2]

Rupture of chordae tendineae is the most common cause of acute MR. Papillary muscle rupture and infective endocarditis may also cause severe acute MR.[3-9] The most common causes of acute and chronic MR are summarized in Table 1. The management and indications for surgical intervention are different in acute versus chronic MR. Two representative case presentations will emphasize the clinically significant differences between acute and chronic MR.

Chronic Mitral Regurgitation

Case Presentation

A graphic presentation of the patient's history is shown in Fig. 1.

A 55-year-old white male had mitral valve reconstructive surgery in May 1989. His cardiac history began in 1975 when he had an abnormal stress electrocardiogram as a part of a routine evaluation for employment. A cardiac catheterization

Table 1

Common Causes of Mitral Regurgitation

Chronic
- Mitral valve prolapse associated with floppy mitral valve – isolated or a part of recognized connective tissue disorder syndromes (e.g. Marfan syndrome, Ehlers-Danlos syndrome)
- Rheumatic carditis
- Mitral annular calcification
- Coronary artery disease
- Dilated cardiomyopathy
- Hypertrophic cardiomyopathy
- Congenital

Acute
- Severe papillary muscle ischemia or rupture
- Infective endocarditis
- Chordae tendineae rupture

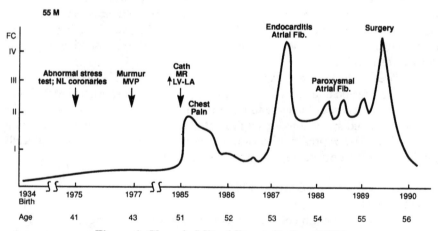

Figure 1. Chronic Mitral Regurgitation: MVP

Natural history of a patient with mitral valve prolapse (MVP) and chronic mitral regurgitation (MR). Note the long natural history. NL normal; cath, cardiac catheterization; LV, left ventricle; LA, left atrium; Fib, fibrillation; M, male.

was performed which was reported "normal" at that time. He remained asymptomatic.

In 1977 a "new" murmur was noted on a routine examination and was attributed to MVP. He developed chest pain in 1985 and presented for the first time to The Ohio State University Hospitals (OSUH) for further evaluation. Cardiac catheterization was performed which revealed normal coronary artery anatomy, increased LV and LA size, normal LV systolic function, MVP with a floppy mitral valve and

Table 2

Chronic Mitral Regurgitation Hemodynamic Data		
	1985	**1989**
RA pressure (mm Hg)		
Mean	5	10
A	5	9
V	9	14
Pulmonary artery pressure (mm Hg)		
Systolic	45	36
Diastolic	20	17
PCW pressure (mm Hg)		
Mean	18	14
A	18	10
V	35	20
LV pressure (mm Hg)		
Systolic	110	124
Diastolic	16	10
Aortic pressure (mmHg)		
Systolic	110	124
Diastolic	65	76
CI (l per min/BSA, green dye)	4.10	4.39
LV-EDVI (cm^3/BSA)	182	220
LV-ESVI (cm^3/BSA)	70	75
LV ejection fraction (%)	62	66
CI (l per min/BSA, angiographic)	7.84	11.01
Regurgitant fraction (%)	48	60
LV end-systolic stress (kdynes/cm^2)	140	165
End-systolic stress/LV-ESVI	2.0	2.2

RA, right atrium; PCW pulmonary capillary wedge; LV, left ventricular; CI, cardiac index, EDVI, end-diastolic volume index, ESVI, end-systolic volume index; BSA, body surface area.

severe MR. Cardiac catheterization data are shown in Table 2. A radionuclide exercise test demonstrated good exercise tolerance, a resting ejection fraction of 58% which increased to 72% with exercise.

In November 1986 the patient developed "flu-like" symptoms (chills, dry cough, myalgias, anorexia). He was treated in December 1986 with oral erythromycin without improvement. In January 1987 he reported having nightly fever up to 102°F, nightly sweats and palpitations. He denied dyspnea, orthopnea, paroxysmal nocturnal dyspnea, or edema. Dental procedures had been performed in October 1986 with oral antibiotic prophylaxis prior to the dental work.

He returned to the OSUH for further evaluation and therapy. The diagnosis of infectious endocarditis was confirmed when blood cultures were positive for Streptococcus sanguis, and he received a 6-week course of intravenous antibiotics. At the time of admission his rhythm was atrial fibrillation with rapid ventricular response. Digitalis therapy was associated with conversion to sinus rhythm. An echocardiogram demonstrated a redundant mitral valve with vegetations on the atrial surface of the posterior mitral valve leaflet. He was maintained on digitalis therapy and discharged. He returned to full-time work as an executive vice-president of a local company. Between January 1987 and February 1989 he had two episodes of atrial fibrillation for which he came to the emergency department of the OSUH. The first episode converted spontaneously without additional therapy. After the second episode of atrial fibrillation, therapy with quinidine was initiated.

In April 1989 the patient had another episode of atrial fibrillation which was associated with mild shortness of breath and he was admitted to the hospital for two days. The physical examination during this admission revealed a pleasant 55-year-old man in no distress. His height and arm span were 72", with an upper segment to lower segment ratio of 0.92. His blood pressure was 120/80 and his heart rate was 84 beats/min and irregular. The jugular venous pressure was normal with slightly increased V wave. The carotid pulse was brisk (Fig. 2). The cardiac apex was in the sixth intercostal space at the mid-clavicular line; it was sustained and diffusely enlarged (Fig. 3). A loud grade IV-V/VI apical systolic murmur masked the first heart sound and radiated to the left axilla and left sternal border. An LV S3 gallop was present (Fig. 2 and 3). A soft murmur of tricuspid regurgitation was heard at the lower left sternal border and was increased in intensity with inspiration. The lungs were clear, and there was no peripheral edema or hepatosplenomegaly. The electrocardiogram on admission showed atrial fibrillation, increased precordial voltage, and ST&T wave changes to which digitalis and quinidine may add (Fig. 4). At the time of discharge the electrocardiogram showed sinus rhythm (Fig. 4). The chest x-ray showed slightly increased cardiac size with clear lung fields (Fig. 5).

The echocardiogram demonstrated increased LV and LA size, MVP and a voluminous and redundant mitral valve (Fig. 6). Doppler and color Doppler echocardiography demonstrated severe MR (Fig. 7). Because of the frequency of

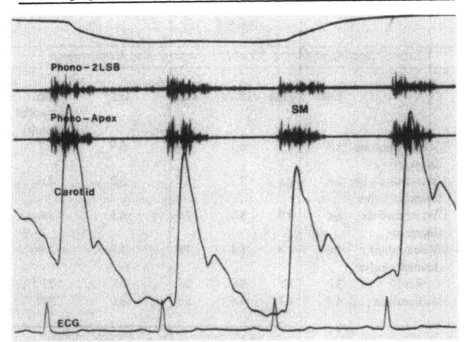

Figure 2

Phonocardiogram (phono) obtained from the second intercostal space left sternal border (2LSB) and from the cardiac (apex), carotid arterial pulse (carotid), and electrocardiogram (ECG). Note the holosystolic murmur (SM) and the rapid carotid upstroke.

the episodes of paroxysmal atrial fibrillation and progressive LV and LA enlargement, mitral valve surgery was recommended.

Cardiac catheterization performed prior to surgery demonstrated large LV and LA size, floppy mitral valve, and severe MR (Fig. 8). The coronary arteries were normal. A patent foramen ovale with a small left-to-right shunt was also demonstrated. The hemodynamic findings are summarized in Table 2. Reconstructive mitral valve surgery and closure of the atrial septal defect were performed. The mitral valve reconstruction included chordal repair and use of annuloplasty ring. Doppler and color Doppler echocardiography were used during the operation to assess surgical results. Postoperative atrial arrhythmias were treated medically. He was discharged with digitalis and quinidine.

Six months after the operation (December 1989) he was asymptomatic. Physical examination included normal jugular venous pressure, clear lungs, and no peripheral edema. The first heart sound was decreased in intensity with normal splitting of the second heart sound and no murmurs in any body position (Fig. 9).

Table 3

Chronic Mitral Regurgitation: Serial Echocardiographic Measurements						
	1985	**1986**	**1987**	**1988**	**1989**	**1989** (6 months postop)
LV end-diastolic diameter	5.7	5.7	6.1	6.0	6.8	5.7
LV end-diastolic diameter index	2.6	2.6	2.7	2.7	3.0	2.6
LV end-systolic diameter	3.6	3.9	4.0	4.3	4.3	3.6
LV end-systolic diameter index	1.6	1.8	1.8	1.9	1.9	1.6
%Δ D	37	32	34	28	37	37
LA diameter	4.7	4.7	4.6	5.5	6.0	5.1

LV, left ventricular, %ΔD, % fractional shortening of the LV internal diameter, LA, left atrial.

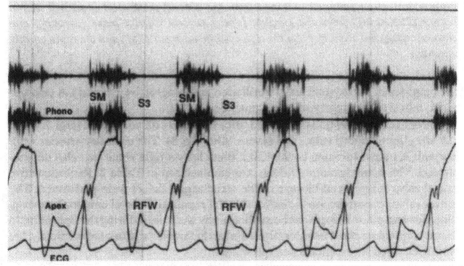

Figure 3

Phonocardiogram recorded at cardiac apex (phono), apex cardiogram (apex), and electrocardiogram (ECG). The apex impulse is sustained with an exaggerated rapid filling wave (RFW). An S3 gallop (S3) which coincides with the RFW was also recorded on the phono.

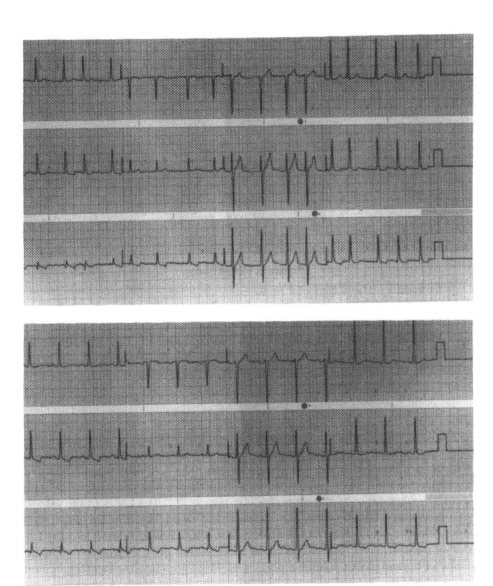

Figure 4
Upper panel: Atrial fibrillation with ST and T wave changes especially in the inferolateral leads. Lower panel: Sinus rhythm with ST and T wave changes in the inferolateral leads.

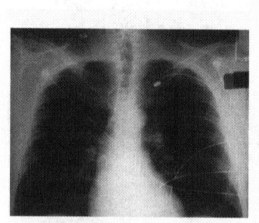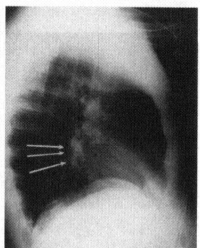

Figure 5. Chest X-ray
Note mild cardiomegaly with clear lung fields. Left atrial enlargement is also seen in the lateral view (arrow).

The echocardiogram demonstrated increased LV and LA size and thickened mitral valve; there was no MVP (Fig. 10). Doppler echocardiogram demonstrated trivial MR and trivial tricuspid regurgitation. Serial echocardiographic measurements are shown in Table 3.

Pathophysiology

Clinical progression in patients with chronic MR is usually gradual permitting adaptative compensatory mechanisms.[1,6] During ventricular systole, part of LV volume is ejected into the low- pressure LA. The LA dilates gradually and accommodates this extra volume load; as a result there is only minimal or moderate increase in LA pressure during ventricular systole.[10-12] The LV diastolic volume also increases gradually, since in addition to the blood flow from the pulmonary veins, blood ejected into the LA during ventricular systole returns into the LV during diastole. As a result of this gradual dilatation the LV ejects two or more times its normal stroke volume a portion of which goes into the LA (regurgitant volume).

Figure 6. Echocardiogram Apical Four-Chamber View
Upper: note marked thickening of the mitral valve (MV). Lower: note mitral valve prolapse (MVP). LV, left ventricle; LA, left atrium.

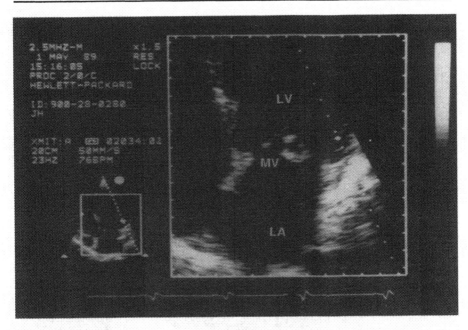

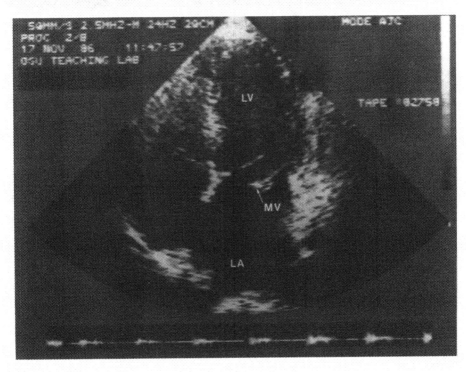

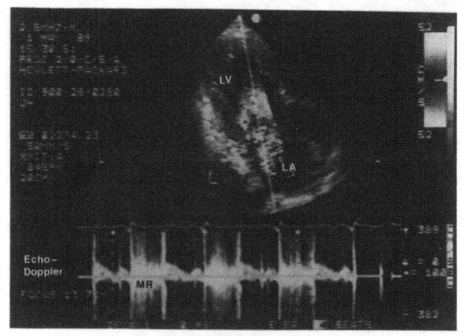

Figure 7. Doppler Echocardiogram
Mitral regurgitation (MR) is shown. LV, left ventricle; LA, left atrium.

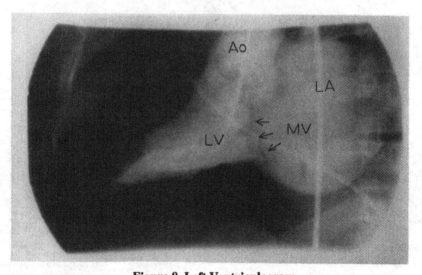

Figure 8. Left Ventriculogram
Note the large left atrial (LA) size. Mitral valve (MV) thickening is also shown. LV, left ventricle; Ao, aorta.

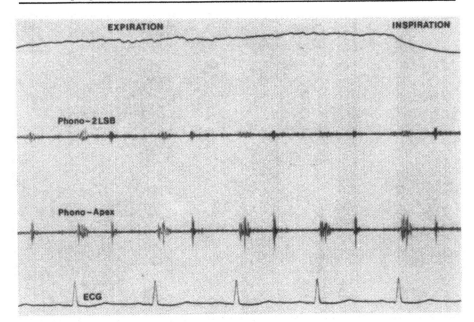

Figure 9

Phonocardiogram obtained from the second intercostal space (phono-2LSB) and from the cardiac apex (phono apex) simultaneously with electrocardiogram (ECG) six months after surgery. Note the absence of heart murmur. (Compare with the phono before surgery in Fig. 2.)

Chronic LV and LA dilatation result in increased diastolic compliance of these chambers. Thus, the LV diastolic and LA systolic and diastolic pressures remain relatively normal despite the large volumes.

Since the LV ejects blood into the low-pressure LA in addition to that ejected into the aorta, LV ejection is rapid and brief with a supernormal ejection fraction prior to the development of LA and LV muscle dysfunction. Since LV diastolic and LA pressures are relatively normal, there is little or no pulmonary congestion; the patient often complains of fatigue rather than dyspnea on exertion (Fig. 11).

Diagnostic Evaluation

Physical Findings. Patients with chronic MR have physical findings that are related to the severity of MR and to underlying etiology of the disorder.

MVP is a very common cause of chronic MR. Since MVP represents a spectrum of mitral valve disease and may be progressive, the physical findings in patients with MVP depend on the degree of mitral valve dysfunction. Early in the course of the disease a mitral nonejection click may be present; as the mitral valve abnormality

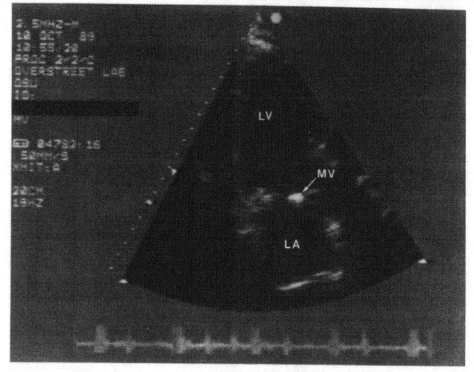

Figure 10
*Echocardiogram obtained six months after surgery: thickening of the mitral valve is
still present; mitral valve prolapse, however, is not seen. LV, left ventricle; LA, left
atrium; MV, mitral valve.*

progresses a late systolic murmur with or without click, and later a holosystolic
murmur may be heard[1] (Fig. 12).

The case presentation (Fig. 1) summarized the physical findings for patients with
chronic MR. For completeness, the physical findings in patients with chronic and
significant MR are described briefly.

The arterial pulse is brisk but the amplitude is usually low.

Abnormalities of the jugular venous pressure become apparent late in the
disease; an exaggerated A wave may be present when right ventricular dysfunction
develops. The presence of accompanying tricuspid regurgitation may be reflected
by a systolic V wave and high jugular venous pressure.

The apex impulse may be displaced to the sixth intercostal space and laterally
in patients with LV enlargement; the apex impulse may be hyperdynamic, diffuse,
and sustained. A parasternal lift may be present which reflects systolic LA expan-

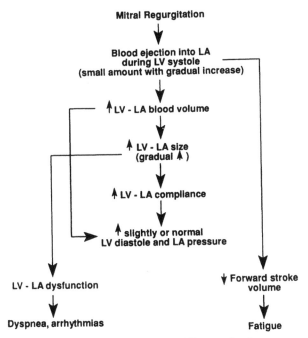

Figure 11. Chronic Mitral Regurgitation

Pathophysiologic mechanisms. Schematic presentation. LA, left atrium, LV, left ventricle; ↑, increase; ↓, decrease.

sion from the regurgitant volume into the LA. This should be distinguished from the parasternal lift present in patients with right ventricular enlargement.[13]

The characteristic auscultatory findings include a high-frequency holosystolic murmur beginning with the first heart sound. The intensity of the murmur is usually constant through systole and does not change with respiration; the murmur is best heard at the apex and radiates to the axilla. The intensity of the first heart sound is usually diminished.[13] Because of the abbreviation of the duration of systole, premature closure of the aortic valve may occur and results in wide splitting of the second heart sound. A ventricular (S3) gallop is audible at the apex. As a general rule, if the S3 gallop is accompanied by a loud MR murmur, ventricular function may be preserved, but if the ventricular gallop is accompanied by a soft murmur,

MVP: DYNAMIC SPECTRUM & NATURAL PROGRESSION

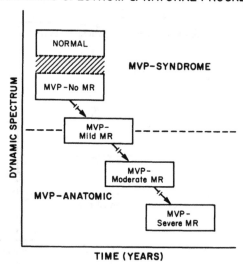

Chronic Mitral Regurgitation (MR):
Natural History - Precipitating Factors

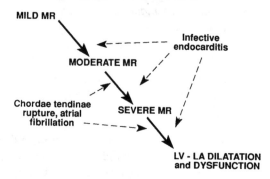

Figure 12

Upper panel: The dynamic spectrum, time in years, and the progression of mitral valve prolapse (MVP) are shown. A subtle gradation (cross-hatched area) exists between the normal mitral vavle and valves that produce mild MVP without mitral regurgitation (No MR). Progression from the level MVP (No MR) to another level may or may not occur. (From Boudoulas and Wooley[1] with permission.) Lower Panel: Natural history and precipitating factors in chronic MR. Schematic presentation. LV, left ventricle: LA, left atrium.

LV dysfunction is usually present. An apical diastolic mitral rumble may be present, reflecting the large blood volume flowing through the mitral valve early in diastole.

Laboratory Findings. When sinus rhythm is present the electrocardiogram may show abnormal P waves consistent with LA involvement; findings consistent with LV enlargement may also be present. The chest x-ray in patients with MVP and connective tissue disorders may show scoliosis, pectus excavatum, and straight back.[1] Cardiomegaly with LV and LA enlargement occur later in the course of the disease. The pulmonary vasculature is usually normal until late, when venous pulmonary hypertension may develop.

Echocardiography may show MVP and a thickened mitral valve; later in the disease it may show LV and LA enlargement, chordae tendineae rupture or flail mitral valve leaflet may be present.[1] Doppler and color Doppler echocardiography will show MR which is mild early and severe later in the course of the disease.[1,14]

Exercise radionuclide angiography provides information about ventricular function at rest and during exercise.

Cardiac catheterization provides valuable diagnostic and prognostic information, particularly before decisions about intensive medical therapy or surgical intervention. Cardiac output, LV pressures at rest and during exercise, intracardiac shunt detection, severity of MR, regurgitant fraction, and coronary anatomy are important determinants. Left ventricular wall stress can be approximated by the Laplace relationship. Stress $= P \times r \, 4/2h$, where P = LV pressure, r = LV radius, and h = LV wall thickness.[12] LV wall radius and thickness can be calculated from left ventriculogram or the echocardiogram.

Natural History

The natural history of chronic MR depends on the etiology. As a general rule, MR progresses gradually. Factors which accelerate the natural course of MR include infectious endocarditis, the development of atrial fibrillation, chordae tendineae rupture, LA and LV dysfunction (Fig. 12).

Since MVP is the most common cause of significant MR which requires surgical intervention in the Western world, the natural history of MVP will be described briefly.

Symptoms and serious complications related to mitral valve dysfunction in patients with MVP include infectious endocarditis, progressive MR that requires medical therapy or mitral valve surgery, ruptured chordae tendineae, thromboembolic phenomena, serious supraventricular or ventricular arrhythmias, atrioventricular conduction defects, congestive heart failure, and death. As a general rule, complications related to MVP increase with age.[1,6,15,16]

To date there are few prospective long-term follow-up studies in adult patients with MVP. Duren et al[17] reported the results of a long-term prospective follow-up study in 300 patients with MVP diagnosed by clinical, cineangiographic, and echocardiographic criteria. All patients had auscultatory findings consistent with

MVP. The ages ranged from 10 to 87 years (mean 42.2 years). The study included all patients with MVP irrespective of clinical condition at the onset, with an average follow-up period of 6.1 years.

The clinical condition remained stable in 153 patients. Twenty-seven of the 153 patients developed supraventricular tachycardia that was controlled with medications; 20 patients developed signs of MR but remained clinically asymptomatic.

Serious complications developed in 100 patients. Sudden death occurred in three, ventricular fibrillation in two, ventricular tachycardia in 56, and infective endocarditis in 18. Twenty-eight patients had mitral valve surgery because of progressive MR; an additional eight patients with severe MR were considered surgical candidates. Eleven patients had cerebrovascular accidents. Although the study population may not be representative for the entire MVP population, the results strongly support the concept that MVP may be associated with significant morbidity and mortality.

Nishimura et al[18] determined prognosis in a prospective (mean 6.2 years) follow-up study in 237 minimally symptomatic or asymptomatic patients with MVP documented by echocardiography. The average age was 44 years (range 10 to 69 years). Sudden death occurred in six patients. In multivariable analysis of echocardiographic factors, the presence or absence of redundant mitral valve leaflets (present in 97 patients) emerged as the only variable associated with sudden death. Ten patients sustained a cerebral embolic event; one had an LV aneurysm with apical thrombus, one had infective endocarditis, six were in atrial fibrillation with LA enlargement, and two were in sinus rhythm. Infective endocarditis occurred in three patients. Progressive MR prompted valve replacement in 17 patients. The LV end-diastolic diameter exceeding 60 mm was the best echocardiographic predictor of the subsequent need for mitral valve replacement. Twenty patients had no clinical auscultatory findings of a systolic click or murmur; none of these patients had any complications during follow-up. The authors concluded that while most patients with echocardiographic evidence of MVP have a benign course, subsets of patients can be identified by echocardiography that are at high risk for the development of progressive MR, sudden death, cerebral embolic events, or infective endocarditis.

Marks et al[19] confirmed Nishimura's data in a retrospective study. Clinical and two-dimensional echocardiographic data from 456 patients with MVP were analyzed. Two groups of patients were compared: those with thickening of the mitral valve leaflet and redundancy and those without leaflet thickening. Complications, or a history of complications (i.e. infective endocarditis, MR, and the need for mitral valve replacement), were more prevalent in those with leaflet thickening and redundancy compared to those without leaflet thickening. The incidence of stroke, however, was similar in the two groups.

Kolibash et al[15] reported the natural history in 86 patients who presented with severe MR. Eighty patients had a preexisting heart murmur first detected at an average age of 34. Patients remained asymptomatic for an average of 25 years before clinical symptoms first appeared. After significant symptoms developed, mitral valve surgery was necessary in most of the patients within 1 year. This rapid deterioration could generally be attributed to chordal rupture or the development of atrial fibrillation. Twenty-eight patients had serial evaluations; these serial studies demonstrated progressive MR, cardiomegaly, and LA enlargement. From this study, it is apparent that a subset of patients with MVP will develop progressive, severe MR.

These long-term follow-up studies in patients with MVP associated with a floppy, myxomatous mitral valve permit several conclusions: (1) serious complications do occur in patients with MVP, (2) MVP patients constitute a non-homogeneous population, (3) complications are directly related to the specific subset of MVP patients included in the study, (4) complications in patients with MVP appear to occur primarily in patients with diagnostic auscultatory findings, and (5) redundant mitral valve leaflets and increased LV size in patients with MVP are associated with a high frequency of serious complications.

The possibility that a patient with MVP will require mitral valve surgery increases with age[7,15,16] (Fig. 13). Male MVP patients required mitral valve surgery more often than did female patients with MVP.

Natural History of Causes of Chronic MR Other Than MVP

Chronic MR may occur in the presence of abnormalities such as dilated cardiomyopathy, hypertrophic cardiomyopathy, rheumatic heart disease, and coronary artery disease[2,20-22] (Table 1). The natural history in these situations depends on the natural history of the underlying disease. The natural course of rheumatic MR associated with mitral stenosis usually is gradual. Certain patients, however, with postinflammatory MR secondary to rheumatic fever develop acute or subacute MR which require early surgical intervention. To date, such reports have come primarily from South Africa and Japan.[4]

MR is present in approximately 20% of patients with coronary artery disease; moderate to severe MR, however, is present in only a small percentage of patients with coronary artery disease.[22] Increasing severity of MR has a progressive negative impact on survival regardless of treatment.

MR is frequent in dilated cardiomyopathy and may contribute to the poor prognosis in this group of patients.[2]

Timing for Surgery

The timing of surgery for MR, particularly in the asymptomatic or mildly symptomatic patient, may be a difficult decision.[12,23] Preservation of LA and LV function are important considerations. If LV dysfunction is mild and contractile reserve still exists, patients will generally experience relief of symptoms or limitations with only a mild fall in LV ejection performance. If LV dysfunction has

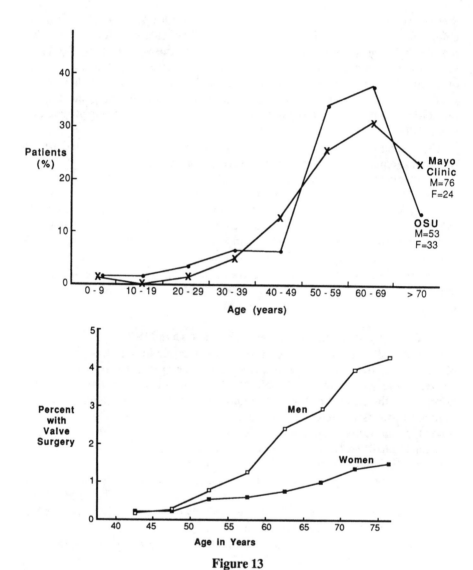

Figure 13

Upper panel: Mitral valve surgery for mitral regurgitation secondary to MVP in relation to age. Data from the Ohio State University (OSU) and Mayo Clinic. (Figure constructed from Refs. 7 and 15). Lower panel: Estimated lifetime risk of mitral valve surgery by age and sex among cohorts diagnosed as having MVP. Age-specific events were calculated from the State of New South Wales, Australia. (From Wilcken and Hickery[16] with permission.) M; male: F, female.

Table 4

Predictors for Suboptimal Response to Mitral Valve Replacement in Patients with Chronic Mitral Regurgitation

---

LV end-diastolic diameter index	$>$ 4.0 cm/m^2
LV end-systolic diameter index	$>$ 2.6 cm/m^2
LV end-diastolic volume index	$>$ 220 cm^3/m^2
LV end-systolic volume index	$>$ 75 cm^3/m^2
LV ejection fraction	$<$ 55%
%ΔD	$<$ 32%
End-systolic stress/end-systolic volume index	$<$ 2.4

LV, left ventricular; %ΔD, % fractional shortening of the LV internal diameter.

become severe, surgery may be associated with a severe fall in ejection performance, persistence of symptoms, and even death from congestive heart failure. Thus, the ideal timing for mitral valve surgery is at the onset of LV dysfunction, when good surgical results should be expected.

Proper timing of mitral valve surgery requires recognition of LV dysfunction before it has become severe. Unfortunately, the clinical evaluation of LV function has been difficult in MR because the lesion causes significant alterations in loading conditions. Indeed in MR, increased preload with decreased afterload results in an augmentation of the ejection performance with a supernormal ejection fraction.[12,24] Good postoperative results have been reported when % shortening of the LV internal diameter (%ΔD) is greater than 32%. Once %ΔD or ejection fraction has fallen into the low normal range, a severe postoperative fall in ejection performance may occur. Thus, preoperative ejection fraction may not be a good predictor of postoperative ejection fraction, but when the ejection fraction is frankly subnormal survival is greatly reduced. Values of LV ejection fraction and end-systolic indexes, which may define patients with poor outlook for benefit from surgery, are: LV ejection fraction $<$ 55%; end-systolic diameter index $>$ 2.5 cm/m^2; end-systolic volume index $>$ 60 mg/m^2; and end-systolic stress/end-systolic volume index $<$ 2.4 (Table 4).[12,24] These are only guidelines and no single value can be used exclusively in deciding when to perform mitral valve surgery. This decision must be made with comprehensive knowledge of the individual patient's natural history, individual indicators of LV function, and the evolving state of mitral valve surgery for MR.

Development of symptoms in chronic MR usually coincides with onset of LV dysfunction. As such, even mild symptoms are probably significant. If symptoms

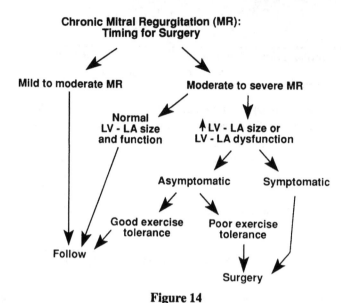

Figure 14

Timing for surgery in patients with chronic MR, based on left ventricular (LV) and left atrial (LA) size and function and exercise tolerance.

are present and ventricular function has begun to decline, surgery should be considered. A question often asked is "how should I manage the asymptomatic patient who is beginning to show signs of LV dysfunction by physical or echocardiographic examination?" It is difficult to recommend surgery for a truly asymptomatic patient. The guidelines for operative intervention, based in part on signs of developing LV dysfunction, are not perfect predictors of outcome. Thus, a poor outcome could occur despite favorable preoperative indexes. Some patients who claim to be asymptomatic have in fact limited their activities to avoid symptoms. In most instances an exercise tolerance test will help delineate normal or reduced exercise tolerance.[25] The patient who is truly asymptomatic, who has normal exercise tolerance in an objective evaluation, and who is beginning to show signs of LV dysfunction by echocardiography requires very close follow-up. If symptoms intervene, LV function continues to worsen or response to medical therapy is limited, mitral valve surgery should be considered (Fig. 14).

Mitral Valve Replacement Versus Reconstructive Surgery

Papillary muscle integrity plays a major role in normal ventricular contraction.[11,12] Removal of the chordae tendineae affects the role of the papillary muscles and decreases overall ventricular performance. Recent studies suggest that mitral valve repair or replacement with chordae tendineae left intact helps preserve postoperative LV function. Mitral valve repair has the advantage of leaving the patient with a native mitral valve instead of a prosthesis, eliminating certain complications associated with prosthetic valve.[8,23,26-28]

The optimal timing for mitral valve surgery has been changing with the evolution of reparative mitral valve surgery with preservation of the papillary muscle complex. The clinician may be inclined to proceed with surgery earlier to preserve LV function when there is a high probability of a mitral reparative procedure rather than a replacement procedure.

Experience with mitral valve repair suggests that localized valve pathology without extensive calcification lends itself to mitral valve repair. Mitral valve replacement, with preservation of at least the posterior papillary muscle, should be performed in those patients with a greatly dilated annulus or severe valve dysfunction, particularly those with extreme calcification. Recent techniques, however, allow reconstructive surgery even in patients with massive mitral annular dilatation. Mitral valve reconstruction in experienced hands appears to be widely applicable with potential for fewer complications. Thus, mitral valve repair should be the goal of both cardiologists and surgeons.

A second factor in the timing of mitral valve surgery is new information about the prognostic implications of chronic atrial fibrillation.[29,30] Atrial fibrillation was thought to be a relatively benign rhythm that could be controlled by digoxin therapy. Recent studies, however, have shown that this rhythm is not benign and is associated with increased long-term mortality, presumably from thromboembolism. Studies from the insurance industry[29] have shown that even in the absence of structural heart disease, individuals with chronic atrial fibrillation do not live as long as those with sinus rhythm. The Framingham study[30] has shown that patients with chronic atrial fibrillation experience more cardiovascular events and do not live as long as those who have normal sinus rhythm. Patients with atrial fibrillation of less than 12 months duration have a high probability of conversion to normal sinus rhythm, but after a year the patient with chronic atrial fibrillation is unlikely to revert to normal sinus rhythm. Thus, the appearance of atrial arrhythmias in a patient with MR suggests LA dysfunction; in those patients further diagnostic studies and the possibility of mitral valve surgery should be considered.

Rarely, mitral valve surgery has been performed in patients with MVP without severe MR, for life-threatening arrhythmias, pain or dyspnea. Analyses of the combined results indicate that the symptoms may improve in some patients but success is not consistent. Because of the small sample size, short follow-up, and incomplete postoperative evaluation, inadequate data are available to formulate conclusions regarding the appropriateness of surgery for these indications, and at present surgery for these indications in patients with MVP must be considered investigational.[8]

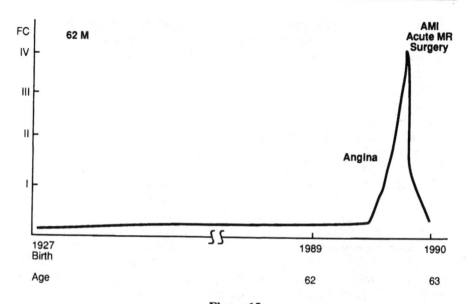

Figure 15

Natural history of the patient with acute mitral regurgitation. Note the acute course of the disease. M, male; AMI, acute myocardial infarction; MR, mitral regurgitation.

Chronic MR: Mitral Valve Surgery for Causes Other Than MVP

Patients with coronary artery disease and MR should undergo cardiac diagnostic studies to delineate coronary anatomy, mitral valve, LA and LV function. Myocardial revascularization with or without mitral valve surgery should be considered with hemodynamic deterioration. It is likely, but not proven, that mitral valve repair is preferable to replacement. Surgical mortality in patients with coronary artery disease and MR is high (between 10 and 30%).[9,22,31] Surgery before hemodynamic deterioration may improve survival; data are lacking at present, however. Nevertheless, at present the long-term prognosis for patients with associated severe LV dysfunction remains poor.

The indications for mitral valve surgery in patients with rheumatic MR are similar to those outlined for MVP. Reconstructive surgery can be performed in certain patients with rheumatic mitral disease and can result in low hospital and late mortality.[26] In certain patients with acute or subacute MR secondary to rheumatic fever, early surgical intervention may be necessary.[4]

Acute Mitral Regurgitation
Case Presentation

A graphic presentation of the patient's history is shown in Fig.15.

A 62-year-old white male transferred to The Ohio State University Hospital on October 17, 1989, with chest pain and dyspnea. He was in good health until one week prior to admission when he first experienced exertional chest pain. He awoke on October 14, 1989, with acute severe anterior chest pain associated with nausea and diaphoresis. A diagnosis of acute myocardial infarction was established at his local hospital. He received tissue plasminogen activator and intravenous nitroglycerin. The pain subsided and he was free of chest pain on October 15, 1989. A two-dimensional echocardiogram showed good LV function and normal mitral valve. The next day the chest pain recurred and was refractory to medical therapy. On October 17, 1989, he developed shortness of breath and was transferred to the University Hospital.

He appeared acutely ill. The venous jugular pressure was normal; there was no peripheral edema. Rales were present in both lungs which covered 50% of the lung fields. His blood pressure was 95/75 and his heart rate was 98 beats/min and regular. The carotid upstroke was brisk with a rapid runoff. Peripheral pulses were normal. A systolic thrill was palpable at the apex. The first heart sound was soft and the second heart sound was widely split. An apical grade IV-V/VI crescendo-decrescendo murmur was heard at the cardiac apex and was radiated to the left sternal border; the murmur terminated prior to the second heart sound. An LV S_4 gallop was heard at the apex. The electrocardiogram was consistent with an inferoposterior myocardial infarction; marked ST segment and T wave depression were present in the lateral precordial leads (Fig. 16). The chest x-ray showed changes consistent with pulmonary edema (Fig. 17).

The clinical diagnosis was acute MR secondary to papillary muscle rupture. An intra-aortic balloon pump was inserted through the left groin; immediately after this he underwent diagnostic cardiac catheterization. The hemodynamic data are shown in Table 5. The LV size was slightly increased; there was mild inferior wall hypokinesis; severe MR was noted (Fig. 18); the LA size was slightly increased. Prominent V waves were noted in the pulmonary capillary wedge pressure tracing.

The patient was taken from the catheterization laboratory to the operating room where he underwent mitral valve replacement. At surgery, the papillary muscle was necrotic with some necrosis of the surrounding endocardium (Fig. 19). The mitral valve was replaced with a #31 Metronic Hall prosthesis. He tolerated the operation remarkably well. Postoperatively he required circulatory support with an intra-aortic balloon pump for 72 hr. He was discharged ten days after surgery in good condition. The discharge electrocardiogram showed sinus rhythm and changes consistent with the inferoposterior myocardial infarction (Fig. 20). The chest x-ray showed mild cardiomegaly and clear lungs (Fig. 21).

Pathophysiology

Patients with acute MR have entirely different clinical presentation than patients with chronic MR. This reflects the unique pathophysiology of acute MR.

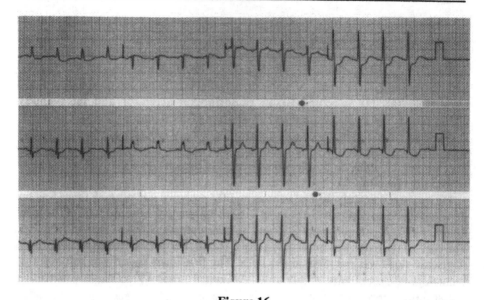

Figure 16
Admission electrocardiogram shows inferoposterior myocardial infarction and marked ST & T wave changes in the lateral leads.

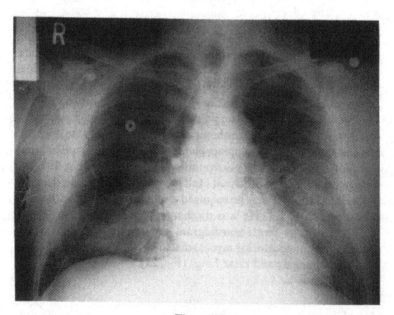

Figure 17
Admission chest x-ray shows pulmonary edema.

The immediate direct effects of regurgitant blood flow into the LA in patients with acute MR are obvious because there is no time for LA adaptation.[13] In severe acute MR, a large regurgitant volume is ejected into the LA during ventricular systole. Since there is no time for the LA and LV to dilate, the large LA volume and consequently the large LV diastolic volume will result in striking elevation of LA and LV diastolic pressures. LA V wave pressures of 60 mm Hg or greater are

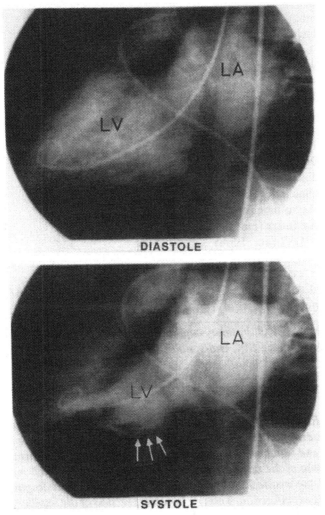

Figure 18. Left Ventriculogram
Upper panel: Diastolic frame. Lower panel: Systolic frame. Note the severe mitral regurgitation with only slightly increased left atrial (LA) size. Segmental contraction abnormality is seen in the inferior left ventricular (LV) wall (arrows).

Table 5

Acute Mitral Regurgitation Hemodynamic Data		
RA Pressure (mm Hg)		
Mean		7
A		8
V		7
Pulmonary artery pressure (mm Hg)		
Systolic		54
Diastolic		27
PCW pressure (mmHg)		
Mean		28
A		23
V		72
LV pressure (mmHg)		
Systolic		98
Diastolic		23
Cardiac output (green dye, l/per min)	4.2	
Cardiac index (l/per min/BSA)	2.2	
Stroke volume (cm^3 per min)		65
Stroke Index (cm^3 per min/BSA)		35
LV-EDVI (cm^3/BSA)		139
LV-ESVI (cm^3/BSA)		53
LV Ejection fraction		62
Cardiac index (angiographic, l/per min/BSA)		13.81/min
Regurgitant fraction		63.5%

RA, right atrium, PCW, pulmonary capillary wedge; LV, left ventricular; EDVI, end-diastolic volume index; ESVI, end-systolic volume index.

Figure 19

Upper panel: Ruptured papillary muscle. The mitral valve posterior papillary muscle rupture was due to recent infarction(arrows). Anterior papillary muscle is not shown. The ruptured end had been previously excised for histology. The muscle is mottled. Note the twisting of the attached chordae tendineae (arrow) which reflects the free movement of the avulsed papillary muscle tip. Lower panel: Ruptured papillary muscle with recent infarction. This is a histologic section of the papillary muscle seen in the upper panel. Endocardium (E) is present at the far left with advanced necrosis of muscle fibers in the center and right portion of the photograph. Between the endocardium and necrotic myocardium is a zone of ischemic myocytes showing cytoplasmic vacuolization or myocytolysis (arrows). Hematoxylin and Eosin, X180.

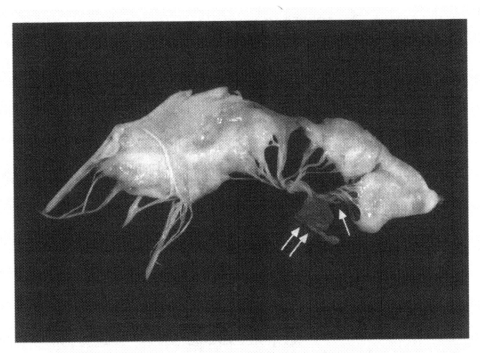

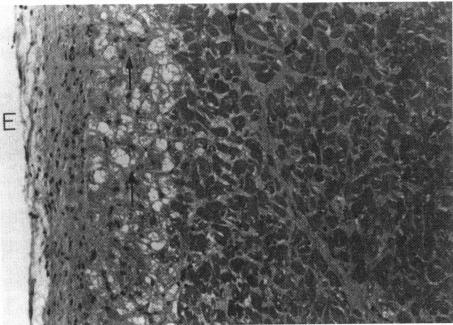

not uncommon. The marked increase in pulmonary venous pressure results in pulmonary congestion and pulmonary edema. The patient complains of severe dyspnea. Since the LV is of normal size and a large amount of blood goes into the LA during ventricular systole, the forward LV stroke volume is markedly diminished. The net result is tissue hypoperfusion, low cardiac output, hypotension and shock (Fig. 22).

Diagnostic Evaluation

The etiology of most common causes of acute MR is shown in Table 1. Distinguishing the three most common types of acute MR (papillary muscle rupture, infective endocarditis, chordae tendineae rupture) clinically is reasonably straightforward.[3,7,31-33]

Acute myocardial infarction often results in transient or permanent mild MR. Papillary muscle rupture or significant papillary muscle dysfunction results in severe MR; this usually leads to death in hours or a few days, unless surgical correction is possible.

Patients with infective endocarditis usually have other systemic manifestations of the disease; MR usually is mild to moderate in severity, but occasionally, especially in patients with preexisting MR, severe MR may occur.

Rupture of chordae tendineae is the most common cause of acute MR in an otherwise healthy person. Thus, rupture of chordae tendineae should be suspected in the absence of other obvious causes.

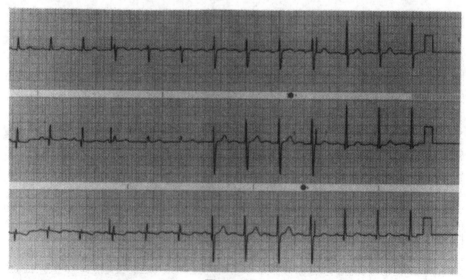

Figure 20
Discharge electrocardiogram shows inferoposterior myocardial infarction, sinus rhythm, and nonspecific ST and T wave changes.

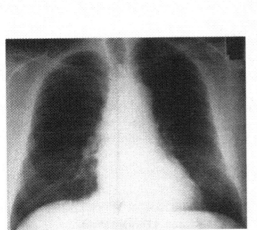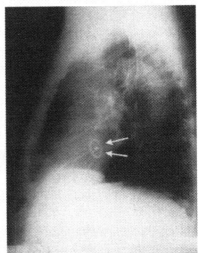

Figure 21

Discharge chest x-ray shows mild cardiomegaly with clear lung fields. The prosthetic valve is also seen (arrows).

Physical Findings. The case presentation of the patient with acute MR incorporated many of the significant physical findings of patients with acute MR. The physical findings in a patient with severe acute MR usually include an LV S_4 gallop; an S_3 gallop may also be present. However, since acute MR is associated with sinus tachycardia, a summation gallop is commonly heard.

The systolic murmur has several characteristics that distinguish it from the holosystolic murmur of chronic MR. The murmur may peak in midsystole and diminish in intensity before the second heart sound (Fig. 23). If the mitral regurgitant jet is directed toward the intra-atrial septum and impinges on the aortic root, the murmur may radiate toward the base of the heart and appear loudest in the second and third left intercostal space at the left sternal border. The result is a crescendo-decrescendo systolic murmur that seems to disappear before the second heart sound and may be heard best at the base of the heart. Although these findings may suggest valvular aortic stenosis, the carotid pulse rises rapidly and is short in duration, and the murmur does not usually radiate into the neck. The wide splitting of the second heart sound due to early aortic closure is also inconsistent with LV outflow tract obstruction.[5,13] In the case of anterior papillary muscle or chordae tendineae rupture, the murmur may radiate posteriorly to the spine.

Laboratory Findings. The electrocardiogram may show acute myocardial infarction and/or myocardial ischemia in patients with acute ischemic MR related to myocardial infarction or severe ischemia.

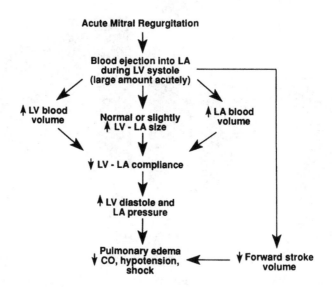

Figure 22

Pathophysiologic mechanisms in acute mitral regurgitation. Schematic presentation. LV, left ventricle; LA, left atrium; CO, cardiac output; ↑, increase; ↓, decrease.

Chest x-ray shows normal or slightly increased heart size with pulmonary congestion or pulmonary edema.

The echocardiogram usually shows normal or slightly increased LV and LA size with normal function. Papillary muscle, chordae tendineae rupture or flail leaflet may be seen. EchoDoppler and color Doppler echocardiography shows severe MR; the direction of the regurgitant flow can also be evaluated.

Cardiac catheterization with left ventriculography shows severe MR into a slightly enlarged LA chamber. LA pressure is elevated and a large V wave is present in the LA pressure recording; LV diastolic pressure is high. The LV size may be normal or only slightly increased. An LV segmental contraction abnormality may be present. Coronary arteriography defines the coronary artery pathology responsible for the acute myocardial infarction and the severity of the coronary artery disease.

Differential Diagnosis. The sudden appearance of a new systolic murmur accompanied by shortness of breath in the middle-aged patient should raise the strong suspicion of acute severe MR. Infective endocarditis or myocardial infarction can usually be identified on the basis of the clinical history and the physical examination. If infection and ischemic causes are excluded, rupture of the chordae ten-

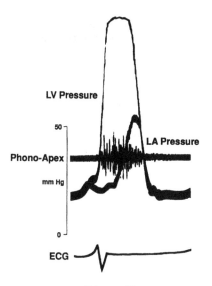

Figure 23

Simultaneous recordings of left ventricular (LV) and left atrial (LA) pressures with external phonocardiogram obtained from the cardiac apex (phono-apex) in a patient with acute mitral regurgitation. Note the large V wave in the LA pressure tracing. As the LA pressure increases during LV systole the systolic pressure gradient diminishes and the intensity of the systolic murmur decreases.

dineae is the most likely diagnosis. So-called "spontaneous" rupture occurs in the presence of chordal structural abnormalities usually associated with MVP or the Marfan syndrome.

Physicians who are not familiar with the syndrome of acute MR may be confused by the presence of acute interstitial pulmonary congestion in a patient with relatively normal LV and LA size. To the inexperienced ear, the murmur — which decreases in intensity before the second heart sound and radiates to the base of the heart — may seem to suggest ventricular outflow obstruction. Awareness of the fine points of the differential diagnosis of MR may be critical, since time is of the essence.

In the presence of acute myocardial infarction, acute MR must be differentiated from the rupture of the ventricular septum. Doppler and color Doppler echocardiography should distinguish MR from ventricular septal rupture.[34] Cardiac catheterization with left ventriculography may be used to define the structural abnormality, coronary pathology, the magnitude of left to right shunt and pulmonary vascular resistance in the presence of rupture of the ventricular septum.

Natural History

In cases of severe acute MR, the patient's clinical status deteriorates rapidly despite "good" medical management and usually leads to death without surgical intervention. The natural history of other causes of acute MR (without myocardial infarction) depends on the etiology, the degree of mitral valve dysfunction, the severity of the MR and the functional status of the LV and LA. Patients with less severe MR, especially with MR secondary to infective endocarditis, may progress less rapidly, respond to medical therapy, and may not require emergency surgical intervention. The same is true in certain patients with chordae tendineae rupture when the MR is not severe and the patient remains in sinus rhythm.

Timing for Surgery

Patients with acute severe MR, pulmonary congestion and hypotension require emergency surgical intervention. Any delay will result in irreversible clinical deterioration. Mitral valve reconstructive surgery is preferable when feasible, but mitral valve replacement may be necessary in certain circumstances. Patients with less severe acute MR without pulmonary congestion or tissue hypoperfusion may be managed medically without emergency surgical intervention. Decisions about surgical therapy should be based on the patient's symptoms, clinical status, the presence of atrial fibrillation, LV and LA size and function as discussed above in patients with chronic MR. Reperfusion therapy with thrombolysis or angioplasty has been successful in restoring valve competence in patients with less severe ischemic acute MR.[9,22,31]

Acute MR: Timing for Surgery of Causes Other Than Papillary Muscle Rupture

Hemodynamically unstable patients with acute MR should be considered for emergency surgery regardless of the etiology. Occasionally, emergency surgery may be necessary in hemodynamically stable patients with infective endocarditis who have extensive floating mitral valvular vegetations with a threat of embolism[3]; however, data about these patients are limited at present.

Comments

Two patients, one with chronic MR and one with acute MR, were presented and discussed. The clinical presentation, pathophysiology and management are entirely different in patients with chronic MR versus patients with acute MR.

Chronic MR, as a general rule, is characterized by a long natural history. A heart murmur is present for many years before the patient becomes symptomatic. There is a progressive enlargement of LV and LA size with gradual alterations of LV filling and LA pressures. Progressive LA and LV chamber enlargement due to volume overload may lead to progressive LV and LA dysfunction without surgical intervention.

Infective endocarditis, chordae tendineae rupture, and onset of atrial fibrillation accelerate the natural progress of the disease, increase the degree of MR, and initiate or precipitate symptoms. The development of symptoms, atrial fibrillation, progressive LV and LA dilatation, early signs of LV dysfunction, and increased LV end-systolic stress should prompt surgical intervention. It should be emphasized that LV dysfunction in patients with significant MR may be masked because of increased preload and decreased afterload. For these reasons, exercise stress testing should be performed in asymptomatic patients with MR and early signs of LV dysfunction in order to subjectively evaluate exercise tolerance and ventricular function. If exercise tolerance is good, the patient should be followed closely and surgery should be considered if symptoms progress or deterioration of LV performance occurs. The increasing use of mitral valve repair coupled with the realization that chronic atrial fibrillation leads to decreased long-term survival has and will continue to influence the timing and type of surgery. The intraoperative use of echo-Doppler and color Doppler has enhanced surgical results.[35]

Sudden disruption of mitral valve integrity results in acute, massive MR in the presence of relatively normal LV and LA size. This results in a marked increase in LA and pulmonary capillary wedge pressure with the development of pulmonary edema. In addition, because of the relatively normal LV size in the presence of significant MR, the forward stroke volume is decreased significantly; this will result in a significant decrease in tissue perfusion, hypotension, and shock. For these reasons, emergency cardiovascular evaluation followed by emergency surgical intervention is indicated in patients with severe acute MR.

References

1. Boudoulas H, Wooley CF: Mitral Valve Prolapse and the Mitral Valve Prolapse Syndrome. Mount Kisco, NY, Futura Publishing Co Inc, 1988.
2. Keren G, Katz S, Strom J, et al. Dynamic mitral regurgitation. An important determinant of the hemodynamic response to load alterations and inotropic therapy in severe heart failure. Circulation. 1989;80:306-313.
3. Stulz P, Pfisterer M, Jenzer HR, et al: Emergency valve replacement for active infective endocarditis. J Cardiovasc Surg. 1989; 30:20-26.
4. Marcus RH, Sarels P, Pocock WA, et al: Functional anatomy of severe mitral regurgitation in active rheumatic carditis. Am J Cardiol. 1989;63:577-584.
5. Boudoulas H, Lewis RP, Dervenagas S, et al: Abbreviation of systolic time intervals in acute mitral regurgitation with observations on the effect of mitral valve replacement. Am J Cardiol. 1979;44:595-599.
6. Boudoulas H, Kolibash AJ, Baker P, et al: Mitral valve prolapse and the mitral valve prolapse syndrome: A diagnostic classification and pathogenesis of symptoms. Am Heart J. 1989;118:796-718.
7. Olson LJ, Subramanian R, Ackerman DM, et al: Surgical pathology of the mitral valve: A study of 712 cases spanning 21 years. Mayo Clin Proc. 1987;62:22-34.

8. Cosgrove DM: Mitral valve prolapse: Surgical management: Mitral Valve Prolapse and the Mitral Valve Prolapse Syndrome. Mount Kisco, NY, Futura Publishing Co Inc, Boudoulas H, Wooley CF (eds): 1988, pp 345-74.

9. Replogle RL, Campbell CD: Surgery for mitral regurgitation associated with ischemic heart disease. Circulation. 1989;79(suppl I):122-125.

10. Wisenbaugh T. Does normal pump function belie muscle dysfunction in patients with chronic severe mitral regurgitation? Circulation. 1988;77:515-525.

11. Hansen DE, Sarris GE, Niczyporuk MA, et al: Physiologic role of the mitral apparatus in left ventricular regional mechanics, contraction synergy, and global systolic performance. J Thorac Cardiovasc Surg. 1989;97:521-523.

12. Carabello BA: Mitral regurgitation: Part 1: Basic pathophysiological principles; Part 2: Proper timing of mitral valve replacement. Mod Concepts Cardiovase Dis. 1988; 57:53-58,59-64.

13. Rackley CE, Edwards JE, Karp RB: Mitral valve disease in Hurst WJ (ed): The Heart. New York, McGraw-Hill Information Services Co, 1990, pp 820-851.

14. Bradley JA, Gibson DG: Assessment of the severity of mitral regurgitation from the dynamics of retrograde flow. Br Heart J. 1988;60:134-140.

15. Kolibash AJ, Kilman JW, Bush CA, et al: Evidence for progression from mild to severe mitral regurgitation in mitral valve prolapse. Am J Cardiol. 1986;58:762-767.

16. Wilcken DEL, Hickey AJ: Lifetime risk for patients with mitral valve prolapse of developing severe valve regurgitation requiring surgery. Circulation. 1988;78:10-14.

17. Duren DR, Beeker AE, Dunning AJ: Long-term follow-up of idiopathic mitral valve prolapse in 300 patients: A prospective study. J Am Coll Cardiol. 1988;11:42-47.

18. Nishimura RA, McGoon MD, Shub C, et al: Echocardiographically documented mitral valve prolapse. Long-term follow-up of 237 patients. N Engl J Med 1985;313:1305-1309.

19. Marks AR, Choong CY, Sanfilippo AJ, et al: Identification of high-risk and low-risk subgroups of patients with mitral valve prolapse. N Engl J Med. 1989;320:1031-1036.

20. Tomaru T: The multifactorial etiology of mitral valve prolapse, a new entity of postinflammatory mitral valve prolapse. Herz, 1988;13:271-276.

21. Turri M, Theine G, Bortolotti V, et al: Surgical pathology of disease of the mitral valve with special reference to lesions promoting incompetence. Int J Cardiol. 1989;22:213-219.

22. Hickey M, Smith RL, Muhlbeuer LH, et al: Current prognosis of ischemic mitral regurgitation; Implications for future management. Circulation, 1988;78(suppl I):51-59.

23. Cohn LH: Surgery for mitral regurgitation. JAMA. 1988;18:2883-2887.

24. Zile MR, Gaasch WH, Carroll JD, et al: Chronic mitral regurgitation: Predictive value of preoperative echocardiographic indexes of left ventricular function and wall stress. J Am Coll Cardiol. 1984;3:235-242.

25. Boudoulas H, Wooley CF. Mitral valve prolapse and the mitral valve prolapse syndrome. in Rakel RE (ed): Conn's Current Therapy, WB Saunders Co., pp 236-241.

26. Duran CD, Revnetta JM, Gaite L, et al: Stability of mitral reconstructive surgery at 10-12 years for predominantly rheumatic valvular disease. Circulation. 1988;78(Suppl II): 91-96.

27. Carpentier A, Chauvand S, Fabiani JN, et al: Reconstructive surgery of mitral valve incompetence. J Thorac Cardiovasc Surg. 1980;79:338-348.

28. Galloway AC, Calvin SB, Bauman GF, et al: Current concepts of mitral valve reconstruction for mitral insufficiency. Circulation. 1988;78:1087-1098.

29. Gajewski J, Singer RB. Mortality in an insured population with atrial fibrillation. JAMA. 1981;245:1540-1544.

30. Kannel WB, Abbott RD, Savage DD, et al: Epidemiologic features of chronic atrial fibrillation. N Engl J Med. 1982;306:1018-1022.

31. Peterffy A, Nagy Z, Vaszily M, et al: Valve surgery combined with myocardial revascularization. Scand J Thorac Cardiovasc Surg. 1989;23:25-27.

32. Mann JM, Roberts WC. Rupture of the left ventricular free wall during acute myocardial infarction: Analysis of 138 necropsy patients and comparison with 50 acute myocardial infarctions without rupture. Am J Cardiol. 1988;62:847-859.

33. Baker PB, Bansal G, Boudoulas H, et al: Floppy mitral valve chordae tendinae: Histo pathologic alterations. Hum Pathol. 1988;19:507-512.

34. Patel AM, Miller FA Jr, Khandheria BK, et al: Role of transesophageal echocardiography in the diagnosis of papillary muscle rupture secondary to myocardial infarction. Am Heart J. 1989;118:1330-1333.

35. Czer LSC, Maurer G, Bolger AF, et al: Interoperative evaluation of mitral regurgitation by Doppler color flow mapping. Circulation. 1987;76(Suppl III):108-116.

Case 2

Cystic Fibrosis in Adults

Andrew Libertin, MD and John S. Heintz, MD

Case History

A 21-year-old white female college student was referred for evaluation of an elevated sweat chloride test. She had been having chronic cough for the past two years, which had gradually increased in severity, and chronic sinus congestion for which she had been seeing an allergist. On further questioning, it was apparent that she had suffered from frequent cough and lingering colds over much of her life. Treatment prior to referral consisted of hyposensitization shots over the previous two years. At the initiation of her therapy, she had normal x-ray and pulmonary function tests. Treatment prior to referral had included the intermittent use of Rondec TR, Vancenase, a Proventil inhaler, and intermittent antibiotics. Just prior to referral her allergist obtained a sweat chloride test because of her poor response to therapy. This was elevated and she was referred for further evaluation and treatment.

She was hospitalized at age 18 months for croup and had childhood infectious diseases including colds, measles, mumps, and chickenpox. She reported allergies to penicillin, which caused unconsciousness; sulfa drugs, which caused nausea and rash; and environmental allergies which included grass, molds, dust, pollen, and trees. Menarche was at age 14. Thalassemia minor was incidentally identified when she was tested for presumed mononucleosis. Her siblings include a half-sibling and one full sibling, neither of whom has any significant medical complaints.

Physical Examination. Weight was 54.7 kg, which is the 35th percentile, and height 169.9 cm, which is approximately the 85th percentile. Vital signs were normal. Examination of the nasal mucosa demonstrated inspissated mucus in the left nostril. The throat was slightly red but otherwise normal. The neck had scattered small lymph nodes. Chest examination demonstrated decreased breath sounds but was otherwise clear. Cardiac examination was normal. Extremities demonstrated no cyanosis or clubbing. Examination was otherwise normal.

Laboratory Data. Repeat sweat chloride test had a value of 90. Other chemistries were normal. Chest x-ray demonstrated a peribronchiolar thickening. There was a mild pectus excavatum deformity. Lung volumes appeared to be normal. Initial throat culture was normal. Pulmonary function testing demonstrated a vital capacity of 73% of predicted. FEV1 was 73% of predicted. The FEV1 to FVC ratio was 80. FEF 25-75 was 67% of predicted, and FEF 50 was 68% of predicted with FEF 75 being 34% of predicted. The ratio of residual volume to total lung capacity was 47%. Pulse oximetry demonstrated 97% saturation. These demonstrated moderate obstructive pulmonary disease with a moderate degree of air trapping.

Course since the Diagnosis. The diagnosis of cystic fibrosis was made. Therapy with a Beconase inhaler was initiated and Proventil aerosol treatment was continued with instruction in chest physiotherapy at home. A course of oral cephalosporin was initiated for chronic sinus infection. Repeat pulmonary function tests on this treatment regimen improved over the following months. The forced vital capacity increased to 95% of predicted and FEV1 increased to 104% of predicted. FEF 50 increased to 107% of predicted and FEF 75 increased to 78% of predicted. The throat cultures began to grow *Staphylococcus aureus* which has persisted in repeat throat cultures. Additional therapy with oral contraception and a multivitamin has been added since the initial diagnosis.

This young woman has remained quite active, reporting only mild shortness of breath from time to time while she figure skates.

Discussion

Epidemiology. Cystic fibrosis (CF) is a multisystem, autosomal recessive disorder with a gene frequency in Caucasians of 1:20 and an incidence of 1:2,000. It is the most common lethal autosomal recessive disorder in the white population.[1,2] CF is much less common in black (1:17,000) and Asian populations.[3]

Pathophysiology. Biochemical, cellular, and genetic research support a unifying hypothesis that a mucosal defect causing chloride impermeability results in abnormal ion and water transport across cell membranes. Quinton first demonstrated that impermiabilty to chloride ion in ductal epithelium results in abnormal electrolyte reabsorption in CF patients.[4,5] Other studies have confirmed anion impermeability in airway and secretory-coil epithelium.[6,7] More recently, the mucosal defect has been associated with cAMP-induced activation of chloride channels which transport ions across cell membranes.[8] The failure of these chloride channels to open in the presence of the cAMP-dependent protein kinase suggests that the defect is within the chloride channel itself or in an associated regulatory protein.[9]

Genetic research has provided invaluable information regarding this abnormally functioning anion channel. In 1985, the CF gene was localized to the long arm of chromosome 7, band 31.[1,3] Collaborative research from the laboratories of Tsui,

Riordan, and Collins in 1989 identified the CF gene as a large locus consisting of approximately 250,000 bp. Approximately 79% of the mutations in CF correspond to the deletion of a single 3bp codon in this locus. The result is an abnormal gene product (a 1480-amino-acid polypeptide) which lacks a phenylalanine at position 508. The polypeptide's proposed structure is characteristic of a transmembrane protein. It has been termed the cystic fibrosis transmembrane conductance regulator (CFTR). It is proposed that the genetically defective CFTR is directly responsible for abnormal ion transport in CF. Further study is needed to determine whether the CFTR is the chloride channel itself or a protein regulating ion channel activity through protein kinase phosphorylation.[10-12]

Anion channel impermeability impacts on many organ systems in CF by altering the physical properties of exocrine gland secretions. In sweat ducts, chloride channel impermeability results in defective electrolyte reabsorption and excessive chloride and sodium loss. Defective electrolyte transport from respiratory epithelium into the lumen, however, results in mucus with reduced water content and lower concentrations of sodium and chloride.[2] The secretions are subsequently more viscid. Pancreatic, biliary, cervical, and male reproductive secretions are similarly more viscid.

System Pathology. The mucus in CF is deficient in water, is excessively glycosylated and contains increased numbers of sulfated glycoproteins.[13] Inspissated mucus impairs mucus clearance and causes airway obstruction. Furthermore, the accumulation of viscid mucus produces airway inflammation and stimulates the proliferation of goblet cells.[2] Chronic infection in CF causes airway inflammation and potentiates mucus hypersecretion. All of these factors contribute to the development of progressive obstructive lung disease which is characterized by bronchiolectasis, bronchiectasis, fibrosis, and cyst formation.

Even though up to 10% of patients have no clinical evidence of pancreatic insufficiency, the pancreas is almost always abnormal, and ductal obstruction by viscous exocrine secretions results in autodestruction of the pancreas by trapped pancreatic enzymes. Ductal dilatation, pancreatic fibrosis, and pancreatic insufficiency often follow and result in malabsorption of fat. Destruction of the islet cells may sometimes result in hyperglycemia.

Involvement of the hepatobiliary tree is variable. Ductal obstruction can cause focal, then diffuse, biliary cirrhosis. Other gastrointestinal tract involvement includes hyperplasia of mucous glands within the intestines.

Males have greater than a 95% azoospermia rate due to obstructive atrophy of the vas deferens, epididymis, and seminal vesicles. Females have viscid cervical mucus, but no other significant reproductive abnormalities.

Diagnosis. The onset and severity of symptoms vary markedly in CF. This is likely a consequence of different alleles in the population and variable genetic penetrance.[1,3] Specifically, evidence supports that pancreatic sufficiency is determined by the effect of different mutant alleles in the CF gene product.[3,12] The diagnosis of CF is made in approximately 80% by age five, but approximately 5% are diagnosed during adulthood.[14] Pulmonary disease occurs in over 99% of patients, and those presenting with only respiratory tract symptoms are diagnosed later than those with concurrent malabsorption.[14,15] Recurrent pulmonary infections are a hallmark of CF. Cough, dyspnea, and wheezing are the predominant pulmonary symptoms. Early sputum colonization with *Staphylococcus aureus* and *Haemophilus influenzea* is common, and by the time of death approximately 80% of patients are colonized by strains of mucoid *Pseudomonas aeruginosa*.[14] In recent years, *Pseudomonas cepacia* has become a dreaded pathogen which may cause accelerated clinical deterioration in some patients. Pulmonary disorders in adolescents or young adults, which are suggestive of CF include: recurrent pneumonia or bronchitis, staphylococcal pneumonia, chronic cough, chronic bronchitis, colonization with mucoid pseudomonas, or radiographic evidence of bronchiectasis. Other common respiratory tract disorders of patients diagnosed during adulthood include chronic sinusitis and nasal polyposis.

Patients with gastrointestinal-related symptoms are usually diagnosed early with bowel obstruction in infancy called meconium ileus, or with malabsorption in childhood. A common presentation in older patients is pancreatitis, despite a history of apparently intact exocrine pancreatic function. CF should be considered in the differential diagnosis of pancreatitis when chronic cough is present, or if no other etiology is apparent. Cholelithiasis in an adolescent without a history of hemolytic anemia may also be a presentation of CF. Signs and symptoms of cirrhosis such as hepatosplenomegaly, varices, or ascites are an uncommon initial presentation of CF. CF has also presented as bowel obstruction known as meconium ileus equivalent or as rectal prolapse.

Classically, the diagnosis of CF requires the coexistence of characteristic pulmonary or pancreatic disease or a family history of CF **and** the demonstration of abnormal sweat electrolyte studies.[16] Confirmation of abnormal sweat electrolytes, on at least two separate occasions, is essential. The quantitative pilocarpine iontophoretic technique is the most widely accepted sweat electrolyte study. Sweat is collected following local stimulation, and the chloride concentration is determined by chloridometric titration. In the appropriate clinical setting, a value of greater than 60 mEq/liter is considered diagnostic. Other disorders which can produce an elevated sweat electrolyte concentration, but which are clinically distinct from CF, include adrenal insufficiency, nephrogenic diabetes insipidus, hypothyroidism, fucosidosis, and hypoparathyroidism.

The diagnosis can be elusive in patients with subtle clinical symptoms or in patients with recognized variants of CF where sweat electrolytes are indeterminate or even normal.

Other studies can be helpful in equivocal cases. The 72-hr quantitation of fecal fat may document pancreatic insufficiency in patients without clinical steatorrhea. Prior to the identification of the CF gene mutations at a DNA sequence level, DNA

Table 1

Criteria for Cystic Fibrosis Diagnosis in Atypical Patients

- **Major criteria**
    1. Sweat chloride 60 mEq/liter before age 20 years (80 mEq/liter in adults)
    2. Chronic obstructive pulmonary disease with pseudomonas airway infection
    3. Unexplained obstructive azoospermia

- **Minor criteria**
    1. Sweat chloride 40 mEq/liter before age 20 years (60 mEq/liter in adults.
    2. Family history of classic cystic fibrosis
    3. Exocrine pancreatic insufficiency before age 20 years
    4. Unexplained chronic obstructive pulmonary disease before age 20 years
    5. Unexplained azoospermia (without scrotal examination)

---

analysis was able to detect the CF gene only in situations where gene comparison could be made to a family member having CF. With the current knowledge of CF genetic mutations, 46% of patients without a family history can be diagnosed by gene analysis. Almost 70% of the CF carriers can be identified with a probe for the mutation at amino acid position 508.[12]

Obstructive azoospermia is also supportive of a diagnosis of CF. Stern evaluated obstructive azoospermia as a diagnostic criterion. He proposed extending the diagnosis of CF to patients fulfilling either two major, or one major and one minor criterion as listed in Table 1.[17] The patient's two criteria must involve two different organ systems.

Because of the clinical heterogeneity in CF patients may be undiagnosed until adolescence or even adulthood. This is most often the case in patients without clinical evidence of pancreatic insufficiency. CF should be included in the differential diagnosis of various symptoms in adolescents and adults. Those signs and symptoms with indications for sweat electrolyte testing are listed in Table 2.

Assessment: The goals of therapy for those with CF are: achieve and maintain optimal functional status for the stage of disease present, recognize and manage complications, and finally, prepare the patient and significant others for death when that point is reached. For those with newly diagnosed CF, a comprehensive

Table 2

Common Presentations of Cystic Fibrosis in Adolescents and Adults

Respiratory infections with *Staphylococcus*
  or *Pseudomonas*
Bronchiectasis
Recurrent bronchitis/pneumonia
Pansinusitis
Nasal polyposis
Hemoptysis
Clubbing
Pancreatic insufficiency
Pancreatitis (unexplained)
Cirrhosis — portal hypertension
Cholecystitis
Rectal prolapse
Heat prostration
Obstructive azoospermia

baseline evaluation must be made. Once done, a program of lifelong surveillance and management is undertaken and complications dealt with as they come.

Initial assessment and management include both medical and social realms. The reality that CF is a fatal disease is discussed, though not always comprehended, and the potential for a prolonged and productive life offered to the patient and his family.

Education, age-appropriate concerns, and emotional and financial support systems are all best discussed openly and early on. The primary physician should initiate contact with the nearest CF center, although these centers urge the family physician to maintain his relationship to the patient as well. The involvement of a known and trusted caregiver will facilitate family and patient understanding and acceptance of the disease.

Medical assessment is through a combination of clinical evaluation and testing, with the most important being pulmonary and nutritional status. The presence of cough and amount of sputum production are assessed with baseline sputum or swab throat culture to determine the nature of the colonizing bacteria. The chest x-ray is very seldom normal, even with minimal symptoms, and can be scored on the Brasfield chest x-ray scale,[18] or as part of the more inclusive Schwachman and Kulczycki scale.[19] Baseline pulmonary function testing also aids in determination of initial states and should improve with therapy. The pattern is that of small airway obstruction with FEF 25-75 almost invariably decreased, residual volume to total lung capacity elevated, and prominent V:Q mismatching.[2] Growth and sexual maturation provide data about nutritional status in the adolescent while in the adult, weight is the easiest, and in most cases a sufficient, measure of overall nutritional status. The degree of pancreatic insufficiency and malabsorption is gauged grossly by stool characteristics such as stool frequency, odor, and visible oil, with tests such as the CCK-secretin and l-benzoyl-l-tyrosy-p-aminobenzoic acid (BT-PABA) tests reserved for more careful quantitation if need be.[20] Since fat-soluble vitamins are malabsorbed, determination of prothrombin time is useful initially while others recommend measurement of vitamin E.[21] Other initial laboratory work that may be helpful is a fasting glucose and an arterial blood gas.

Management. Once the initial assessment is completed, a beginning management plan is possible. The well patient may need no more than education and institution of routine care such as chest physiotherapy, bronchodilators and nutritional measures. However, commonly the patient will be ill enough to justify hospitalization for both education and therapy. Characteristics that would prompt admission would be deteriorating functional status, weight loss, fever, or increasing sputum.

Outpatient and inpatient therapy have a number of basic principles in common. Chest physiotherapy (CPT) for the mobilization of secretions has long been a mainstay of therapy, and an area where noncompliance has been a particular problem due to the time it requires, especially in adolescence.[2] A number of researchers have attempted to prove or disprove its efficacy and improve on the results. Kerrebijn showed no change in pulmonary function tests with CPT, whereas Desmond showed deterioration in function when CPT was omitted.[22,23] A recent large study compared CPT and a forced expiratory/cough technique (FET), over three years and found CPT useful in preventing decline in pulmonary function.[24] Vibrating percussors are commonly used by adults and older children. Appropriate exercise also functions well and some believe that it can obviate the need for CPT, at least in the mild to moderately impaired patient.[25] In short, evidence currently indicates that some form of pulmonary toilet should be included in the care of all but the most asymptomatic patients, to improve clearance of secretions.

A variety of aerosols may be helpful, and are commonly used. Bronchodilators should be assessed with pulmonary function tests. They improve function in some patients, and actually worsen it in others. In some patients they may be most useful intermittently for worsening symptoms. Mucolytics such as *N*-acetylcysteine have fallen out of favor at many centers, due to bronchospasm, tracheitis and hemoptysis, but are still used elsewhere. It may be tried as the 5% solution, and combined with a bronchodilator if bronchospasm ensues, but should be discontinued if this persists in spite of bronchodilator therapy.[26] Typically, aerosols are used before CPT, and the combination is used two times per day on a routine basis.

Maintenance antibiotic therapy is variable from center to center. Some place patients on antistaphylococcal therapy regardless of symptoms. Others treat based on sputum or throat cultures, whereas still others withhold therapy until symptoms worsen. A reasonable choice is to treat worsening symptoms very promptly, based on the results of routinely obtained cultures.[26] Worsening symptoms of sinusitis are treated with Augmentin, trimethoprimsulfamethoxazole, oral cephalosporins, or ciprofloxacin, with more aggressive therapy reserved for resistant symptoms.

The use of steroids is controversial. The presence of allergic bronchopulmonary aspergillosis, diagnosed by the normal criteria, is a clear indication for steroids, with severe reactive airway disease also occasionally calling for steroids, which may be systemic or inhaled.[26] At least one trial has shown decreased morbidity and improved lung function and growth with alternate-day prednisone therapy. Confirmation with further studies will be needed before this becomes standard care.[27] Nasal polyps are responsive to topical steroids with surgery reserved for resistant, troublesome lesions.

Long-term management requires frequent follow-up, with visits every two months appropriate. Ongoing psychosocial assessment is extremely important with attention paid to both the patient and the family. Items that need to be followed on an ongoing basis include cough, stool characteristics, weight, school or work, family response to the patient's chronic illness, counseling as to fertility, adoption, and genetics, and the patient's affect with particular attention to the possibility of depression. A close, trusting relationship with the patient facilitates the expression of concerns, with the type of issue divulged appearing to follow a particular pattern over time: first, concerns about the illness itself and work or school activities, and, as much as two years later, family and emotional problems.[28] Often these disclosures are to a nurse or social worker, and physicians should encourage these relationships.

Nutritional counseling is ongoing. Most patients develop some degree of malabsorption, often manifested as steatorrhea. The dose of pancreatic enzyme is titrated, with four capsules with meals, and two with snacks often being adequate. In spite of this, patients require 130-150% of expected calories. If weight maintenance is a problem, then supplements should be used. Occasionally, nighttime nasogastric feedings with hydrolyzed formula are necessary.[26] Hyperalimentation is rarely used in adults. By no means should nutritional problems be ignored, as doing so may be a fatal mistake. Patients should take a double dose of a multivitamin daily. Those with prolongation of PT or chronic antibiotic therapy require vitamin K.[26] A variety of concerns relating to vitamin E deficiency have been raised, including a syndrome of peripheral neuropathy, nystagmus, and impaired posterior column sensation. Vitamin E supplementation in those with steatorrhea at a dose of 100-200 units water-miscible alpha-tocopherol per day is reasonable. An alternative is to measure serum vitamin E levels and treat those who are low.[21,29]

Pulmonary function is followed in a variety of manners, with cough, sputum production, pulse oximetry and activity tolerance being followed semimonthly. Chest radiographs and PFTs should be followed semiannually and as needed for changes in symptoms. Throat and sputum cultures obtained at each visit are important to follow changes in colonization and antibiotic sensitivity. Influenza vaccine must be administered annually.

Exercise is emerging as an important adjunct to other therapies. Patients with mild to moderate lung dysfunction have normal peak work capacity, with only those with severe lung dysfunction having diminished peak capacity, oxygen desaturation, and clinical deterioration with exercise.[30] Contraindications to vigorous exercise include: esophageal varices, cor pulmonale, extensive bronchiectasis, and massive hemoptysis. Exercise goals should be concrete and realistic, with reasonable guidelines being a heart rate of 70-85% of patient's own peak rate for up to 30 min several times per week.[25]

Abstinence from drugs, excessive alcohol and even cigarettes should not be assumed and should be specifically addressed at some point.

Complications

Infection. Signs of increased airway infection may be seen as fever, increased sputum production, or dyspnea. However, signs are often more subtle, with weight loss or malaise being the most prominent symptoms. Infection should always be treated very promptly. Traditionally, infection is treated in hospital with high-dose antibiotics appropriate to the specific infectious agent, which is generally readily obtainable, or already known from the last routinely obtained sputum. A combination of two antibiotics should be used. Dosages used are higher than normal, because of increased renal clearance and the need for adequate penetration into bronchial secretions, and the duration of therapy is usually two to three weeks, though this is varied depending on symptoms. Table 3 lists commonly used antibiotics. Serum levels should be followed with the highest safe levels maintained. Often, although the organism may be resistant to all antibiotics, an empiric combination often is found which is effective.[31] Therapy for *H. influenzae* and *S. aureus* is often successfully pursued with oral antibiotics.[14] CPT and aerosol treatments are increased in frequency. These treatments for infectious exacerbations have usually been undertaken in the hospital setting, but the advent of home IV therapy has spurred the increasing acceptance of therapy at home for those with a well-known response to therapy and those not sufficiently ill to require hospitalization.[32] Mild to moderate exacerbations are occasionally treated with aerosolized aminoglycosides (40-120 mg in 3 cc total volume TID after CPT), ceftazidime (1 gm in 3 cc total volume after CPT), or ticarcillin (1 gm) over a 4-16 week period at home. Resulting bronchospasm should be detected and treated. Long-term multi-center trials are currently being done to assess efficacy.[33] The place of aerosolized antibiotics in CF is controversial. Colonization with *Pseudomonas cepacia* is

Table 3

Antibiotic Dosages for Patients with Cystic Fibrosis

Antibiotic	Daily Dose[a] (mg/kg/day)	Dosing Interval (hours)
Methicillin, IV	200	4-6
Nafcillin, IV	150	4-6
Dicloxacillin, PO, IV	50-100	4-6
Cloxacillin, IV	100-200	4-6
Gentamicin/tobramycin IV	10-20[b]	6-8
Amikacin, IV	15-30[c]	6-8
Netilmycin, IV	10-12	6-8
Aztreonam, IV	200	6-8
Piperacillin, IV	350-450	4-8
Ticarcillin/clavulinate, IV	350-450	4-8
Imipenen, IV	45-100	6-8
Ceftazidime, IV	150-200	6-8
Azlocillin, IV	350-450	4-8
Carbenicillin, IV	400-600	4-8
Ciprofloxacin, IV, PO	15-30	8-12

Adapted from Strandvik[31] and M. Hoppe, (personal communication, Columbus Children's Hospital).
[a]Maximum dose is the maximum recommended adult dose
[b]Peak serum levels = 8-12, trough serum levels
[c]Peak serum levels = 25-35, trough serum level

increasingly found. Several patterns of *P. cepacia* colonization are seen: (1) chronic asymptomatic carriage, (2) clinical deterioration with recurrent fever, weight loss, and repeated hospital admissions, and (3) rapid, usually fatal progression of disease in those who had previously done well.[34] Isolation of those with *P. cepacia* colonization from those who are free of it is helpful, and antibiotic therapy is usually empiric as it is an organism resistant to virtually all antibiotics.

Hemoptysis. Hemoptysis is common, with blood streaking occurring in a majority of patients at some point.[14] Therapy for this is generally intensification of therapy for infection, and is usually self limited. Expectoration of larger amounts, such as 30-60 cc, requires hospitalization, and of massive quantities, such as 300-2,500 cc, is life-threatening, resulting from erosion of bronchial arteries. Therapeutic options include bronchoscopy, surgical resection of the affected lobe, or arterial embolization.[26] Vitamin K should be given as well, 5 mg twice per week.[35]

Pneumothorax. Pneumothorax occurs frequently (18.9% at Brompton Hospital), with increasing rates with aging.[36] Expectant management with very close follow-up is acceptable with less than 10% pneumothorax, with tube thoracostomy indicated for larger ones.[26] Up to 30% of these events are tension pneumothoraces, and mortality was reported as 15.2% in one center's experience.[26,36] Prolonged tube drainage (greater than 5-7 days) results in high morbidity secondary to infection, impaired cough and emotional deterioration, and the recurrence rate is extremely high; therefore, consideration of pleurodesis, either surgically or medically, after 7 days of persistent air leak or with the first recurrence is reasonable. Some physicians feel medical pleurodesis is usually unsuccessful, and would counsel a surgical approach instead,[36] however, implications for future transplant candidacy and/or pulmonary disease precluding anesthesia favor medical pleurodesis.

Cor Pulmonale. Persistent hypoxia can eventually lead to pulmonary hypertension and cor pulmonale. Onset may be delayed with the use of oxygen at night for sleep hypoxia, and the use of daytime oxygen for oxygen saturation less than 90%. The definitive studies remain to be done. Frank failure may be precipitated by pulmonary exacerbations, and responds poorly to digoxin and vasodilators. Therapy consists primarily of oxygen and diuretics for now. Future modalities may include calcium channel blocking agents, aerosolized disodium cromoglycate, and theophylline.[37]

Intestinal Obstruction. Abdominal pain should not be taken lightly. Intestinal secretions are viscid and obstruction and intussusception well described.[37] Incomplete obstruction may be treated with mineral oil, N-acetylcysteine and/or hypertonic enemas. Total obstruction may require surgery.[26]

Pancreatic Dysfunction. The pancreas of, probably, all patients with CF is abnormal, even in those with adequate exocrine function. Although survival is generally better in those without pancreatic insufficiency, it is precisely these people most at risk for acute pancreatitis.[20,38] This should be treated as pancreatitis as treated in those without CF.[2] Further, evidence is accumulating that up to 38% of infants with CF have exocrine sufficiency, with this percentage eventually decreasing to approximately 15% with increasing age. Exocrine pancreatic function is therefore a changing process, necessitating occasional reevaluation for insufficiency.[38]

Diabetes Mellitus. Diabetes may develop, usually in the teens or later, with about an 11% occurrence. With increasing population age the rate of development of diabetes appears to be increasing as well. A minority require insulin, with most doing well on diet or oral hypoglycemic agents.[14]

Liver Cirrhosis. A small percentage of patients will develop cirrhosis and portal hypertension (1%).[14] Bleeding from varices can occur with therapy consisting primarily of sclerosis, avoiding surgery if at all possible.[26]

Fluid and Electrolyte Abnormalities. Dehydration, metabolic alkalosis and hypoelectrolytemia are potential problems, but occur primarily in children, with adults rarely suffering these complications.[2] Prompt, appropriate therapy is necessary if they do occur, with the setting of exertion and/or heat suggesting the diagnosis.

Pregnancy. Although amenorrhea secondary to poor health or low body fat content is common, pregnancy is also possible. There are increased rates of unsuccessful pregnancies, but those that carry to term demonstrate no excess malformations. Lung function deteriorates during the third trimester, but in those whose prior health was good, most recover well. However, those beginning pregnancy with severe pulmonary disease or low weight decline, and recover very poorly. Oral contraceptives are well tolerated and effective.[14,26] Almost 100% of males are infertile, with very few exceptions. Data for genetic counseling are presented in Table 4. A more precise antenatal diagnosis is possible with chorionic villous sampling and gene-linkage studies.

Table 4

Calculated Risk of a Pregnancy to Yield an Individual with Cystic Fibrosis[a]

Parents	Risk
● General white population	1:2000
● Previous child with cystic fibrosis	1:4
● One parent has cystic fibrosis; other has negative family history	1:40
● One parent is a known carrier; other has negative family history	1:80
● One parent is an unaffected sibling of a person with cystic fibrosis; other with negative family history	1:120
● One parent has a niece or nephew with cystic fibrosis; other has negative family history	1:120-1:160

Adapted from Scanlin, in Pulmonary Diseases and Disorders, 1988.[26]
[a]Assumed carrier rate of 1:20

Prognosis. Although CF is a fatal disease, survival is much longer than in midcentury. Antibiotics and improved diagnosis have certainly been the main contributing factors, with many people feeling that centralized CF centers have also contributed. At present, 50% of patients can expect to reach 25 years of age.[2] Most patients die of lung disease. Huang et al studied 142 patients and found that at age 18, low clinical score (on previously mentioned scales), low weight percentile and colonization with *P. cepacia* portended a poor prognosis, with clinical score best predicting survival for five more years, and low weight, with *P. cepacia* colonization, best predicting shorter term survival. Conversely, high clinical scores, high weight percentile and colonization with *S. aureus* alone predicted survival beyond 23 years of age, with intact pancreatic function also suggesting better performance.[39] Heart-lung transplantation has been performed with success, and may offer a partial solution in the future. Of 35 patients transplanted between 1985 and 1988 by Drs. Yacomb and Wallworth, there were 8 deaths by November 1989. Double lung transplantation has also been successfully performed. These procedures have many of the limitations common to most transplantations, but offer hope to certain CF populations.[40]

In spite of progressive fatal disease, many patients hold jobs, or successfully pursue higher educational goals, and should be encouraged to do so.

Preterminal Management

As the patient's health begins an inexorable decline, frank discussion about approaching death is important, as is encouraging the patient to resolve important affairs. Nonetheless, short-term optimism is appropriate. At death, the physician can help minimize discomfort for both the patient and family with his or her presence and sedation. Acute respiratory failure in an otherwise well functioning patient should be aggressively treated, with mechanical ventilation being entirely appropriate.

Summary

CF is currently universally fatal, but identification of the gene and a hypothetical membrane protein conformation, and the success of heart-lung transplantation offer long-term hope. In the meantime, improved management has resulted in prolongation of life to the point that the internist may well be asked for advice or even be the patient's primary caregiver. We hope that this review at least gives you a start.

References

1. Buchwald M, Tsui LC, Riordan J: The search for the cystic fibrosis gene. Am J Physiol. 1989;257:L47-L52.
2. Boat T: Cystic fibrosis, in Murray J, Nadel J (eds): Textbook of Respiratory Medicine. Philadelphia, WB Saunders Co, 1988, pp 1126-1152.

3. Kerem BS, Buchanan JA, Durie P, et al: DNA marker haplotype association with pancreatic sufficiency in cystic fibrosis. Am J Hum Genet. 1989;44:827-834.

4. Quinton PM: Chloride impermeability in cystic fibrosis. Nature. 1983;301:421-422.

5. Quinton PM, Bigman J: Higher bioelectric potentials due to decreased chloride absorption in the sweat glands of patients with cystic fibrosis. N Engl J Med. 1983;308:1185-1189.

6. Knowles MR, Stutts MJ, Spock A et al: Abnormal ion permeation through cystic fibrosis respiratory epithelium. Science. 1983;221:1067-1070.

7. Sato K, Sato F: Defective beta adrenergic response of cystic fibrosis sweat glands in vivo and in vitro. J Clin Invest. 1984;73:1763-1771.

8. Frizzell RA, Rechkemmer G, Shoemaker RL: Altered regulation of airway epithelial cell chloride channels in cystic fibrosis. Science. 1986;233:558-560.

9. Li M, McCann JD, Liedtke CM: Cystic AMP-dependent protein kinase opens chloride channels in normal but not cystic fibrosis airway epithelium. Nature. 1988;331:358-360.

10. Rommens JM, Iannuzzi MC, Kerem B, et al: Identification of the cystic fibrosis gene: Chromosome walking and jumping. Science. 1989;245:1059-1065.

11. Riordan JR, Rommens JM, Kerem B, et al: Identification of the cystic fibrosis gene: Cloning and characterization of complementary DNA. Science 1989;245:1066-1073.

12. Kerem B, Rommens JM, Buchanan JA, et al: Identification of the cystic fibrosis gene: genetic analysis. Science. 1989;245:1073-1080.

13. Frates RC, Kaizu T, Last JA: Mucus glycoproteins secreted by respiratory epithelial tissue from cystic fibrosis patients. Pediatr Res. 1983;17:30-34.

14. Penketh ARL, Wise A, Mearns MB, et al: Cystic fibrosis in adolescents and adults. Thorax. 1987;42:526-532.

15. Gaskin K, Gurwitz D, Durie P, et al. Improved respiratory prognosis in patients with cystic fibrosis with normal fat absorption. J Pediatr. 1982;100:857-862.

16. Wood RE, Boat TF, Doershuk CF: State of the art: Cystic fibrosis. Am Rev Respir Dis. 1976;113:833-878.

17. Stern RC, Boat TF, Doershuk CF: Obstructive azoospermia as a diagnostic criterion for the cystic fibrosis syndrome. Lancet. 1982;1:1401-1403.

18. Brasfield D, Hicks G: The chest roentgenogram in cystic fibrosis: a new scoring system. Pediatrics. 1979;63:24-29.

19. Schwachman H, Kulczycki L: Long term study of one-hundred five patients with cystic fibrosis. J Dis Child. 1958;96:6-15.

20. Biller J, Grand R: Pancreatic disorders in childhood, in Sleisenger M, Fordtran J (eds): Gastrointestinal Disease: Pathophysiology, Diagnosis, Management, ed 4. Philadelphia, WB Saunders Co, 1988, pp 1789-1813.

21. Bye A, Muller D, Wilson J, et al. Symptomatic vitamin E deficiency in cystic fibrosis. Arch Dis Child 1985. 60:162-164.

22. Kerrebijn KF, Veentjer R, Bonjet VD, et al. The immediate effect of physiotherapy and aerosol treatment on pulmonary function in children with cystic fibrosis. Eur J Respir Dis. 1982;63:35-42.

23. Desmond KJ, Schwenk FW, Thomas E, et al: Immediate and long term effects of chest physiotherapy in patients with cystic fibrosis. J Pediatr. 1983;103:538-542.

24. Reisman J, Rivington-Law B, Corey M, et al: Role of conventional physiotherapy in cystic fibrosis. J Pediatr. 1988;113:632-639.

25. Stanghelle JK: Physical exercise for patients with cystic fibrosis: A review. Int J Sports Med 1988;9 (suppl):6-18.

26. Scanlin TF, in: Fishman AP (ed): Pulmonary Diseases and Disorders, ed 2. New York McGraw-Hill, 1988, pp 1273-1294.

27. Auerbach HS, Williams M, Kirkpatrick JA, et al: Alternate day prednisone reduces morbidity and improves pulmonary function in cystic fibrosis. Lancet 1985;2:686-688.

28. Brissette S, Zinman R, Reidy M: Disclosure of psychosocial concerns of young adults with a dvanced cystic fibrosis (CF) by a nurse home visiting program. Int J Nurs Stud. 1988;25:67-72.
29. Cynamon HA, Milou DE, Valenstein E, et al: Effect of vitamin E deficiency on neurologic function in patients with cystic fibrosis. J Pediatr. 1988;113:636-640.
30. Kollberg H: Cystic fibrosis and physical activity: An introduction. Int J Sports Med. 1988;9(Suppl):2-5.
31. Strandvik B: Antibiotic therapy of pulmonary infections in cystic fibrosis: Dosage schedules and duration of treatment. Chest. 1988;95(Suppl 2):146S-149S.
32. Kuzemko JA: Home treatment of pulmonary infections in cystic fibrosis. Chest. 1988;94(Suppl 2):162S-166S.
33. Hodson M: Antibiotic treatment: Aerosol therapy. Chest.1983; 94(Suppl 2):156S-160S.
34. Hiby N., Hemophilus influenza, Staphylococcus cepaci aureus, Pseudomonas cepacia, and Pseudomonas aeruginosa in patients with cystic fibrosis. Chest. 1988;94(Suppl 2):97S-102S.
35. Stern RC: The primary care physician and the patient with cystic fibrosis. J Pediatr. 1989;114:31-36.
36. Penketh A, Knight RK, Hodson M, et al: Management of pneumothorax in adults with cystic fibrosis. Thorax. 1982;37:850-853.
37. Gotz M, Burghuber O, Salzer-Muhar U, et al: Cor pulmonale in cystic fibrosis. J R Soc Med. 1989; 82C (Suppl 16):26-31.
38. Durie P, Forstner G: Pathophysiology of the exocrine pancreas in cystic fibrosis. J R Soc Med. 1989;82(Suppl 16):2-10.
39. Huang NN, Schidlow DV, Palmer J, et al: Clinical features, survival rate, and prognostic factors in young adults with cystic fibrosis. Am J Med 1987;82:871-879.
40. Geddes D, Hodson M: The role of heart and lung transplantation in the treatment of cystic fibrosis. J R Soc Med. 1989;82(Suppl 16):49-53.

Case 3

Thrombotic Thrombocytopenic Purpura

Donald E. Thornton, MD. and Earl N. Metz, MD, FACP

Case History

A 32-year-old carpenter was in vigorous good health until about two months before his admission to the hospital when he began to be aware of increasing fatigue and some loss of appetite. A few weeks later, he developed shortness of breath with exertion and some cough. He did not seek medical attention, however, until the onset of numbness and tingling in his right arm and leg. He was hospitalized and additional history included the absence of fever, chills, significant weight loss, or muscle weakness. His physician did note the presence of scleral icterus and multiple ecchymoses of the skin. The initial laboratory evaluation included a hemoglobin concentration of 6.3 g/dl and a platelet count of 28,000μl. Numerous fragmented red cells (schistocytes) were noted in the peripheral blood film. His reticulocyte count was elevated at 11%. The lactic dehydrogenase concentration in the serum was markedly elevated at 3,275 units and the fibrinogen concentration was slightly reduced at 125 mg/dl. The prothrombin and partial thromboplastin times were normal. A bone marrow aspiration was performed and demonstrated increased megakaryocytes and erythroid hyperplasia. Therapy was begun with prednisone, aspirin, dipyridamole, and red cell transfusions but three days later his platelet count had not improved and he developed expressive aphasia. Arrangements were made for transfer to The Ohio State University Hospital.

Physical examination at the time of admission to our hospital showed a muscular, healthy-appearing young man with a blood pressure of 154/64 mm Hg, a regular pulse of 52 beats/minute, and a normal temperature. He displayed severe expressive aphasia. Additional physical findings included the presence of multiple ecchymoses and petechiae over the extremities as well as small bilateral scleral hemorrhages. His neck was supple. There was no enlargement of superficial lymph nodes. The lungs were clear. The cardiovascular and abdominal examinations were unremarkable. There was no palpable enlargement of spleen or liver. The rectal examination was normal and the stool gave a negative reaction to guaiac testing.

His peripheral pulses were all present and symmetrical. On neurologic examination the deep tendon reflexes and plantar responses were normal. Motor strength and cutaneous sensation were intact but he displayed slurred speech and an expressive aphasia.

Laboratory Data. Laboratory studies at the time of transfer included a hemoglobin concentration of 9.2 g/dl, a white blood cell count of 13,200/μl and a platelet count of 36,000/μl. The differential white cell count included 3 myelocytes, 3 metamyelocytes, 1 band, 73 segmented neutrophils, 18 lymphocytes, and 4 monocytes. The reticulocyte count was elevated at 8.2% and marked fragmentation of red blood cells was again found in the peripheral blood film. A Coombs test was negative. The prothrombin and partial thromboplastin times were again normal and the fibrinogen concentration was 107 mg/dl. Fibrin split products were present in a dilution of 1 to 160. The LDH concentration was greater than 4,000 units. Serum creatinine was 1.9 mg/dl and the blood urea nitrogen was 38 mg/dl. Serum electrolytes and transaminases were normal but total bilirubin was elevated at 2.3 mg/dl with a direct reacting fraction of 0.3 mg/dl. Serum protein electrophoresis was normal. The urinalysis gave a 2 + reaction for protein and the sediment showed red and white blood cells but no casts. Chest x-ray and electrocardiogram were normal. The clinical picture was thought to be compatible with thrombotic thrombocytopenic purpura and, because of his rapidly worsening neurologic status, he was begun immediately on a program of plasma exchange. Approximately 2500 ml of plasma was removed via plasmapheresis and replaced with fresh frozen plasma on the evening of transfer. The following morning his speech was remarkably improved and only slight slurring of his words persisted. Over the next six days, he received a total of five similar plasma exchanges and his neurologic status returned completely to normal. After three exchanges, his platelet count was 105,000/μl and rose further to 300,000/μl on the day of discharge. He returned home taking prednisone, aspirin, and dipyridamole. These drugs were tapered slowly as an outpatient and he remains well off all medications one year after the onset of his illness.

Discussion

This case emphasizes many of the classic features of thrombotic thrombocytopenic purpura (TTP). This is a syndrome which was once almost uniformly fatal and now within recent years is associated with full recovery in over 75% of cases. It is for this reason, its life-threatening yet curable nature, that it is important to recognize the early signs and symptoms associated with this disorder.

Clinical Features. TTP is a relatively rare disorder which in its classic form is characterized by the clinical pentad of fever, thrombocytopenia, microangiopathic hemolytic anemia, neurologic dysfunction, and renal insufficiency. Since Moschowitz originally described the first case[1] many additional cases have been reported and now number several hundred. Most symptoms at presentation are related to altered neurologic function or some form of hemorrhage. Other non-specific symptoms include fatigue, myalgias, nausea, abdominal pain and fever. A majority of patients will have had symptoms for one week or less prior to presentation but occasionally, like the above patient, symptoms will have been present for several weeks or months. In general, females are more frequently affected than males (3:2) and the median age of involvement is in the mid thirties.[2]

Fever is frequently present either on the initial exam or at some point during the course of the illness and is usually less than 102°. Superimposed infections as sources of fever are rarely identified. Thrombocytopenia is usually evident on the physical exam in the form of petechial or purpuric rashes but serious bleeding such as retinal hemorrhages, gross hematuria, vaginal bleeding, and/or gastrointestinal bleeding have also been reported on the initial exam. As a result of brisk hemolysis, anemia can be severe and the skin can be pale and mildly icteric. The neurologic deficit can range from transient, focal dysfunction to global cerebral disorders such as coma or generalized seizures.

Microangiopathic hemolytic anemia and thrombocytopenia are the dominant laboratory abnormalities. The peripheral blood smear reveals a normochromic normocytic anemia with evidence of increased peripheral destruction in the form of schistocytes, burr cells and helmet cells (Fig. 1). Increased reticulocytes and nucleated red cells are also evident. The anemia can be quite severe with a concentration of hemoglobin less than 6.0 g/dl in as many as a third of the cases.[3] Consistent with the increase in red cell destruction an indirect hyperbilirubinemia is common as well as an increase in the LDH. The Coombs test is rarely positive. In more than half the cases, the platelet count is less than $50,000/\mu l$ at presentation and will usually fall to less than $10,000/\mu l$ during the course of the illness. Leukocytosis is also common with counts of $20,000/\mu l$ being common. The differential white blood cell count usually reveals a left shift with frequent immature granulocytes present. A bone marrow aspirate is consistent with the peripheral blood picture in that erythroid hyperplasia and increased megakaryocytes are present in an otherwise normal marrow.

The skin bleeding time is usually prolonged, consistent with the degree of thrombocytopenia. The prothrombin time, fibrinogen and fibrin split products are usually normal but may in rare cases be abnormal. In general, there should be no or little data to support disseminated intravascular coagulation of the more common type and if present is indicative of a poor outcome. Renal impairment is evident in both a urinalysis and in the serum creatinine and BUN. Proteinuria and hematuria are present in 80% of cases and elevations of creatinine are usually less than 3.0 mg/dl. Biopsy of various tissues will reveal a characteristic diffuse hyaline thrombosis of the terminal arterioles and capillaries. There is typically an absence of inflammatory response in the involved arterioles. These hyaline deposits will be evident in most tissues at autopsy. Diagnostic tissue, however, can be easily

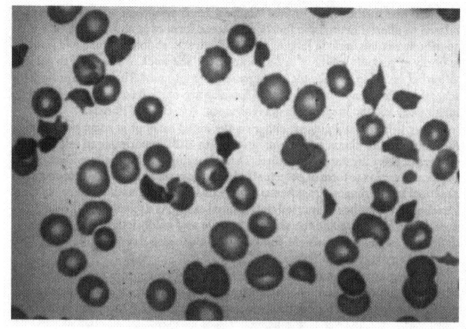

Figure 1. Blood Film Typical of TTP
The presence of fibrin strands in arterioles causes shearing and fracturing of the red cell membrane and leads to hemolysis. In some instances the membrane of the red cell fragments are resealed and these survivors of the fibrin encounter can be seen in the peripheral blood film in the form of helmet-shaped cells and microspherocytes (schistocytes).

obtained from biopsies of the bone marrow, skin, gingiva, or lip. It is believed that these hyaline deposits represent various stages of platelet thrombi with layers of fibrin.

Differential Diagnosis. In cases which display all five of the classic findings the diagnosis of TTP is not difficult. The diagnosis can be made on clinical grounds as we did in the case presented. This patient presented with neurologic symptoms, thrombocytopenia, obvious microangiopathic anemia, and after his transfer to our hospital, renal insufficiency was evident. Atypically, fever was not observed at any time during his course. Nevertheless, the diagnosis of TTP was obvious on the basis of this type of presentation and the need for tissue biopsy confirmation of the diagnosis was not necessary. However, many cases do not present such classic findings. Sometimes the severity of the patient's condition and the fear that other treatable conditions exist make it necessary to establish the diagnosis with tissue biopsy.

Late in the course of severe TTP, evidence of disseminated intravascular coagulation (DIC) can exist and it may be difficult to distinguish the primary problem, DIC versus TTP. The differential diagnosis is actually rather limited. Adult hemolytic-uremic syndrome (HUS) is generally considered a variant of TTP with the distinguishing feature of more prominent renal involvement and less CNS symptoms. Consideration should also be given to systemic lupus erythematosus (SLE) which can have similar symptomatology with some evidence of microangiopathic hemolytic anemia and thrombocytopenia. More commonly, however, in SLE the anemia is the result of Coombs-positive hemolysis or chronic inflammation. Although ANA titers can be present in TTP, titer levels are usually more significantly elevated in SLE. Occasionally some textbooks include idiopathic autoimmune hemolytic anemia (AIHA), idiopathic thrombocytopenia purpura (ITP), or Evan's syndrome (the combination of AIHA and ITP) in the differential diagnosis of TTP. These disorders should not be confused with TTP since microangiopathy, CNS symptoms, or renal insufficiency are not part of ITP, AIHA, or Evan's syndrome.

Although these patients usually present with a severe multisystem illness and may be confusing at first, the differential diagnosis shrinks considerably when the peripheral blood film is examined. Fragmented red blood cells should be readily apparent and the differential then includes only those conditions characterized by mechanical hemolytic anemia. Those conditions include primarily mechanical heart valves, HUS, giant hemangiomas (Kasabach-Merritt syndrome), and a rare patient with widely disseminated carcinoma. Whether or not HUS should be separated out from TTP is debatable.

Tissue biopsy and demonstration of hyaline thrombi in terminal arterioles and capillaries provides a definitive diagnosis of TTP but a patient who presents seriously ill with evidence of mechanical hemolytic anemia, CNS involvement, and renal insufficiency should probably be started on plasmapheresis without delay for additional diagnostic tests.

Pathophysiology. Multiple reports exist in the literature attempting to correlate previous disease states with a subsequent episode of TTP. In general, most patients have no antecedent illness and no consistent associations have been evident. Etiologic roles have been suggested for bacterial or viral infection, environmental factors, pregnancy, malignancy, collagen vascular disorders and genetic predispositions. Some of these deserve special note. For example, a nursing home outbreak of infection with *E. coli* O157:H7 was associated with several cases of an illness indistinguishable from sporadic, idiopathic TTP.[4,5] Second, reports of recurrent mechanical hemolytic anemia in siblings and response to plasma infusion suggest that, indeed, heritable factors may play a role in some cases.[6,7] Evidence of SLE has been reported with an incidence as high as 10%. Other rheumatologic disorders have been associated with TTP including rheumatoid arthritis, Sjogren's syndrome and polyarteritis nodosa. Recently there have been reports of TTP following the treatment of various malignancies. Both HUS and TTP have been described following treatment with mitomycin. Several of the reports of chemotherapy-induced TTP implicate the drug since tumor burden at the time of TTP was reported as small.[5] No general themes can be deduced from this diverse group of factors except that a common immune mechanism must be elicited by these disorders that can, in turn, elicit abnormal thrombosis. Circulating immune complexes have not been consistently isolated from patients, however, nor has immune complex deposition been consistently detected in involved capillaries.[8]

The platelet-fibrin thrombus found in terminal arterioles and capillaries would suggest two possible initial events. First, an agent might be present that can induce vascular endothelial injury which, in turn, induces platelet activation and subsequent fibrin deposits and vessel occlusion. Second, an agent could be present that can induce platelet aggregation as the primary event which would then lead to vessel occlusion and thrombus formation. These two mechanisms are not mutually exclusive and might each play a partial role. Endothelial cell injury can be produced by several factors including IgG, IgM, complement, endotoxin, drugs, viruses, and tumor necrosis factor. Over the last decade most of the attention has focused on the biochemical and molecular events involved with platelet aggregation. Siddiqui and Lian isolated a plasma protein from a patient with TTP that agglutinates platelets.[9] This protein was absent from the same patient upon recovery, was absent from several other normal controls and could be inhibited when mixed with normal plasma or IgG.[10] Since his first description of this platelet-aggregating protein, Lian has also found other patients with a similar protein, suggesting that a subset of patients might have this as a mechanism for their disease process. von Willebrand factor has also been implicated as the abnormal platelet agglutinator in TTP. Unusually large vWF multimers have been isolated from several patients with chronic relapsing TTP and in at least one patient with acute TTP.[11] These multimers are larger than the largest von Willebrand multimers seen in normals. The plasma concentration of these multimers decreases with disease exacerbation but returns upon remission. This has suggested the presence of a "cofactor" required to bring about aggregation and could potentially be produced during an inflammatory process or pregnancy. Wu et al have detected an accelerated loss of prostacyclin in a patient with TTP.[12] Prostacyclin is an arachidonic acid metabolite which inhibits platelet aggregation. They demonstrated the loss of a prostacyclin binding protein which protects prostacyclin from hydrolysis and inactivation. Also, it has been demonstrated that prostacyclin production is depressed in normal endothelial tissue exposed to TTP plasma. In summary, the search for the common pathway which leads to thrombus formation in TTP is ongoing and has focused on agents which can induce vascular endothelial injury or accelerate platelet aggregation.

Treatment. Controlled trials investigating the treatment of TTP are not available primarily because of the rarity of the illness and the fact that the acute and severe nature of the problem does not lend itself to controlled trials. Although several different treatment modalities have been tried, the mainstay of therapy is plasma exchange. Prior to the institution of plasma exchange the mortality of TTP was reported to be in the range of 90%. Whole blood exchange transfusion was first reported to produce a remission by Rubenstein in 1959.[13] This was subsequently confirmed by other studies to induce remission in almost 50% of cases. Plasma exchange began in the late 1970s and was quickly noted to effect remissions in almost 80% of cases. Bukowski reviewed the collected experience at the Cleveland Clinic and the literature and reported 37 of 45 responses (82%).[14] Although most of the reported cases used multimodality therapy along with plasma exchange, six patients at the Cleveland Clinic received plasma exchange alone with five responses.

The goal of treatment is to effect one plasma volume exchange with fresh frozen plasma. Although reports indicate that simple plasma infusion may reverse mild cases, plasmapheresis is the treatment of choice if the resources are available. Plasmapheresis and replacement with fresh plasma should continue until normalization of the CNS and improvement in the platelet count and serum LDH. Anemia and evidence of microangiopathy may take longer to fully normalize and do not require complete resolution before decreasing the intensity of the plasmapheresis. If improvement does not become evident with plasmapheresis, then the volume of exchange can be increased or other modalities can be instituted. Plasmapheresis should be gradually tapered to a three times weekly schedule and then twice weekly. It should be noted that the use of plasmapheresis is designed to fulfill two goals, both the removal and replacement of unknown factors.

Plasma exchange has been credited with the markedly improved remission rate with TTP but relapses have been reported following remission. Recently Rose and Eldor described a 40% (12 of 30) relapse rate following plasmapheresis in 30 patients who survived their initial episode of TTP.[15] Relapses occurred anywhere between 1 and 140 months and episodes of relapse appeared relatively less severe than initial episodes. However, 2 of the 12 died with the subsequent episodes. Two patients had as many as five relapses. Triggering events were also consistent in that one patient had two episodes both occurring with pregnancies, one patient had recurrence associated with surgical procedures (although she also had a third episode unrelated to any event), and one patient had multiple episodes related to repeated episodes of streptococcal tonsillitis. In most patients the presenting signs and symptoms were similar to the initial presentation although several had only laboratory evidence of a microangiopathic hemolytic anemia and thrombocytopenia.

The use of other medications or therapeutic maneuvers is somewhat more controversial since data are lacking concerning their effectiveness. Most hematologists would institute glucocorticoids at the time of diagnosis in the range of 1-2 mg/kg of prednisone daily in order to reduce the inflammatory response to tissue injury. The efficacy of antiplatelet drugs such as aspirin, dipyridamole, sulfinpyrazone, or dextran is somewhat unclear.[16,17] Most reports on the use of these agents utilize at least one other modality and therefore a clearcut benefit has not been established. However, based on the theoretical antithrombotic effect, most clinicians utilize at least one antiplatelet agent and may choose two such as a combination of aspirin and dipyridamole.

Patients who fail to improve after maximal plasmapheresis, steroids, and antiplatelet agents require further intervention. Vincristine is probably the next choice in medical management.[18] Several reports have indicated benefit with vincristine, 2 mg iv/wk. Improvement has been noted after the failure of plasmapheresis, steroids, and antiplatelet agents with one injection to a total of four or five treatments. At least one paper suggests that the use of vincristine will lessen the rate of relapse.[19] Finally, with regard to medical management, anecdotal accounts from several sources exist concerning the use of intravenous immunoglobulin in cases of TTP. These are truly single cases, and intravenous immunoglobulin should be used cautiously.[20]

Splenectomy should be considered when all medical modalities and maximal plasmapheresis have been utilized. Prior to the acceptance of plasmapheresis, splenectomy along with high-dose corticosteroids gained the support of several investigators as the treatment of choice. Several reports noted rapid neurologic improvement within hours of splenectomy and hematologic remission evident within several days of the splenectomy.[21,22] The exact rate of improvement following splenectomy in a large series has not been recorded but Bukowski in his review places the response to steroids and splenectomy at 50%. The decision to proceed to splenectomy is usually difficult in light of the severity of illness in most patients who have failed to improve with maximal medical support but the temporal relationship betweem splenectomy and clinical improvement supports the idea that splenectomy can be an effective treatment in some cases.

Summary. TTP is a syndrome described by the classic pentad of fever, microangiopathic hemolytic anemia, thrombocytopenic purpura, neurologic abnormalities and renal dysfunction. The diagnosis can usually be made on clinical evidence. The pathological lesion responsible for the multisystem disorder is hyaline thrombi composed of platelets and fibrin in terminal arterioles and capillaries distributed throughout most tissues. Diagnostic biopsy may be required in atypical cases and thrombi are evident in gingival, skin, or bone marrow biopsies. Once a uniformly fatal illness, over the last decade the use of plasmapheresis with plasma replacement has become the cornerstone of treatment with remission rates approaching 80%. Steroids and antiplatelet drugs are also commonly used along with plasmapheresis.

References

1. Moschowitz E: An acute febrile pleiochromic anemia with hyaline thrombosis of terminal arterioles and capillaries; an undescribed disease. Arch Intern Med. 1925;36:89-93.
2. Amorosi E, Ultmann O: Thrombotic thrombocytopenic purpura: Report of 16 cases and review of the literature. Medicine. 1966;45:139-159.
3. Kennedy S, Zacharski L, Beck J: Thrombotic thrombocytopenic purpura: Analysis of 48 unselected cases. Semin Thromb Hemostasis. 1980;6:341-347.
4. Carter AO, Borczyk AA, Jacqueline AK, et al: A severe outbreak of Escherichia coli 0157:H7-associated hemorrhagic colitis in a nursing home. N Engl J Med. 1987;317: 1496-1500.
5. Griffin PM, Ostroff SM, Tauxe RV, et al: Illness associated with Escherichia coli O157:H7 infections. A broad clinical spectrum. Ann Intern Med. 1988;109:705-712.
6. Byrnes JJ, Moake JL: Thrombotic thrombocytopenic purpura and the haemolytic uraemic syndrome: Evolving concepts of pathogenesis and therapy. Clin Haematol. 1986;15:413-442.
7. Lyman NW, Michaelson R, Viscuso RL, et al: Mitomycin-induced hemolytic-uremic syndrome: Successful treatment with corticosteroids and intense plasma exchange. Arch Intern Med. 1983;143:1617-1618.
8. Brain Mc, Neame PB: Thrombotic thrombocytopenic purpura and hemolytic uremic syndrome. Semin. Hemostasis Thromb. 1982;8:186-196.
9. Siddiqui F, Lian E: Novel platelet-agglutinating protein from a thrombotic thrombocytopenic purpura plasma. J Clin Invest. 1985;76:1330-1337.
10. Siddiqui F, Lian E: Platelet-agglutinating protein P37 from a thrombotic thrombocytopenic purpura plasma forms a complex with human immunoglobulin G. Blood. 1988;71:299-304.
11. Moake JL, Byrnes JJ, Troll JH, et al: Unusually large plasma Factor VIII: von Willebrand factor multimers in chronic relapsing thrombotic thrombocytopenic purpura. N Engl J Med. 1982;323:1432-1435.
12. Wu KK, Hall ER, Rossi EC, et al: Serum prostacyclin binding defects in thrombotic thrombocytopenic purpura. J Clin Invest. 1985;75:168-174.
13. Rubenstein MA, Kagagn BM, MacGulviray MH, et al: Unusual remission in a case of thrombotic thrombocytopenic purpura syndrome following fresh blood exchange transfusion. Ann Intern Med. 1959;51:1409-1419.
14. Bukowski RM, Hewlett JS, Reimer RR, et al: Therapy of thrombotic thrombocytopenic purpura: An overview. Semin Thromb Hemostasis. 1981;7:1-8.
15. Rose M, Eldor A: High incidence of relapses in thrombotic thrombocytopenic purpura: Clinical study of 38 patients. Am J Med. 1987;83:437-444.
16. Amorosi E, Karpatkin S: Antiplatelet treatment of thrombotic thrombocytopenic purpura. Ann Intern Med. 1977;86:102-107.
17. Rosove MH, Ho WG, Goldfinger D: Ineffectiveness of aspirin and dipyridamole in the treatment of thrombotic thrombocytopenic purpura. Ann Intern Med. 1982;96:27-33.
18. Gutterman LA, Stevenson TD: Treatment of thrombotic thrombocytopenic purpura with vincristine. JAMA. 1982;247:1433-1436.
19. Sennett ML, Conrad ME: Treatment of thrombotic thrombocytopenic purpura: Plasmapheresis, plasma transfusion and vincristine. Arch Intern Med. 1986;146:266-267.
20. Wong P, Itoh K, Yoshida S: Treatment of thrombotic thrombocytopenic purpura with intravenous gamma globulin. N Engl J Med. 1986;314:385.
21. Goldenfarb PB, Finch SC: Thrombotic thrombocytopenic purpura: A ten year survey. JAMA. 1973;226:644-647.
22. Cuttner J: Splenectomy, steroids, and dextran 70 in thrombotic thrombocytopenic purpura. JAMA. 1974;227:397-402.

Case 4

Thyroid Abnormalities in Hyperemesis Gravidarum

Douglas Myers, MD and Ernest L. Mazzaferri, MD, FACP

Case History

A 29-year-old white woman, physician's wife, who was pregnant for the first time was admitted to the Obstetrics service at University Hospitals with protracted nausea, vomiting and dehydration. She was known to be at six weeks gestation with a twin pregnancy that had been achieved with use of exogenous gonadotropins.

Her nausea and vomiting had started several weeks earlier and had progressed to the point that she was unable to ingest any solid food and could only take small amounts of liquids. Despite having received several liters of intravenous fluids at home, her weight decreased from 105 pounds to 95 pounds, she developed extreme weakness, and developed orthostatic symptoms. She was admitted from the out-patient clinic with a diagnosis of hyperemesis gravidarum.

Routine blood studies obtained on the obstetrics inpatient service were normal except for a serum potassium of 3.3 mmole/liter, a blood urea nitrogen of 28 mg/dl, and ketonuria. Screening thyroid function tests disclosed a total thyroxine (T_4) of 20.2 μg/dl (normal 3.5-11), thyroid hormone binding ratio (THBR) of 1.09 (normal 0.7-1.25), free T_4 index (FT_4I) of 18.5 (normal 3.5-11), and thyrotropin (TSH) 0.12 μU/ml (normal 0.2-5.0, lower detection limit 0.01). Her β-hCG was within the expected range. A medical consultation was requested.

The medical consultant found that the patient was receiving intravenous rehydration and potassium supplementation. Upon interviewing the patient further it was found that, other than having asymptomatic mitral valve prolapse documented in the past, she had no previous medical illnesses. There was no history of thyroid illness or recent symptoms of heat intolerance, palpitations, diarrhea or tremors.

Physical Examination. She was a thin, pale female who did not appear anxious, agitated or in severe distress. Vital signs revealed a supine blood pressure of 110/70 mm Hg and resting heart rate of 72. Upon standing, her blood pressure fell to 95/60 mm Hg and her heart rate rose to 88. She was afebrile. She had no evidence of lid lag or proptosis and her thyroid gland was not palpably enlarged. Her cardiac examination disclosed a midsystolic click without a murmur and her abdominal exam was unremarkable. The skin showed no abnormalities, and the neurological examination was not remarkable. She had no tremor.

Hospital Course. Because, in the opinion of the attending obstetricians and medical consultants, she had no signs of thyrotoxicosis, antithyroid therapy was not initiated. The patient's symptoms abated and she improved gradually after 8 liters of replacement fluid therapy, and she was discharged. Within 10 days, however, her vomiting and dehydration recurred and she was readmitted to University Hospital. Her examination and laboratory tests were unchanged from her first hospitalization, including persistent elevation of her FT4I and suppression of basal serum TSH concentrations. Because of a further weight loss, persistent hypokalemia and a low serum albumin, total parenteral nutrition via a central venous catheter was started. She once again improved, and was discharged with instructions for continued home parenteral nutrition on a nightly basis.

Discussion

The patient under discussion presented with the two perplexing problems of severe hyperemesis gravidarum and abnormal thyroid function tests suggesting thyrotoxicosis. Several important questions are posed by this patient's clinical problem. Was she thyrotoxic? Is there a relationship between her hyperemesis gravidarum and the abnormal thyroid function tests? Did she require antithyroid drug treatment? Is she or her child at increased risk of developing thyroid disease in the future?

Thyrotoxicosis is a rare event during pregnancy, developing in only about two of every 1,000 pregnant women.[1] Even pregnant patients with Graves' disease in remission do not usually develop an exacerbation of thyrotoxicosis that requires therapy.[2] However, when thyrotoxicosis does occur during pregnancy it can result in spontaneous abortion, premature labor, and fetal death.[1] Although severe thyrotoxicosis is usually easily diagnosed, recognizing mild or moderate thyrotoxicosis during pregnancy is another matter. Severely thyrotoxic patients tend to have multiple symptoms, including weakness, fatigue, dyspnea, palpitations, profuse sweating, heat intolerance, anxiety, nervousness, and emotional lability.[3] Some of these features may be seen in normal pregnancy and can be confused with simple anxiety.[1]

The pregnant women who fails to gain weight, displays muscle weakness and has severe heat intolerance should be suspected of having thyrotoxicosis. Physical signs that accompany this disorder which are particularly helpful in establishing the diagnosis during pregnancy include goiter, hyperkinetic behavior, fine tremor, eyelid retraction, stare, warm moist skin, fine hair, a rapid pulse, wide pulse pressure, and a hyperdynamic precordium with a systolic murmur. Although goiter is often attributed to pregnancy itself, this is a rare finding which should prompt a search for thyroid dysfunction. In the United States, the most common cause of thyrotoxicosis during pregnancy is Graves' disease, an autoimmune disorder characterized by diffuse goiter, infiltrative eye signs, and pretibial myxedema. Although thyrotoxic Graves' disease can occur in the absence of goiter, this is uncommon and should raise serious question about the diagnosis. The patient under discussion had no symptoms of thyrotoxicosis except for weight loss which could be attributed to her pernicious vomiting, and she had none of the physical findings of Graves' disease, including goiter. Accordingly, the diagnosis of thyrotoxicosis was questioned.

The laboratory diagnosis of thyrotoxicosis is confirmed by demonstrating elevated serum *free* (unbound) thyroid hormone levels, the physiologically active component of thyroid hormone in the circulation. In severely thyrotoxic patients both serum *free* T_4 and T_3 are usually elevated, but in mild thyrotoxicosis both may be barely elevated.[3] Sometimes only the serum T_3 is elevated, a condition termed T_3 toxicosis, but almost never is the T_4 alone high in thyrotoxicosis.[3] Unfortunately, a number of nonthyroidal illnesses, drugs, and certain physiologic conditions alter thyroid function tests in a way that may lead to an erroneous diagnosis of thyrotoxicosis. Typically, nonthyroidal illness lowers the serum T_3 concentration, even in patients with concurrent thyrotoxicosis. Less commonly, nonthyroidal illness elevates the serum T_4 alone, a condition termed euthyroid hyperthyroxinemia which may be confused with thyrotoxicosis. An isolated serum T_4 elevation thus should not be accepted as face value evidence of thyrotoxicosis.

Thyroid function tests are altered by normal pregnancy in a way which may lead to diagnostic confusion in the patient suspected of having concurrent thyrotoxicosis. Early in normal pregnancy, the rise in estrogens stimulates hepatic thyroid-binding globulin (TBG) production.[1] As a result, serum TBG levels begin to rise within the first month of gestation and continue to climb throughout pregnancy. By the fifth gestational week, thyroid function tests are altered and remain modified until 6 to 12 weeks after delivery.[1] In normal pregnancy, total serum T_4 typically rises by 2-4 μg/dl and total serum T_3 increases by 65 to 95 ng/dl.[1] Elevations in serum thyroid hormone concentrations caused by high serum TBG concentrations normally do not elevate serum *free* hormone levels and the patient does not develop thyrotoxicosis. During pregnancy, however, possibly as the result of thyroidal stimulation by hCG, free serum thyroid hormone concentrations rise slightly during the first trimester, gradually returning to normal by the third trimester as hCG levels drop.[1] Nonetheless, pituitary TSH secretion remains detectably unaltered and basal serum TSH levels remain normal throughout pregnancy, correctly confirming the patient's euthyroid status.

Serum *total* T_4 values above 15 μg/dl in the pregnant woman suggest thyrotoxicosis, and elevated serum free hormone levels confirm this diagnosis. However, radioimmunoassays (RIA) using T_4 (or T_3) analogues designed to measure free hormone concentrations may be misleading during pregnancy.[1] Likewise, calculated free hormone estimates (free T_4 or T_3 index) derived from the total hormone (total T_4 or T_3) and THBR may be erroneous during pregnancy, and are altered by non-thyroidal illness.[a]

The serum TSH measurement can be used to diagnose thyrotoxicosis because, with rare exceptions, high serum thyroid hormone concentrations suppress pituitary TSH secretion. Baseline serum TSH levels are depressed and the pituitary will not release TSH in response to thyrotropin-releasing hormone (TRH). Older, less sensitive TSH RIAs, however, could not distinguish between normal and suppressed basal serum TSH concentrations, and a TRH[b] stimulation test was required to identify equivocal thyrotoxicosis. Newer TSH immunometric (IMA) assays, which are at least tenfold more sensitive than the older RIAs, can reliably distinguish between normal and suppressed basal serum TSH concentrations, thus making TRH testing unnecessary. The serum TSH IMA concentration in euthyroid subjects, including normal pregnant women, is usually between 0.5 and 5.0 μU/ml and the lower detection limits are between 0.1 and 0.01 μU/ml, depending upon the TSH IMA kit used. About 90-95% of thyrotoxic patients have undetectable basal TSH concentrations, while the others have low but detectable TSH values.[3] Even though non-thyroidal illness may lower serum TSH IMA concentrations, an undetectable TSH is strong evidence for thyrotoxicosis.[3]

Thus the diagnosis of thyrotoxicosis sometimes can be difficult during pregnancy because the signs and symptoms of thyrotoxicosis may be mistaken for the normal physiologic changes of pregnancy, and diagnostic tests can be misleading. Added to this is the recently recognized fact that thyroid function tests are abnormal in pregnant women who develop hyperemesis gravidarum.[4] However, the patient under discussion had a low but detectable serum TSH IMA, raising serious question about the diagnosis of thyrotoxicosis.

---

[a]*Tests that reflect thyroid hormone binding to plasma proteins as the T_3 resin uptake test (T_3RU) are now collectively called the thyroid hormone binding ratio (THBR). The free T_4 index is calculated from the total T_3 index from the total T_3 and THBR, but the exact method of calculation critically influences the result (see Letter to the Editor. Revised nomenclature for tests of thyroid hormone and thyroid-related proteins in serum. J Clin Endocrinol Metab. 1987;64(5):1089-1093).*

[b]*The TRH test is performed by giving an intravenous bolus of 400 μg TRH with measurement of serum TSH concentrations at 9, 30, and 60 min. The peak increment in serum TSH concentrations after TRH in normal subjects varies considerably, ranging from 2 to 32 μU/ml, and occurs from 10 to 45 min after TRH administration. The basal serum TSH concentration is below the assay detection limits and fails to rise with TRH in thyrotoxic patients. The TRH test, however, is expensive, often causes side effects, and is no longer necessary in most patients when TSH IMA is measured.*

Nausea and vomiting are commonly seen in the first three months of pregnancy, occurring in up to 50% of pregnant women.[5] However, hyperemesis gravidarum[6] — defined as several weeks of vomiting resulting in weight loss[7] — is seen in less than 1% of pregnancies. Although the exact etiology of hyperemesis gravidarum is unknown,[8] thyroid functional abnormalities have been implicated as a cause of this problem.

Rarely, nonpregnant patients have nausea and vomiting as the main presenting feature of thyrotoxicosis.[9] In pregnancy, several case reports[4,10,11,12] have implicated thyrotoxicosis as the cause of hyperemesis gravidarum. However, more recently, a number of studies[6,7,13-15] have demonstrated that up to 73% of patients[3] with hyperemesis have transient elevations of serum T_4 concentrations.

The first series of patients with hyperemesis gravidarum and abnormal thyroid function tests was reported in 1982 by Bouillon et al.[7] During their episode of hyperemesis gravidarum, 24 of 33 (73%) pregnant women had an elevated free T_4 index, either alone or with a high serum free T_3 index. In five patients who were tested, no increase in serum TSH concentrations occurred in response to TRH injection. Hyperthyroxinemia returned to normal in one to several weeks, whether or not it was treated with antithyroid drugs. A lower birth weight was observed in the pregnancies complicated by hyperemesis gravidarum and elevated serum free T_4 concentrations, but the abortion rate and duration of pregnancy were not discernably influenced.

In other studies the incidence of hyperthyroxinemia in patients with hyperemesis gravidarum has been reported to range from 33% to 44%.[6,13-15] Even in some pregnant women with mild morning sickness, serum free T_4 rises above, and TSH falls below, normal limits.[16] In pregnant women with hyperemesis gravidarum, no difference in pregnancy outcome, including birth weight, was noted in subjects with and without hyperthyroxinemia by one group,[14] while another[7] reported lower birth weights when mothers were hyperthyroxinemic. Indeed, whether or not patients with hyperemesis gravidarum and hyperthyroxinemia with suppressed pituitary TSH secretion are actually thyrotoxic at a tissue level remains enigmatic. However, if this represents occult thyrotoxicosis, it does not affect the fetus in the same devastating way as overt thyrotoxicosis as shown in the study by Sugure[17] in which fetal mortality in untreated thyrotoxicosis approached 50% and, even with therapy, was about 15%.

The pathogenesis of hyperthyroxinemia in women with hyperemesis gravidarum is not clear. Although controversial, there is evidence that very high levels of β-hCG can stimulate the thyroid follicle to secrete thyroid hormone. Elevated β-hCG levels, as occur in trophoblastic neoplasms, correlate directly with elevated maternal serum T_4 concentrations,[18] an observation which is controversial.[19] One study[6] of pregnant women with hyperemesis gravidarum showed elevated serum β-hCG levels in those with elevated serum thyroxine levels. Similar findings were reported in another study[16] of pregnant women with milder nausea.[16] Nevertheless, a causal relationship between elevated β-hCG and hyperthyroxinemia can only be inferred from these studies.

Whatever the underlying mechanism, it is clear that the thyroid gland of women with hyperemesis gravidarum is being stimulated by a TSH-like substance, which is perhaps hCG, and not by TSH itself. Bober et al[13] showed that 8 of 10 hyperemesis gravidarum patients with elevated FT_4 levels also had suppressed serum TSH levels. All 10 had an impaired TSH response to TRH stimulation similar to that which occurs in thyrotoxicosis. Suppressed basal and TRH-stimulated serum TSH concentrations indicate that pituitary TSH secretion had been suppressed by hyperthyroxinemia in these patients, an observation confirmed by others.[7,16]

Since overt thyrotoxicosis in pregnancy may coincide with, or cause, hyperemesis gravidarum[4,10,11] it is important to differentiate the two. However, at present there is no certain method for differentiating euthyroid hyperthyroxinemia caused by hyperemesis gravidarum from thyrotoxicosis in pregnancy complicated by pernicious vomiting. Several authors have suggested that erythrocyte zinc levels might differentiate the two. The erythrocyte zinc level has been found to be low in thyrotoxicosis[20-22], but it is normal in hyperthyroxinemic women with hyperemesis gravidarum.[23,24] Circulating erythrocytes take time to change their zinc concentrations and transient hyperthyroxinemia would not be expected to change their zinc concentrations. It is thus not surprising that patients with hyperemesis gravidarum have normal erythroctye zinc concentrations. Further studies must be performed if this test is to become clinically helpful.

At present, the most reliable features that differentiate thyrotoxicosis from hyperemesis gravidarum with hyperthyroxinemia are bedside signs such as goiter, infiltrative ophthalmopathy, or other clear signs of thyrotoxicosis such as a markedly hyperdynamic precordium, muscle weakness, and clear thyrotoxic changes in the skin and its appendages. A TSH IMA below the assay detection limits, ordinarily a strong sign of thyrotoxicosis, may not be reliable in this situation.

An approach to this problem is summarized in Fig. 1. Although not without its uncertainties, along with close followup, true cases of thyrotoxicosis usually can be identified and differentiated from hyperemesis gravidarum with hyperthyroxinemia. Using this approach, antithyroid medications will not be given while thyrotoxic women will be promptly treated.

Our patient presented with hyperemesis gravidarum and laboratory evidence of hyperthyroidism. Because she had no palpable thyroid gland and no clinical evidence of thyrotoxicosis, she was treated conservatively with antiemetics and rehydration. After about 8 weeks of parenteral nutrition, she gained weight, her hyperemesis resolved, and for the remainder of her pregnancy she was able to eat and drink without difficulty. However, because of preterm labor at 20 weeks gestation, she was readmitted to the hospital when it was discovered that one of the fetuses had expired. The preterm labor was halted successfully. At that time her total T_4 was 13.3 μg/dl, the FT_4I was 10.4, and her TSH was 3.4 μU/ml. She was

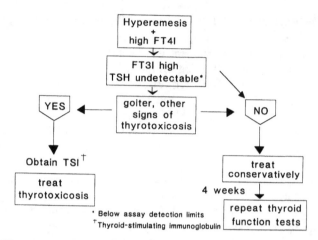

Figure 1. Evaluation of Hyperemesis with High Serum FT4I

placed on terbutaline and remained at bed rest until a healthy boy was delivered at 37 weeks gestation. There was no evidence of thyroid abnormalities in either mother or son at the time of delivery.

This patient's ordeal appears to be consistent with numerous cases of hyperemesis gravidarum that have recently been reported. Most authors have advocated conservative treatment (i.e., no antithyroid medications) unless there is clinical evidence of thyrotoxicosis. Although the pathogenesis of this disorder is not known, it may be due to a thyroid-stimulating substance, perhaps hCG, that appears early in pregnancy which may also cause nausea and vomiting. Further studies are needed to help clarify the pathogenesis of this syndrome.

References

1. Mazzaferri E: Thyrotoxicosis in pregnancy. in Zuspan FP, Quilligan EJ (eds): Current Therapy in Obstetrics and Gynecology. Philadelphia, WB Saunders Co, 1990.
2. Dozeman R, Kaiser FE, Cass O, et al: Hyperthyroidism appearing as hyperemesis gravidarum. Arch Intern Med. 1983;143:2202-2203.
3. de los Santos ET, Mazzaferri E. Medical management of thyrotoxicosis. Postgrad Med. 1990;87:277-294.
4. Amino N, Tanizawa O, Mori H, et al: Aggravation of thyrotoxicosis in early pregnancy and after delivery in Graves' disease. J Clin Endocrinol Metab. 1982;55:108-112.
5. Evans A, Li T, Selby C, et al: Morning sickness and thyroid function. Br J Obstet Gynaecol. 1985;93:520-522.

6. Swaminathan R, Chin R, Lao T, et al: Thyroid function in hyperemesis gravidarum. Acta Endocrinol (Copenh agen.) 1989;120:155-160.

7. Bouillon R, Naesens M, Van Assche F, et al: Thyroid function in patients with hyperemesis gravidarum. Am J Obstet Gynecol. 1982;143:922-926.

8. Masson G, Anthony F, Chau E. Serum chorionic gonadotrophin (hCG), schwangerschaftsprotein 1 (SP1), progesterone and oestradiol levels in patients with nausea and vomiting in early pregnancy. Br J Obstet Gynaecol. 1985;92:211-215.

9. Rosenthal FD, Jones C, Lewis SI: Thyrotoxic vomiting. Br Med J. 1976;2:209-211.

10. Valentine B, Jones C, Tyack A: Hyperemesis gravidarum due to thyrotoxicosis. Postgrad Med J. 1980;56:746-747.

11. Jeffcoate WJ, Bain C: Recurrent pregnancy-induced thyrotoxicosis presenting as hyperemesis gravidarum. Br J Obstet Gynaecol. 1985;92:413-415.

12. Lao T, Cockram C, Chin R, et al: Transient hyperthyroidism in hyperemesis gravidarum. J Soc Med. 1986;9:613-615.

13. Bober S, McGill A, Tunbridge W. Thyroid function in hyperemesis gravidarum. Acta Endocrinol (Copenhagen). 1986;111:404-410.

14. Lao T, Chin R, Chang A. The outcome of hyperemetic pregnancies complicated by transient hyperthyroidism. Aust NZ J Obstet Gynaecol. 1987;27:99-101.

15. Chin R, Lao T. Thyroxine concentration and outcome of hyperemetic pregnancies. Br J Obstet Gynaecol. 1988;95:507-509.

16. Mori M, Amino N, Tamaki H, et al: Morning sickness and thyroid function in normal pregnancy. Obstet Gynecol 1988;72:355-359.

17. Sugure D, Drury MI. Hyperthyroidism complicating pregnancy: Results of treatment by antithyroid drugs in 77 pregnancies. Br J Obstet Gynaecol. 1980;87:970-975.

18. Norman R, Green-Thompson R, Jialal I, Hyperthyroidism in gestational trophoblastic neoplasia. Clin Endocrinal (Oxford) 1981;15:395-401.

19. Amir D, Osathanondh R, Berkowitz R, et al: Human chorionic gonadotropin and thyroid function in patients with hydatidiform mole. Am J Obstet Gynecol. 1984;150:723-728.

20. Bremner WF, Fell GS: Zinc metabolism and thyroid status. Postgrad Med J. 1977; 53:143-145.

21. Nishi Y, Kawate R, Usui T: Zinc metabolism in thyroid disease. Postgrad Med J. 1980; 56:833-837.

22. Swaminathan R, Segall NH, Chapman C, et al: Red-blood-cell composition in thyroid disease. Lancet. 1976;2:1382-1385.

23. Lao T, et al: Erythrocyte zinc in differential diagnosis of hyperthyroidism in pregnancy: a preliminary report. Br Med J. 1987;294:1064.

24. Lao T, Chin R, Mak Y, et al: Plasma zinc concentration and thyroid function in hyperemetic pregnancies. Acta Obstet Gynecol Scand. 1988;67:599-604.

Case 5

Solitary Pulmonary Nodule

Jeffrey E. Weiland, MD

Case History

A 49-year-old female bank executive presented to Ohio State University Hospitals for a routine physical. She had not seen a physician since her last child was born (age 38) but she was due for a promotion which required a physical examination. She denied any physical complaints. She had a forty pack-year history of smoking. Her past medical history was only remarkable for three pregnancies resulting in healthy term deliveries. She was born and raised in a small town in Ohio but had lived in an urban setting for the past 20 years.

Physical Examination. She was a healthy-appearing middle-aged white woman in no respiratory distress. Her temperature was 98.8°F, pulse rate 80, respiratory rate 16, and blood pressure 110/76 mm Hg. Examination of the head and neck, lymph nodes, and breasts was normal. Lung examination revealed normal breath sounds bilaterally. Cardiac and abdominal findings were normal. There was no bony tenderness, and the neurologic and pelvic examinations were normal.

Laboratory Data. The pertinent laboratory values were: hematocrit 39.5%, hemoglobin 13.2 g/dl, white cell count 6500/mm^3, with a normal differential. The serum electrolytes were normal. The serum aspartate aminotransferase (SGOT) was 32 IU/liter, alanine aminotransferase (SGPT) 7 IU/liter, lactic dehydrogenase (LDH) 190 IU/liter, alkaline phosphatase 86 IU/liter, and glutamyl transpeptidase (GGT) 20 IU/liter. Her PA and lateral chest radiographs are shown in Figures 1 and 2. A chest CT scan is shown in Figure 3.

Discussion

The evaluation of an asymptomatic individual with a solitary pulmonary nodule should proceed along two parallel lines of investigation. The first should address the question: Is the lesion benign or malignant? Unless a finding establishes with absolute certainty that a lesion is benign, the investigation must proceed. The

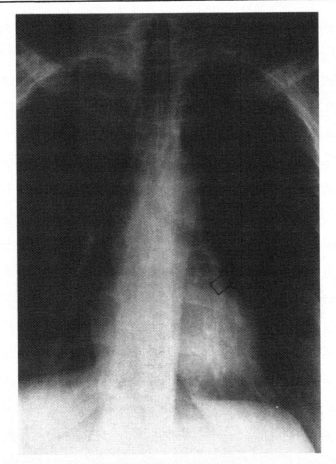

Figure 1. Standard Posterior-Anterior Chest Roentgenogram
Reveals a 1 cm soft tissue nodule in the left midlung field (arrow). There is no obvious calcification.

second question is: Has the disease spread beyond the chest? An affirmative answer obviously alters the course of subsequent investigative efforts.

Is the lesion benign or malignant? Approximately 20% of all solitary pulmonary nodules encountered in a general medical clinic will prove to be malignant.[1] Unfortunately, few historical points or clinical tests can accurately separate benign from malignant disease. The age of the patient and the individual's smoking habits are the two most useful historical points. Less than 1% of solitary pulmonary nodules in patients under 35 years of age are malignant and therefore, most lesions in this age group can safely be observed. The incidence of malignancy rises progressively and peaks in the fifth to sixth decade. Tobacco is an important risk, with over 90% of bronchogenic carcinomas probably directly linked to cigarette smoking. There is an association between the degree of tobacco exposure and risk.[2] Smokers with greater than 25 pack-years have a 10- to 15-fold greater risk of lung cancer,[3] and risk progressively declines after smoking cessation. Cancer risk in former smokers decreases to near the risk for nonsmokers after 10 to 15 years of abstinence.[4]

Two radiographic criteria are extremely useful in establishing the benign nature of a solitary pulmonary nodule. The first relates to the presence or absence of calcification and can usually be adequately assessed on the plain film of the chest. Central, diffuse, laminar or popcorn calcifications only occur in benign nodules. If

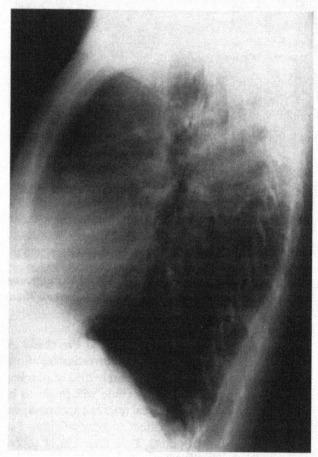

Figure 2. Standard Left Lateral Chest Roentogenogram
Demonstrates the soft tissue nodule in the anterior segment of the left lobe.

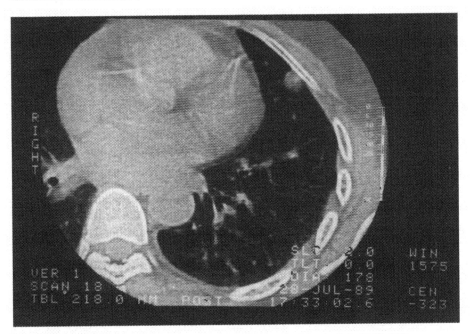

Figure 3. Computed Tomographic Scan at the Level of the Left Hilum
The nodule is better delineated but this study fails to demonstrate any pattern of calcification which would suggest a benign etiology.

the plain film reveals that a lesion is clearly calcified or clearly of soft tissue density, no further roentgenographic studies are needed. If there are questions about the presence of calcium or the density of a nodule, computerized tomography (CT) is sometimes helpful. While CT is no better than standard tomography in detecting calcium, the increased cost of CT is justified by the additional information provided by CT. Specifically, CT may rarely reveal the presence of other nodules not seen on the plain film and will also provide a more accurate assessment of mediastinal adenopathy. The second useful radiographic criterion relates to the nodule's growth rate or doubling time. The doubling time of malignant lesions is between 20 and 400 days.[5] In contrast, benign lesions either grow rapidly (< 30 days) or change little at all. This has led to the axiom that a nodule is benign if it noticeably grows in under 30 days or remains stable for at least 2 years. Unfortunately, growth rates are only helpful if previous films are available or a decision is made to observe the lesion over time.

Of the noninvasive tests available to image pulmonary nodules, only CT has proven to have potential utility in separating benign from malignant disease. It is well known that benign lesions are more dense than malignant lesions and CT scans are fairly accurate in measuring density. Using this principle, two studies have demonstrated that CT can differentiate benign from malignant disease with a fair degree of certainty.[6,7] Unfortunately, these studies have not been reproduced in other centers. This probably relates to the variability between the various CT scanners currently in use.[8] Recently, a lung nodule simulator or phantom has been described which can better standardize the density measurements and can be used with any modern scanner.[9] Initial studies produced results remarkably similar to the earlier studies.[10] However, 1 out of 2 ultimately benign nodules were indeterminate by CT/phantom criteria and there was a false negative. Thus, CT currently is of only modest utility in the evaluation of a noncalcified solitary pulmonary nodule.

Recently, two invasive techniques have come into widespread use in the evaluation of pulmonary nodules. Both transthoracic needle aspiration and transbronchial needle aspiration have demonstrated utility in the diagnosis of malignant disease in the chest.[11,12] The yield of the transthoracic approach is somewhat higher than that of the transbronchial needle biopsy (95% vs 60%) but transbroncial sampling offers the additional advantage of direct visualization of the endobronchial tree. Approximately 10% of respiratory cancers are multicentric and there is also a higher incidence of second primaries, usually in the upper airway. For these reasons, bronchoscopy should be performed prior to resection of any presumed malignant pulmonary lesions. The drawback to both needle aspiration techniques is that it is exceedingly difficult to make a benign diagnosis. Therefore, extending the line of reasoning described above, needle aspiration is rarely useful in assuring a physician or patient that a lesion is benign and can be observed. Several recent reviews of the approach to solitary pulmonary nodules have suggested that by combining CT densitometry with needle aspiration, accuracy of determining a benign diagnosis approaches 90%.[13] Unfortunately, this degree of certainty is highly dependent on the ability of the CT radiographer and the physician performing the aspirate. It is my experience that given the dismal prognosis in the nonsurgical management of lung carcinoma, even a 10% chance of malignancy results in an extremely high level of anxiety in the patient. A course of observation can have a tremendous deleterious effect on the patient's home life.

In summary, the differentiation of a benign from a malignant nodule rests largely on historical (age, smoking habits) and radiographic (calcium pattern, doubling time) information obtainable in the physician's office. Based on these data, if a benign etiology cannot be ascertained with certainty, bronchoscopy should be performed to examine the entire respiratory tract. If evidence of disease outside the chest is lacking, the patient, assuming there is adequate cardiopulmonary reserve, should be referred for thoracotomy and resection.

Has the disease spread beyond the chest? The most common sites of metastases for bronchogenic carcinoma are liver, bone, CNS, adrenal glands, and lymph nodes. Numerous studies have shown that the routine use of radiographic imaging of these organs for the detection of clinically occult metastases is unnecessary and

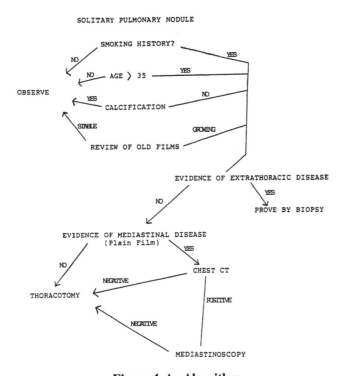

SOLITARY PULMONARY NODULE

SMOKING HISTORY?

NO

NO — AGE > 35 — YES

OBSERVE   NO

YES   CALCIFICATION

STABLE   GROWING

REVIEW OF OLD FILMS

EVIDENCE OF EXTRATHORACIC DISEASE

YES

NO

PROVE BY BIOPSY

EVIDENCE OF MEDIASTINAL DISEASE
(Plain Film)

YES

NO

CHEST CT

NEGATIVE

THORACOTOMY

POSITIVE

NEGATIVE

MEDIASTINOSCOPY

Figure 4. An Algorithm
Depicts a logical approach to the evaluation of a solitary pulmonary nodule.

frequently misleading.[14-16] The incidence of falsely positive bone and liver scans is significant and these findings delay surgery while necessitating a costly, invasive work-up. With the exception of the adrenal gland, the best screen for distant metastases continues to be a good history and physical examination with screening blood tests. Any abnormalities should be followed up with appropriate radionuclide or CT imaging. The adrenal glands are best evaluated by including them on chest CT scans. However, controversy exists regarding the role of chest CT in the staging of bronchogenic carcinomas. In addition to distant metastases, staging of bronchogenic carcinoma should also include an assessment of disease spread within the chest. Pleural and, with the exception of well-differentiated squamous cell carcinoma, mediastinal involvement preclude surgical resection of bronchogenic carcinomas. In practice, occult mediastinal involvement is probably the most common cause of unresectability at the time of surgery. While it is clear that CT is superior to plain films or standard tomograms in detecting enlarged lymph nodes in the mediastinum,[17] normal sized lymph nodes may contain microscopic foci of tumor and this has resulted in a false-negative rate of up to 33% in some studies.[18] Thus, the gold standard for staging of the mediastinum is mediastinoscopy. Unfortunately, this technique requires general anesthesia and is therefore expensive and not without risk. In addition, solitary pulmonary nodules in the peripheral two-thirds of the chest have a very low incidence of mediastinal metastases that are roentgenographically occult. Taken together, solitary nodules in the periphery of the lung do not require staging of the mediastinum unless there are abnormalities on the plain film. When mediastinal abnormalities are evident on the plain film, or the suspicious lesion arises in the central one-third of the chest, evaluation of the mediastinum should be performed, first with chest CT. Any suspicious lymph nodes should be evaluated by mediastinoscopy prior to thoracotomy.

Summary. The clinician's goal in the approach to a solitary pulmonary nodule must be to minimize unnecessary thoracotomies for benign disease while at the same time avoiding unnecessary delays in potentially curative surgery. An algorithm for this approach is depicted in Fig. 4. In the case presented above, previous films were not available. There was no evidence of extrathoracic spread and her mediastinum was normal on the plain film. A bronchoscopy was essentially normal and a transbronchial biopsy revealed only mild inflammatory changes. Routine pulmonary function testing revealed adequate pulmonary reserve. Because of her age and smoking history, she was referred for thoracotomy and wedge resection. This revealed a well-differentiated adenocarcinoma of the lung. Mediastinal nodes were negative for tumor. Her recovery was uneventful. She is currently two years out with no evidence of recurrence and she has stopped smoking.

References

1. Lillington GA. Systematic diagnostic approach to pulmonary nodules, in Fishman AP (ed): Pulmonary Diseases and Disorder. New York, McGraw-Hill Book Co. Inc., 1988, pp 1945-1954.

2. Doll R, Peto R: Cigarette smoking and bronchial carcinoma: Dose and time relationships among regular smokers and lifelong non-smokers. J Epidemiol Community Health. 1978; 32:303-313.

3. Doll R, Peto R: Mortality in relation to smoking: 20 year's observations on male British doctors. Br Med J 1976;2:1525-1536.

4. Smoking and Health. A report of the Surgeon General. Washington DC, US Department of Health, Education and Welfare, Publ. No. (PHS) 79-50066, 1979.

5. Mizuno T, Masaoka A, Ichimura H, et al: Comparison of actual survivorship after treatment with survivorship predicted by actual tumor-volume doubling time from tumor diameter at first observation. Cancer. 1984;53:2716-20.

6. Siegelman SS, Zerhouni EA, Leo FP, et al: CT of the solitary pulmonary nodule. Am J Roentgenol. 1980; 135:1-3.

7. Proto AU, Thomas SR. Pulmonary nodules studied by computed tomography. Radiology. 1985;156:149.

8. Zerhouni EA, Spivey JF, Morgan RH, et al: Factors influencing quantitative CT measurements of solitary pulmonary nodules. J Comput Assist Tomogr. 1982;6:1075-1087.

9. Zerhouni EA, Boukadoum M, Siddiky MA: A standard phantom for quantitative CT analysis of pulmonary nodules. Radiology. 1983;149:767.

10. Zerhouni EA, Stitik FP, Siegelman SS, et al: CT of the pulmonary nodule: A cooperative study. Radiology. 1986;160:319-327.

11. Khouri NF, Stitik FP, Erozan YS, et al: Transthoracic needle aspiration biopsy of benign and malignant lung lesions. Am J Roentgenol. 1985;144:281.

12. Shure D, Fedullo PJ: Transbronchial needle aspiration of peripheral masses. Am Rev Respir Dis 1983;128:1090-1092.

13. Khouri NF, Meziane MA, Zerhouni EA, et al: The solitary pulmonary nodule. Assessment, diagnosis, and management. Chest. 1987;91:128-133.

14. Hooper RG, Beechler CR, Johnson MC: Radioisotope scanning in the initial stage of bronchogenic carcinoma. Am Rev Respir Dis. 1978;118:279.

15. Ramsdell JW, Peters RM, Taylor AT, et al: Multiorgan scans for staging lung cancer. Correlation with clinical evaluation. J Thorac Cardiovasc Surg. 1977;73:653.

16. Turner P, Haggith JW: Preoperative radionuclide scanning in bronchogenic carcinoma. Br J Dis Chest. 1981;75:291.

17. Baron RL, Levitt RG, Sagal SS. Computed tomography in the preoperative evaluation in bronchogenic carcinoma. Radiology. 1982;145:727.

18. Underwood GH Jr, Hooper RG, Axelbaum SP, et al: Computed tomographic scanning of the thorax in the staging of bronchogenic carcinoma. N Engl J Med. 1979;300:777-778.

Case 6

Acute Pericarditis

James Bacon, MD

The entire breadth of acute pericardial illness encompasses a diverse and long list of etiologies.[1-3] Clinicians deal with the types of pericardial disease most likely to present to their specialty and practice setting. Cancer specialists are most frequently exposed to malignant pericardial disease, thoracic surgeons are experienced in the management of traumatic and postoperative pericardial disease, and nephrologists commonly treat uremic or dialysis-associated pericarditis. Tertiary care centers may be involved in the evaluation or treatment of the more acute pericardial illnesses (i.e. tamponade) as well as the coordination of long-term care of chronic pericardial disorders. What is the role of the general internist? This case report and the following discussion will focus upon primary acute idiopathic pericarditis (no obvious cause on initial presentation), in which the general internist is more likely to be initially involved. The goals for this chapter are to (1) discuss the presenting features of acute idiopathic pericarditis, (2) establish a differential diagnosis, (3) recommend a reasonable diagnostic approach in reference to the extensive list of causes, and (4) suggest guidelines for therapy and follow up.

Case History

D.E., a previously well 43-year-old white man, presented to our hospital after a one-week illness characterized by sore throat and chest tightness. During this period, his pain progressively worsened and was exacerbated by inspiration and relieved with sitting forward. His past medical history was unremarkable. There was no history of clinical illness or exposure to tuberculosis, but a tuberculin skin test had been positive in the past. There had been no significant medical illnesses or major operations. He denied illicit drug use and was on no medication at the time of presentation. He was divorced, heterosexual, and employed as a printer. His work environment did not include any obvious exposure to toxic chemicals. He seemed to be at increased risk for the development of coronary artery disease, since his father had undergone coronary bypass grafting.

Physical Exam. The patient appeared uncomfortable. His respiratory rate was 22/min with rapid shallow breaths, supine blood pressure 120/80 mm Hg, without pulsus paradoxus, heart rate 80 beats/min, and temperature was 99.0°. The head and neck exam was normal. The pharnyx was without erythema or exudate. No cervical or supraclavicular lymphadenopathy was palpable. The lungs were clear to auscultation. His cardiac exam demonstrated a two-component pericardial friction rub, heard in both supine and sitting positions. No other abnormal cardiac auscultatory findings were present. No jugular venous distension was noted. The abdominal and skin exams were unremarkable. The remainder of the physical exam was normal.

Laboratory Studies. Routine electrolytes, blood urea nitrogen, creatinine, and glucose were normal. The white blood cell count was $11,600/mm^3$ with 85% neutrophils, 9% lymphocytes, 4% monocytes and 1% eosinophils. Hemoglobin, hematocrit, platelet count and coagulation parameters were all within normal limits. Liver function tests were normal. Antinuclear antibody and rheumatoid factor tests were negative.

The admission chest radiograph demonstrated a normal cardiac silhouette. No pleural effusion was present. No evidence of acute or chronic parenchymal lung disease was present. The electrocardiogram demonstrated normal sinus rhythm. Significant J-point elevation with a normal-appearing ST segment was present in leads I to III, aVF, and V2 through V6. The changes were consistent with acute pericarditis.

Hospital Course. The patient was admitted to a telemetry unit. His pain responded dramatically to therapy with indomethacin, 50 mg three times a day. No arrhythmias or other complications developed. A 2D echocardiogram demonstrated a small pericardial effusion, with no evidence of pericardial thickening or constriction. Over a course of two days the patient's symptomatology improved and he was discharged on indomethacin to be followed as an outpatient.

Subsequent Course. The patient did well initially, but approximately ten days after discharge his symptoms of chest pain returned. He had also developed dyspnea with moderate levels of exertion. On presentation he appeared in distress. His blood pressure was 115/70 mm Hg with a 12 to 15 mm Hg pulsus paradoxus, jugular venous pressure was increased, with prominent x descents. A soft pericardial friction rub was present. Pertinent laboratory studies included an elevated white cell count of $14,900/mm^3$ with a normal differential. The cardiac silhouette was enlarged on chest radiography. There was evidence of mild pulmonary venous congestion. He was readmitted for further therapy and evaluation.

Second Hospital Course. A 2D echocardiogram now demonstrated a large pericardial effusion. Due to his moderate distress, a therapeutic pericardiocentesis was performed at the time of right and left heart catheterization. Prior to pericardiocentesis, hemodynamic studies demonstrated near equilibration of pressures. Right atrial mean pressure was 12 mm Hg, right ventricular end-diastolic pressure

14 mm Hg, pulmonary artery diastolic pressure 15 mm Hg and left ventricular end diastolic pressure 15 mm Hg. Approximately 200 cc of serosanguinous fluid was removed by subxyphoid percutaneous pericardiocentesis, and repeat hemodynamic study showed no further equilibration of pressures.

Laboratory Studies. The total protein level of the pericardial fluid was 5.1 gm/dl. The total white cell count was 2400/mm^3, and the glucose level was 65 gm/dl. The pericardial fluid was cultured for viruses, bacteria (including acid-fast studies), and fungi. All cultures were subsequently negative. The acid-fast smear was also negative. Serum fungal (aspergillus, blastomyces, coccidioides, histoplasma) titers were all negative. Coxsackie neutralizing antibody titers were negative.

Hospital Course. The patient clinically improved following pericardiocentesis. He remained on anti-inflammatory medication in the form of indomethacin. Computed tomography of the chest demonstrated no abnormalities except for a minimally thickened pericardium. Following several days of observation, he showed no clinical deterioration and was discharged to outpatient follow-up. Four weeks following discharge he was doing well. Repeat Coxsackie titers remain negative.

Discussion

The wide spectrum of disease processes which cause pericarditis requires an initial broad approach when considering etiology. Acute idiopathic pericardial disease[4] is defined by the presence of pericarditis (with or without cardiac tamponade) in the absence of known causes. Many of these cases will subsequently be shown to be of viral etiology. Bacterial causes are rare. However, in the majority of patients the cause will remain unknown[4] with present diagnostic techniques. The purpose of this scheme is to allow a specific approach to be outlined with reference to the patient described in this case report: a previously healthy individual who presents with acute pericarditis.

Presenting Features
History and Physical. This patient presented with classic acute pericarditis. The diagnostic historical and physical exam features of his first presentation were chest pain and the presence of a pericardial friction rub. Chest pain typically occurs in most cases of primary acute pericarditis.[1,5] A smaller unknown percentage of patients with acute idiopathic pericarditis may present not with pain but with evidence of systemic venous congestion and cardiac tamponade. Chest pain in acute pericarditis has a characteristic pattern. It most commonly begins acutely and may become progressively worse. It is typically described as sharp but occasionally dull, located over the left precordium, and it radiates classically to the left trapezius ridge.[1] Radiation to the elbows or lower arms occurs infrequently.

One of the most important descriptors of pericardial pain is its relation to motion. Typically, pericarditis is described by exacerbation of pain with deep breathing, supine position, chest rotation, or swallowing, and is relieved by sitting up and leaning forward.

The presence of a pericardial friction rub may be the only sign of acute pericardial inflammation.[2] The rub is best heard near the left lower to mid sternal border with the patient sitting forward and during deep inspiration.[6] With careful auscultation (i.e., a quiet room) the rub in most patients is three components: an atrial sound (presystolic) as well as systolic and diastolic components will be heard.[6] It is not unusual, however, to only hear a two-component rub (as in this case) or even a single systolic rub. The ventricular systolic component is the loudest and most noticeably heard, and at times may be mistaken for a systolic murmur. The character of the rub is typically described as superficial, scratchy, rough, or more vividly as "the crunch of footsteps on cold snow."[3] The presence of a pericardial friction rub is variable.[2,5] If not present initially, repeating the exam several hours later may be helpful, particularly if the diagnosis is strongly suspected. Pericardial rubs are probably due to friction between inflamed surfaces of visceral and parietal pericardium or between parietal pericardium and adjacent pleura. This latter cause may explain why rubs can still be audible even in the presence of a large pericardial effusion.[6]

As in the case report above, many patients with acute idiopathic pericarditis may give a history of a preceding upper respiratory infection. This varies from 28%[2] to as high as 58%.[7] The incidence of a preceding upper respiratory illness may be higher in the patient who eventually is diagnosed with postviral pericarditis. Typically this infection will precede the onset of chest pain (reflecting pericarditis) by one to four weeks. The absence of this history, however, does not exclude a postviral etiology.

Electrocardiogram

The electrocardiographic (ECG) changes that occur with acute pericarditis have been extensively studied and described.[8-11] Spodick has formulated four stages of ECG changes that typically evolve in pericarditis.[9,10] Stage 1 consists of elevation of the ST segment junction (J point) with the ST segment maintaining a normal concave upward appearance. These changes are most obvious in leads I, II, aVL, aVF, and V3-6. ST segment depression may be seen in aVR and occasionally in lead V1. Stage 1 changes usually develop within hours of the onset of symptoms, and evolve to Stage 2 changes in one to two days. Stage 2 is characterized by return of the ST segment junction to baseline and by flattening of the T wave. Stage 3 changes, which may be seen several days to weeks following the episode of pericarditis, are noted by T wave inversion without loss of R wave height or presence of abnormal Q waves. Stage 4 is described as the return to the prepericarditis baseline ECG tracing. In Spodick's original study, all four stages occurred in nearly half of the patients.[9] This entire sequence may evolve in a matter of days, but typically occurs over a a period of several weeks.

Analysis of the PR segment has become critical in the diagnosis of pericarditis.[8] Spodick has again demonstrated PR segment depression (using the TP segment as baseline) in 82% of patients with classic Stage 1 criteria for acute pericarditis. (In the case described only minimal PR segment depression was noted.) The presence of PR segment depression is highly sensitive for the diagnosis of acute pericarditis, but of unknown specificity.[10]

The origin of the ECG changes in pericarditis reflect myocardial involvement with the pericardial inflammatory process.[12] The pericardium is electrically silent on the surface ECG. The ST segment shifts occur due to areas of electrical potential differences between the inflamed superficial epicardial surface and normal myocardial layers. The PR segment depression is due to atrial myocardial inflammation which causes the atrial repolarization wave, which is normally "lost" in the QRS complex, to appear earlier in the PR segment and depress it.[12]

The role of the surface ECG in the "diagnosis" of acute pericarditis is fundamental but at times confusing. Clearly in the patient with chest pain consistent with pericardial origin and a pericardial friction rub on physical exam, the ECG is the "test most likely to give diagnostic information."[2] However, in a series of 44 patients with the clinical diagnosis of acute pericarditis, 43% (19 patients) were found to have atypical ECG patterns.[11] Of these 19 patients, all of whom had friction rubs, 7 had no ST segment changes and 3 had no ECG changes of any kind. Of the total group of 44 patients, 4 patients had PR segment depression as the only sign of pericarditis. Thus, the surface ECG lends supportive diagnostic information only and in the absence of typical ECG changes the diagnosis may still be made if in the physician's judgement other evidence (chest pain, friction rub) of pericarditis is present. In some instances, serial ECGs may be diagnostic. In particular, the patient with acute pericarditis may be difficult to differentiate from the "normal variant" ECG pattern until a follow-up tracing shows further evolution typical for pericarditis.

Chest Radiograph

The chest radiograph is usually normal in acute pericarditis.[1,2] Enlargement of the cardiac silhouette occurs in the presence of moderate to large pericardial effusions of at least 200 cc. Some patients may have an associated left pleural effusion or pulmonary infiltrate. A baseline chest film is important in the initial diagnostic evaluation of the previously healthy patient with acute pericarditis primarily to further exclude tuberculosis or metastatic disease as potential causes.

Differential Diagnosis — Major

The major differential diagnostic problems arise when the patient with acute pericarditis presents with chest pain and an abnormal ECG but without a pericardial friction rub on first evaluation. In these instances it is critical to exclude other causes of chest pain with an abnormal ECG. One of the most urgent problems for consideration is whether an acute myocardial infarction is present. Other important differential diagnostic considerations include acute aortic dissection, pneumothorax, pulmonary embolus, and angina (usually of the "variant" type).

The immediate diagnosis of an acute myocardial infarction is critical for the delivery of thrombolytic therapy which has been shown to significantly improve long-term survival. This diagnosis, in the urgent setting, is based upon chest pain and ECG changes consistent with transmural myocardial injury. The chest pain of myocardial ischemia or infarction is usually quite different from pericardial pain.[1,2] Pericardial pain is typically positional (aggravated by supine position and relieved by sitting forward) and exacerbated by motion or breathing. Infarct pain usually is not influenced by motion of the thorax nor relieved by any peculiar position. While the quality of pericarditis is described as sharp and pleuritic by most patients, infarct pain is typically described as a pressure or tightness sensation. The response to sublingual nitroglycerin may be helpful; the patient with ischemia or infarct may note temporary relief or lessening of discomfort, but the patient with pericarditis usually does not obtain relief with nitrates. The immediate past history would also be important in this differential. The patient with acute infarct may have a preceding pain pattern suggestive of unstable or preinfarction angina. Pericarditis usually begins acutely without any previous symptoms of chest pain.

The ECG distinction between acute pericarditis and acute myocardial infarction is not always easy, but obviously is a critical step. Fortunately, important differences have been described.[13-15] In pericarditis, inflammation is usually diffuse rather than localized. ST segment elevation is therefore present in most leads (except aVR) and produces an ST segment vector which closely parallels the mean QRS vector. In acute infarction, the ST segment elevation occurs in the leads corresponding to the segment of myocardial injury, and may be associated with reciprocal changes (ST depression) in the electrically opposite leads. Reciprocal ST depression is unusual in acute pericarditis. Early ST changes in acute pericarditis are described as being concave upward, in distinction to the elevated, convex ST segment of acute infarction. The Q-T interval can also be used as a discriminator. In infarction it is prolonged, in pericarditis it may be normal or shortened. Finally, though not helpful in the acute setting, serial ECG changes clearly distinguish between these two entities. In pericarditis, ST segments quickly return to baseline before T wave inversion, and without abnormalities in R wave height or development of pathologic Q waves. In the evolution of myocardial infarction, ST segments may remain elevated as T wave inversion occurs along with the development of abnormal Q waves or loss of R wave height.

The discrimination between these two disease states requires careful clinical evaluation and interpretation of ECGs. The development of thrombolytic therapy for use in infarction has made it critical to establish diagnosis as accurately as possible.

The evaluation for the other potential differential diagnoses listed above needs also to proceed promptly, and again historical features as well as findings on the physical exam are quite helpful diagnostically. The patient with an acute aortic dissection usually has a history of hypertension. The ECG may show ST elevation, but evidence of left ventricular hypertrophy is usually present. The pain of dissection is described as tearing and typically radiates into the back. There may be physical exam evidence of compromised peripheral pulses. Pneumothorax should be quickly diagnosed by the findings of diminished breath sounds in one lung and also by chest x-ray. The patient with pulmonary embolism presents with chest pain and dyspnea, symptoms which may be present in acute pericarditis. However, the findings of hypoxemia, presence of a pleural friction rub and an abnormal lung perfusion scan should lead to the correct diagnosis of pulmonary embolus. Hyperacute ST elevation, as seen in the patient with primary coronary vasospastic disease, may mimic changes seen in pericarditis. These ST changes, however, are usually well-localized to a specific ECG area and may quickly revert to baseline after treating the patient with nitroglycerin.

Differential Diagnosis – Acute Pericarditis

Once the diagnosis of acute pericarditis has been made, a broad outline of possible etiologies should be considered (Table 1). As mentioned above, a wide variety of disease states are associated with pericarditis and pericardial effusion. Many of these diagnoses can be excluded with the initial history, physical exam and laboratory evaluation.

History

A thorough history is an essential first step in the initial evaluation of a patient with acute pericarditis. Features suggestive of malignancy (e.g. weight loss, abnormal masses, persistent cough, hemoptysis) should be sought. Malignant pericardial involvement may account for up to 5% of cases initially diagnosed as idiopathic pericarditis.[4] A past history of radiation exposure, of previous cardiothoracic surgery, or of chest trauma should be easily obtainable. A history of a myocardial infarction within the past 3 months should lead to the consideration of postmyocardial infarction pericarditis or Dressler's syndrome.[16] Most patients with symptomatic rheumatoid pericarditis have definite or classic rheumatoid arthritis which should be discernible from the history.[17] As with rheumatoid arthritis, extracardiac manifestations are usually present when pericardial involvement complicates other rheumatic diseases. In one study, only 6% of patients with systemic lupus erythematosus presented with pericarditis as the initial clue to their illness.[1] Finally, a complete drug history is needed to exclude iatrogenic pericardial disease. Procainamide, hydralazine, and phenytoin are commonly prescribed therapeutic agents known to produce pericarditis via a lupuslike reaction.

Table 1

Acute Pericarditis*

Infection
    Viral (Coxsackievirus, Adenovirus, Echovirus)
    Bacterial (Staphylococcus, Strepococcus, Mycobacterium)
    Fungal (Histoplasma, Coccidioides, Cryptococcus)
Immunologic
    Systemic lupus erythematosus
    Rheumatoid arthritis
    Scleroderma
Cardiac Disease
    Acute myocardial infarction
    Post myocardial infarction
    Aortic dissection
Neoplasm
    Primary
    Metastatic (Breast, Lung, Lymphoma)
    Irradiation
Metabolic Disease
    Hypothyroidism
Renal Disease
    Uremia
    Dialysis associated
Iatrogenic
    Post surgical
    Cardiac instrumentation
Drugs
    Procainamide
    Hydralazine
    Isoniazid
    Others
Idiopathic

*This is not meant to be an all encompassing list. Examples of particular etiologies within a category are given in parentheses.

Physical Examination

The physical exam in a patient with acute pericarditis should be done in a directed manner, searching for clues of a systemic illness and providing an impression of the overall "sickness" of the patient. Any evidence of malignancy (e.g. lymphadenopathy, breast masses) creates the suspicion of malignant pericardial disease. Patients with malignant pericardial disease often present with cardiac tamponade; findings of systemic venous congestion, pulsus paradoxus and hemodynamic instability should strongly suggest this diagnosis.[18] Patients should be carefully examined for abnormal skin or joint findings which may suggest underlying rheumatic tissue disease. Clinical evidence for hypothyroidism would be critical, patients with myxedema commonly have pericardial effusions and on occasion have presented with cardiac tamponade.[19] Most patients with purulent pericarditis have signs of significant systemic toxicity.[20] Many pyogenic infections spread to the pericardium from local sources or systemically via bacteremia, rarely is the pericardium the primary site of a bacterial infection. The most common routes of infection to the pericardium are from pulmonary, hematogenous, or intracardiac sources.[20] Clinical evidence for pneumonia, pleural effusion or endocarditis in the patient with pericarditis would heighten the consideration of a purulent etiology. Pericarditis occurring after cardiac surgery is usually caused by incompletely understood immunologic mechanisms, but can be purulent.

Laboratory Tests

No single laboratory test in the patient with acute pericarditis will be diagnostic. Test selection and interpretation are best guided by the clinical impression obtained from the directed history and physical exam. The complete blood count typically shows an elevated white blood cell count with neutrophilia. However, the white cell count may be entirely normal.[5,21] An elevated blood urea nitrogen or serum creatinine would suggest a uremic cause for the pericarditis. Moderate elevations in the erythrocyte sedimentation rate (ESR) are common but nonspecific. An extremely elevated ESR suggests a rheumatic, infectious, or malignant etiology. Serum transaminases are usually normal in patients with acute idiopathic or postviral pericarditis.[5] Antinuclear antibody and rheumatoid factor tests are usually positive if there is clinical evidence of systemic lupus or rheumatoid arthritis. In patients with lupus and pericarditis, testing for antimyosin antibodies may be appropriate. These antibodies have been associated with the presence of constrictive physiology in these patients.[22] Finally, thyroid studies should be obtained when hypothyroidism is suspected. The role of cardiac enzymes in patients with pericarditis will be discussed in the section concerning hospital management.

When fever or systemic toxicity is present, blood cultures are needed to identify a bacteremic process. In most patients, the evaluation of a possible infectious etiology should be limited to appropriate viral studies. The most common viral causes of acute pericarditis are the enteroviruses (Coxsackie Groups A and B, echovirus).[5,21] In some instances studies for adenoviruses, Ebstein-Barr, hepatitis or influenza may be warranted. A diagnosis of viral pericarditis is made by demonstrating a fourfold or greater increase in serum neutralizing antibody titers within the first month of illness.[2] Virus may occasionally be cultured from the throat or stool in the acute stage of illness.[5] If obtained, pericardial fluid should also be appropriately cultured. However, enteroviruses uncommonly are isolated from pericardial fluid.[21] Other possible tests for more unusual infectious causes would include cold agglutinins for mycoplasma, ASO titer, fungal serologic studies, and a heterophile test for mononucleosis.

The diagnosis of tuberculous pericarditis requires a high index of suspicion. The majority of patients report a protracted illness prior to presenting with pericarditis, or will have evidence of active tuberculosis elsewhere.[23] Sputum and possibly gastric cultures should be obtained in this situation. A tuberculin skin test is not always useful. If negative, some authorities believe a diagnosis of tuberculous pericarditis is unlikely.[24] Other studies, however, have shown a high prevalence (75%) of negative skin tests in patients proven to have tuberculous pericarditis.[25] As in this case study, many patients may have known positive skin tests limiting the diagnostic usefulness in the acute setting.

Pathophysiology

Much of the knowledge concerning the pathophysiology of acute pericarditis has been gained from studies concerning infectious pericarditis, particularly viral pericarditis. Viral infections are typically blood-borne, and usually infect both myocardium and pericardium.[3] Host factors and properties of the infecting virus presumably determine whether myocarditis or pericarditis predominates.[21] The degree of pericardial inflammation depends on the virulence of the agent and in the case of a virus is usually mild. In most cases a limited amount of epicardium is also involved. The tissue damage which occurs is the result of either direct viral damage or is mediated through cytotoxic T lymphocytes which recognize viral antigens on the cell surfaces. The inflammatory response in the epicardium may lead to interstitial edema which in some patients leads to obstruction of lymphatic channels and results in the formation of a pericardial effusion. The parietal pericardium does not have lymphatics.[21] Once this inflammation resolves, the effusion may gradually be reabsorbed. Pathologic changes in the recovery phase may further be characterized by mild fibrosis and adhesions between pericardial surfaces. Fortunately, the healing response to a viral infection rarely leads to chronic pericardial constriction,[3] though a transient phase of pericardial constriction has been reported in patients with effusive acute idiopathic pericarditis.[25]

Natural History

The natural history of acute idiopathic or postviral pericarditis is usually uncomplicated.[1-3,5] In most cases, the illness lasts from two to six weeks. However, as Gold mentions, in some patients the initial illness may persist for several years before resolution.[5] If associated significant myocarditis is present, the acute illness may be much more severe. Death in acute idiopathic pericarditis is rare and usually is associated with underlying structural heart disease or cardiac tamponade.[5] Of particular concern is the development of cardiac tamponade during treatment with anticoagulants, and anticoagulants should not be used in acute idiopathic pericarditis unless overwhelming thrombotic indications require their use.

Acute recurrences mark the natural history in 20% to 25% of patients with acute idiopathic pericarditis. The most common feature of recurrent pericarditis is chest pain, though some patients will present with ECG changes or friction rubs similar to those present in their initial episode.[26] These episodes may be symptomatically less severe than the initial presenting illness. Most recurrences happen within 6 months; however, some may occur years following the first attack. The reason for recurrences is unknown, but may be an immune response to the previous myocardial injury.[2] In a detailed and longitudinal study by Fowler and Harbin, however, no abnormalities were demonstrated in total serum immunoglobulins, total lymphocyte count, ratio of T helper to suppressor cells, or in serum complement levels in patients with recurrent acute pericarditis.[26] The development of massive pericardial effusions, congestive heart failure or constrictive physiology is unusual in patients with recurrences.[1,26]

Management

In managing patients with acute pericarditis the physician is concerned not only with pain relief but also with the possibility of complicating problems. Specific therapy in acute pericarditis is dependent upon specific diagnoses. In the case presented above, no specific etiology was initially found and general measures were prescribed for the treatment of acute idiopathic pericarditis.

Most authorities recommend that the initial pain therapy in patients with acute idiopathic pericarditis be either aspirin or nonsteroidal anti-inflammatory medication.[1] Aspirin, in a dosage of 1 gm every 4 to 6 hours, may be effective only in a limited number of patients. In my opinion, since pain relief should be attempted as quickly as possible for the patient's comfort, indomethacin should be considered as the first choice. At a dosage of 25 to 50 mg three times a day, indomethacin will be successful in alleviating pain in the majority of patients.[1] If patients have a history of upper gastrointestinal tract disease or known intolerance to indomethacin, ibuprofen at a dose of 400 to 600 mg four times a day may be tried initially. This regimen may be associated with fewer gastrointestinal side effects. In general, once symptoms have remitted for 5 to 7 days, the pain therapy can be tapered and discontinued.[1] The total duration of therapy may be 10 to 14 days and in some instances longer.

In a minority of cases, the therapy as described above will be unsuccessful in alleviating symptoms. More aggressive therapy in this setting is controversial.[1,3]

Options include therapy with steroids, primarily prednisone, or therapy with immunosuppressive agents. Also, Imuran, 50 mg three times a day, has been prescribed in some patients.[1] Therapy with prednisone should be avoided within the first two weeks of the illness.[3,21] Also, tuberculous pericarditis should be carefully excluded before beginning steroids. The dosage of prednisone varies; some suggest starting therapy at 20 mg four times a day, decreasing by 25% weekly until the least effective dose is found.[3] Unfortunately, 10 to 20% of patients will relapse when steroid therapy is completely withdrawn.[1] In these patients, the chronic use of prednisone is measured against more aggressive modes of treatment, i.e. pericardiectomy. Colchicine, 1 mg per day, has been shown to improve symptoms and allow the complete withdrawal of prednisone in two patients with relapsing idiopathic pericarditis who were steroid dependent.[27]

The treatment of symptomatic recurrences is similar to the treatment of the first episode. In addition, there may be a role for pericardiectomy in patients who have chronic recurrences over a several year period.[28] The recommendation for pericardiectomy is a difficult one; not all patients will have symptomatic improvement and no predictive variables are known that may suggest which patients will improve after pericardiectomy.

A second aspect in the management of patients with acute pericarditis is hospitalization for rest and observation. Though not all patients with acute pericarditis are admitted to a hospital, in my opinion admission is warranted because of the likelihood of associated myocarditis with the acute illness.[3] In addition, animal studies have demonstrated that stress or exercise enhances the virulence of certain types of viral illness.[21] In the acute stage, patients should have activity restricted until the fever and pericardial friction rub subside. Some conservative authorities recommend that patients should rest for 30 days.[21] However, I believe that a gradual return to more normal activity can proceed sooner if the patient remains asymptomatic after the first 2 to 3 weeks from presentation. Patients need to be followed closely after discharge, and instructed to be aware of the return of any symptoms. The fact that acute idiopathic pericarditis in the majority of patients is a benign, self-limited process is reassuring to most patients and should be an important aspect in the "education" of the patient. Rest is important in the management of recurrent pericarditis; some reviewers suggest that increased activity may prolong the duration of symptoms at the time of relapse.[5]

Patients admitted with acute idiopathic pericarditis should be observed for the occurrence of any arrhythmias. The incidence of arrhythmias in acute idiopathic pericarditis varies between studies but appears to be quite low[12,29] (0 to 15%). Life-threatening arrhythmias are very unusual. Spodick has carefully observed that arrhythmias occurring in patients with pericarditis are usually a marker of intrinsic structural heart disease or are associated with cardiac tamponade.[29] In one study, supraventricular arrhythmias occurred in 3 of 20 patients with idiopathic pericarditis; 2 of these 3 subsequently developed cardiac tamponade. Thus, patients with acute idiopathic pericarditis who developed an arrhythmia should be carefully evaluated for the presence of a pericardial effusion or cardiac tamponade, as well as for any other evidence of structural myocardial or valvular heart disease.

The etiology of arrhythmias in patients with pericarditis is controversial.[3,12] Spodick states that pericardial inflammation is not arrhythmogenic, and the arrhythmia relates more to a structural heart problem or the compressive effects of a pericardial effusion.[12] Inflammation of the atria, as evidenced by PR segment depression, may be the cause of atrial fibrillation or flutter seen in some instances.[3]

It is my opinion that the CK-MB enzyme is not helpful in the initial diagnostic evaluation of the patient with pericarditis, but should be followed in the immediate hospital course. Cardiac enzyme values, primarily creatine kinase (CK) and the MB isoenzyme, are classically described as being normal or only slightly increased in patients with acute idiopathic pericarditis.[2,30] However, instances of moderately elevated CK-MB values have been reported in patients with pericarditis[31] even in the setting of normal total serum CK and myoglobin values. Whether the increase in CK-MB reflects myocardial necrosis is controversial. Some authors state that the enzyme may leak due to changes in membrane permeability of cells on the epicardial surface of the heart involved with the pericardial inflammation and not necessarily cell death.[31] In following serum CK values, normal or only slightly elevated results should be expected. If significant amounts of CK-MB are present, the question of a more serious myocardial involvement should be raised.[32]

Pericardial Effusion

Some degree of a pathologic increase in pericardial fluid probably occurs in most cases of acute pericarditis[2] since the normal amount of fluid is only 15 to 20 cc. The exact incidence of an effusion complicating idiopathic pericarditis (either at presentation or developing in the subsequent course as in the patient presented) is unknown. In the study from Barcelona, the incidence of pericardial effusion was 54% in a series of 231 patients with primary acute pericardial disease. This series included patients with malignant or tuberculous disease.[4] In patients shown to have acute idiopathic pericarditis, the incidence may be slightly lower. Agner and Gallis studied 18 patients with echocardiography and demonstrated effusions in 5 (28%).[19]

The symptoms of a pericardial effusion may be absent or relate to compression of various mediastinal structures. Cough, dyspnea, hoarseness and dysphagia have all been reported.[2] The hemodynamic significance of an effusion will depend upon the rate of accumulation, total volumne of fluid, and physical characteristics of the pericardium. In the case study presented, approximately 200 cc of fluid was removed at the time of pericardiocentesis. Though this is not a large (greater than 350 cc[33]) effusion, the accumulation in a relatively short time period probably accounted for the significant hemodynamic effect.

Pericardiocentesis can be done for both diagnostic and therapeutic reasons. Somewhat paradoxically, patients who require "therapeutic" pericardiocentesis are more likely to have a diagnosis made than when fluid is removed electively for "diagnostic" purposes.[4] This is consistent with previous experience in the literature: patients with malignant effusion are more likely to present with tamponade and require pericardiocentesis.[19]

The size and character of a pericardial effusion may not be helpful with regards to specific diagnoses. Colombo et al studied a group of men presenting with large pericardial effusions.[33] The most common etiologies were malignant, idiopathic and uremic. Of the patients with idiopathic pericarditis and large pericardial effusions, 25% were shown to have hemorrhagic effusions and tamponade. Though not all patients had pericardial fluid analyzed in the study from Duke, no differences between parameters (glucose, total protein, hematocrit, white cell count) measured in the fluid were demonstrated among patients with idiopathic, uremic, malignant, tuberculous, or chronic pericarditis.[19] The presence of a large pericardial effusion in patients with idiopathic pericarditis is not associated with a poor prognosis. In the study mentioned above, only one patient died in follow-up and of a noncardiac cause.[33]

Conclusions

The patient presented remains well several months after his first presentation. His course, though not typical of the majority of patients with acute pericarditis, was not unusual. Most patients follow a benign course, but as in this patient, a more acute illness may evolve requiring an urgent therapeutic procedure or a more extensive evaluation. This review has attempted to cover a wide variety of concerns in the management and evaluation of patients with acute idiopathic pericarditis. Important aspects in the initial presentation, including keys to suspected underlying diseases, should be remembered. A critical approach to differential diagnosis is prudent, particularly in the patient with chest pain and ECG changes. Treatment modes have not changed dramatically for many years and the concern over the use of steroids or the role of pericardiectomy in these patients continues. Hospitalization for rest and observation should be part of routine management. And, as in the case study presented, the ability to manage and evaluate patients with pericardial effusions or tamponade is required in some instances.

References

1. Fowler NO: Acute pericarditis, in Fowler NO (ed): The Pericardium in Health and Disease. New York, Futura Publishing Co, 1985, p 153.
2. Brandenburg RO, McGoon DC: The pericardium, in Brandenburg RO, Fuster V, Giuliani ER, McGoon DC (eds): Cardiology: Fundamentals and Practice. Chicago: Year Book Medical Publishers, Inc, 1987, p 1654.

3. Smith CB: Pericarditis, in Hoeprich PD (ed): Infectious Diseases. Philadelphia, Harper and Row, 1986;p 1157.
4. Permanyer-Miralda G, Sagrista-Sauleda J, Soler-Soler J: Primary acute pericardial disease: A prospective series of 231 consecutive patients. Am J Cardiol. 1985;56:623-630.
5. Gold RG: Post-viral pericarditis. Eur Heart J. 1988;9(Suppl G):175-179.
6. Spodick DH: Acoustic phenomena in pericardial disease. Am Heart J. 1971;81:114-124.
7. Carmichael DB, Sprague HB, Wyman SM, et al: Acute nonspecific pericarditis: Clinical, laboratory and follow-up considerations. Circulation. 1951;3:321-331.
8. Spodick DH: Diagnostic electrocardiographic sequences in acute pericarditis: Significance of PR segment and PR vector changes. Circulation. 1973;48:575-580.
9. Spodick DH: Electrocardiogram in acute pericarditis. Distributions of morphologic and axial changes by stages. Am J Cardiol. 1974;33:470-472.
10. Spodick DH: The normal and diseased pericardium: Current concepts of pericardial physiology, diagnosis and treatment. J Am Coll Cardiol. 1983;1:240-251.
11. Bruce MA, Spodick DH: Atypical electrocardiogram in acute pericarditis: Characteristics and prevalence. J Electrocardiol. 1980;13:61-67.
12. Spodick DH: Electrocardiographic changes in acute pericarditis, in Fowler NO (ed): The Pericardium in Health and Disease. New York, Futura Publishing Co, 1985, p 79.
13. Marriott HJL: Practical electrocardiography. ed 8. Baltimore, The Johns Hopkins University Press, 1988, pp 518-519.
14. Constant J: Learning Electrocardiography. A Complete Course, ed 3. Boston, Little, Brown, and Co, 1987, pp 262-266.
15. Diamond T: The ST segment axis: A distinguishing feature between acute pericarditis and acute myocardial infarction. Heart Lung. 1985;14:629-631.
16. Fowler NO: Post-myocardial-infarction pericarditis (Dressler's syndrome), in Fowler NO (ed): The Pericardium in Health and Disease. New York, Futura Publishing Co, 1985, p 343.
17. Franco AE, Levine HD: Rheumatoid pericarditis. Report of 17 cases diagnosed clinically. Ann Intern Med. 1972;77:837-844.
18. Kerber RE, Sherman B: Echocardiographic evaluation of pericardial effusion in myxedema. Incidence and biochemical and clinical correlations. Circulation. 1975;52:823-830.
19. Agner RC, Gallis HA: Pericarditis. Differential diagnostic considerations. Arch Intern Med. 1979;139:407-412.
20. Klacsmann PG, Bulkley BH, Hutchins GM: The changed spectrum of purulent pericarditis. An 86 year autopsy experience in 200 patients. Am J Med. 1977;63:666-673.
21. Lerner AM: Myocarditis and pericarditis, in Braude AI, Davis CE, Fierer J (eds): Infectious Disease and Medical Microbiology. Philadelphia, WB Saunders Co, 1986 p 1291.
22. Wolf RE, King JW, Brown TA: Antimyosin antibodies and constrictive pericarditis in lupus erythematosus. J Rheumatol. 1988;15:1284-1287.
23. Ortbals DW: Tuberculous pericarditis. Arch Intern Med. 1979;139:231-234.
24. Silber EN, Katz LN: Heart Disease. New York, Macmillan Publishing Co Inc, 1975, pp 996-997.
25. Sagrista-Sauleda J, Permanyer-Miralda G, Candell-Riera J, et al: Transient cardiac constriction: An unrecognized pattern of evolution in effusive acute idiopathic pericarditis. Am J Cardiol. 1987;59:961-966.
26. Fowler NO, Harbin AD: Recurrent acute pericarditis: Follow up study of 31 patients. J Am Coll Cardiol. 1986;7:300-305.
27. De La Serna AR, Soldevila JG, Claramunt VM, et al: Colchicine for recurrent pericarditis. Lancet. 1987;1517.
28. Miller JI, Mansour KA, Hatcher CR: Pericardiectomy: Current indications, concepts and results in a university center. Ann Thorac Surg. 1982;34:40-45.

29. Spodick DH: Frequency of arrhythmias in acute pericarditis determined by Holter monitoring. Am J Cardiol. 1984;53:842-845.
30. Roberts R, Sobel BE: Creatine kinase isoenzymes in the assessment of heart disease. Am Heart J. 1978;95:521-527.
31. Marmor A, Grenadir E, Keidar S, et al: The MB fraction of creatine phosphokinase. An indicator of myocardial involvement in acute pericarditis. Arch Intern Med. 1979;139:819-820.
32. Hashimoto R, Ogata M, Koga Y, et al: Clinical manifestations of acute Coxsackie-B viral myocarditis and pericarditis with a special reference to serum enzyme patterns and long term prognosis. Kurume Med J. 1987;34:19-27.
33. Colombo A, Olson HG, Egan J, et al: Etiology and prognostic implications of a large pericardial effusion in men. Clin Cardiol. 1988;11:389-394.

Case 7

Asthma

Gary C. Kindt, MD

Case History

This was the second Ohio State University Hospitals admission for this 28-year-old woman admitted with one week of increasing dyspnea and wheezing. She reported a history of asthma dating back to childhood, with many hospital admissions up to the age of thirteen. Since that time, she remained in good health, with the exception of a single hospitalization for an acute exacerbation two years prior to admission. She had never required mechanical ventilation. She was in her usual state of health until two weeks prior to admission, when she noted symptoms of an upper respiratory tract infection and a nonproductive cough. During the week prior to admission, she noted increasing dyspnea, especially with exertion, and audible expiratory wheezing. There had been no fever, chills, or chest pain. There was neither a history of sensitivity to aspirin nor a history of hay fever.

Her past medical history was otherwise unremarkable. Her medications included long-acting theophylline, 250 mg twice daily, and an albuterol inhaler, two puffs four times daily. There was no family history of asthma. She was employed as a receptionist at The Ohio State University. She had never smoked. The remainder of her review of systems was unremarkable.

Physical Examination. The patient was an alert, cooperative black woman who appeared in acute respiratory distress. Her vital signs showed: pulse 140, blood pressure 140/80, respiratory rate 36, oral temperature 98.8°F. There were no nasal polyps present. Her chest was somewhat hyperresonant to percussion. Chest auscultation revealed overall decreased breath sounds, marked inspiratory and expiratory wheezing throughout all lung fields, and a prolonged expiratory phase. Her cardiovascular examination as well as the remainder of her general physical examination were unremarkable.

Laboratory Data. Initial arterial blood gases were obtained on room air (ABG #1, Table 1). Her initial PA chest roentgenograph was within normal limits, without evidence of an acute infiltrate (Fig. 1). A complete blood count showed a

Table 1

		Arterial Blood Gases			
ABG #	pH	pO^2 (mm Hg)	pCO^2 (mm Hg)	HCO^3 (mmoles/liter)	O^2 sat %
1	7.34	58	45	27	88
2	7.29	89	51	24	96
3	7.11	554	66	23	99
4	7.40	109	36	23	99

white cell count of $7500/mm^3$ with a normal differential count, hemoglobin of 15.0 gm/dl, and a hematocrit of 44%. The theophylline level was 5.0 mg/liter. A chemistry panel revealed: BUN 9 mg/dl, Cr 1.0 mg/dl, glucose 179 mg/dl, Na 144 mmoles/liter, K 3.7 mmoles/liter, Cl 112 mmoles/liter, and CO_2 content 24 mmoles/liter.

Hospital Course. While in the emergency room, the patient received aerosolized metaproterenol, epinephrine (1:1000) 0.3 ml subcutaneously (two separate dosages), aminophylline 100 mg intravenously, and was begun on supplemental oxygen at 4 liters/min, nasal cannula. She was admitted to the medical intensive

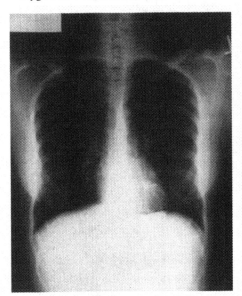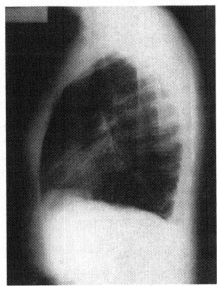

Figure 1. Initial PA and Lateral Chest Roentgenograms

care unit. An aminophylline drip was started and follow-up arterial blood gases were obtained (ABG #2, Table 1). The patient was electively intubated. Repeat arterial blood gases were obtained while the patient received mechanical ventilation: F_IO_2 100%, assist control rate of 14, tidal volume 700 ml (ABG #3, Table 1). The patient was agitated and was subsequently paralyzed with vancuronium. On the following hospital day, arterial blood gases were obtained on an F_IO_2 of 40% (ABG #4, Table 1). On the third hospital day the patient developed roentgenographic signs of progressive left lower lobe collapse despite aggressive pulmonary toilet and postural drainage (Fig. 2).

Bronchoscopy was performed, and thick secretions, obstructing the left mainstem bronchus, were removed by suction. Her respiratory status improved slowly and she was extubated on the seventh hospital day. Left lower lobe atelectasis eventually resolved with aggressive pulmonary toilet, and she was discharged on the fifteenth hospital day. Her medications at the time of discharge included: Long-acting theophylline 400 mg orally twice daily, prednisone 40 mg orally per day in tapering dosages, and an albuterol inhaler two puffs four to six times daily.

Subsequent Course. The patient was seen several weeks after discharge in the pulmonary outpatient clinic. She still noted moderate dyspnea with exertion. Pulmonary function tests were obtained (Table 2) including a flow-volume loop (Fig. 3).

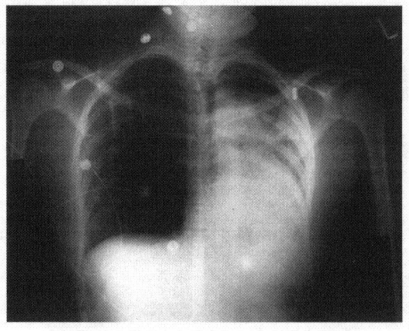

Figure 2. Progressive Left Lower Lobe Collapse

Table 2

Pulmonary Function Tests			
Spirometry Values	Predicted Values	Actual Values[a]	Post Bronchodilator Values
Forced vital capacity (FVC)	2.80 L	2.52 (90%)	3.21(115%)
Forced expiratory volume in 1 second (FEV1)	2.37 L	1.31 (55%)	1.87 (79%)
FEV1 % FVC	>75%	52%	58%
Forced midexpiratory flow rate (FEF 25-75)	3.61 L/sec	0.59 (16%)	0.95 (26%)
Peak expiratory flow rate	5.93 L/sec	2.90 (49%)	2.89 (49%)
Lung Volumes			
Slow vital capacity	2.80 L	2.52 (90%)	
Expiratory reserve volume (ERV)	1.03 L	0.40 (39%)	
Functional residual capacity (FRC)	2.29 L	2.25 (98%)	
Residual volume (RV)	1.26 L	1.85 (147%)	
Total lung capacity (TLC)	4.06 L	4.37 (108%)	
Diffusing Capacity			
Diffusing capacity (DLCO)b	22.77	23.73 (104%)	
Alveolar ventilation (VA)	4.06 L	4.37L (109%)	
DLCO/VA	5.61	5.37 (96%)	

[a]*Numbers in parentheses indicate percent predicted values.*
[b]*Diffusing capacity was measured as the diffusing capacity for carbon monoxide by the single breath method and is measured in units of ml/min/mm Hg.*

Comment: The spirometry indicates a pattern of moderate obstruction with a significant improvement in the FVC and FEV1 following acute bronchodilator challenge suggesting reversibility of obstruction. Elevated RV in the presence of obstruction suggests air trapping. Elevated TLC suggests mild hyperinflation. The diffusing capacity is normal.

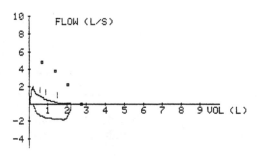

Figure 3. Flow-Volume Loop

Discussion

Differential Diagnosis/Clinical Presentation. The patient presented with a lifelong history of intermittent dyspnea and wheezing and an obstructive pattern on pulmonary function testing. Several frequently encountered disorders are associated with chronic airflow obstruction (Table 3). Less common disorders associated with airway obstruction include α1-antitrypsin deficiency, endobronchial sarcoid, and the carcinoid syndrome. Two cardiovascular disorders which can occasionally present with dyspnea and wheezing are cardiogenic pulmonary edema and pulmonary embolism. Other conditions which can be confused with asthma are those that cause upper airway obstruction (discussed further below).

Table 3

Common Disorders Associated with Chronic Airflow Obstruction
● Asthma
● Chronic Bronchitis
● Emphysema
● Bronchiectasis
● Cystic Fibrosis
● Bronchiolitis

Although physicians cannot agree on a universal definition of asthma, a working definition adopted by the American Thoracic Society states that "asthma is a disease characterized by an increased responsiveness of the trachea and bronchi to various stimuli and manifested by widespread narrowing of the airways that change in severity either spontaneously or as a result of therapy".[1] Status asthmaticus is characterized as an episode of asthma unrelieved by an otherwise usually effective course (1/2 to 1 hour) of bronchodilator therapy. Asthma can generally be classified into two major categories. Extrinsic asthma occurs in atopic individuals and can usually be provoked by a particular agent. Intrinsic asthma occurs in patients who have no evidence of atopy, and usually no clearly identifiable provoking factors.

The patient in this case discussion clearly had a past history, physical exam, and laboratory tests consistent with the diagnosis of asthma. The classic symptoms of asthma are wheezing, cough, chest tightness, and shortness of breath. Wheezing is the most common manifestation on physical exam, often accompanied by a prolonged expiratory phase, hyperresonance to percussion, and occasionally an increased anterior-posterior diameter. As the severity of the obstruction increases, tachypnea and tachycardia are common. A paradoxical pulse (fall in systolic blood pressure during inspiration of greater than 10-12 mm Hg) is found in about half of the patients with severe acute exacerbations.[2] As the severity of the asthmatic attack increases, inspiratory contraction of the accessory muscles of respiration is often found. The disappearance of wheezes can be an ominous sign of marked decreased airflow. Arterial blood gases in mild to moderate asthmatic attacks usually demonstrate hypoxemia with hypocapnea and a mild respiratory alkalosis.[3] As the obstruction progresses, a decrease in effective ventilation can occur resulting in first, normocapnea and subsequently, hypercapnea. This progression may identify patients who require endotracheal intubation and mechanical ventilation.[4] Chest roentgenograms often are normal but may show signs of hyperinflation such as flattened diaphragms or an increased retrosternal airspace on the lateral projection. Pulmonary infiltrates or other abnormalities are uncommon. Sputum exam may show eosinophilia, Charcot-Leyden crystals (degenerated eosinophils), or Curschmann's spirals (bronchiolar casts of cells and mucus).

Diagnostic Studies in Asthma. The use of laboratory testing to confirm the diagnosis of asthma lacks both specificity and sensitivity. Pulmonary function testing (PFTs) including spirometry before and after brochodilators, lung volumes, and diffusing capacity can help establish the diagnosis. Classically, asthma manifests as an obstructive pattern on PFTs (FEV1 % FVC < 75%, decreased peak flow), with a decreased FEV1 and often a decreased FVC, which show improvement in airflow after bronchodilators ($\geq$15% improvement in FVC or FEV1 or $\geq$25% improvement in FEF25-75). Lung volumes will often show signs of hyperinflation (FRC or TLC $\geq$120% of predicted) or air trapping (RV $\geq$120% of predicted). The diffusing capacity is usually normal. Because of the episodic nature of the disorder, the diagnosis of asthma occasionally is suspected on clinical grounds alone. In this setting, bronchoprovocation testing may be useful. Bronchoprovocation is often carried out with serial inhalations of methacholine. Bronchial hyperresponsiveness is defined as a 20% decrease in the FEV1. Mild bronchial hyperresponsiveness in a person without symptoms should not be regarded as asthma.

A flow-volume loop can be useful in the patient in whom upper airway obstruction is suspected. An isolated flattening or plateau pattern of the inspiratory loop, as occurred in the patient in this case study (Figure 3), suggests a variable extrathoracic obstruction. Variable intrathoracic obstruction results in flattening of the expiratory limb of the flow-volume loop and fixed upper airway obstruction results in a plateau of portions of both the inspiratory and expiratory limbs of the flow-volume loop. Tracheal stenosis can complicate endotracheal intubation as probably occurred with the patient discussed.

Pathophysiology. Most of our current understanding of the pathologic findings in patients with asthma is derived from postmortem examinations. Macroscopically, patients who have succumbed to asthma show hyperinflated lungs with mucus plugging of the airways.[5] Microscopic features include: (1) bronchial smooth muscle hypertrophy and hyperplasia, (2) thickening of the epithelial basement membrane, (3) bronchial mucosal edema, (4) desquamation of epithelial cells, (5) eosinophil and other inflammatory cell infiltration, (6) hyperplasia of mucous glands, (7) increased numbers of goblet cells.[6,7] Bronchoalveolar lavage in patients with mild asthma shows slight increases in the percentages of eosinophils and mast cells.[8,9]

The pathogenic processes leading to asthma remain unclear. Various stimuli are known to provoke bronchoconstriction (Table 4). In the allergic-immunologic model of asthma, the mast cell is thought to play an important role. Exposure to

Table 4

Common Precipitating Factors in Asthma
Allergens: inhaled (pollen, mites, dander), ingested (foods)
Drugs: aspirin, cholinergic drugs, β-blockers
Infection: viral respiratory infections
Air Pollution: cigarette smoke, sulfur dioxide
Mediators: histamine
Miscellaneous: emotional upset, exercise, hyperventilation, cold or dry air, aerosols, gastric reflux

an antigen in an atopic individual results in elaboration of specific IgE antibodies which attach to mast cells, circulating basophils, or other cell types. Cross-linking of these surface-bound IgE molecules or binding of IgE immune complexes to cell receptors triggers a sequence of events leading to the release of various chemical mediators capable of producing inflammation and bronchoconstriction.[10] These mediators include: histamine, serotonin, eosinophil chemotactic factor of anaphylaxis, leukotrienes, prostaglandins, thromboxane A2, platelet activating factor, and a neutrophil chemotactic factor.[11] These mediators can, in turn, lead to bronchial smooth muscle contraction (bronchoconstriction), increased mucosal edema, and inflammatory cell influx. Recruited eosinophils release additional mediators, some of which augment the bronchoconstriction, and others which potentially harm the respiratory epithelium.[12]

Another theory of the pathogenesis of asthma postulates that the basic defect is an abnormality of the autonomic nervous system.[13] β2-adrenoceptors, when stimulated, cause relaxation of the bronchial smooth muscle via adenyl cyclase and cyclic AMP.[14] The function of these receptors in asthma may be altered.[15] The role of the -adrenergic system has not been well established, although stimulation of this system in asthmatics may cause airway narrowing.[16] The cholinergic system innervates bronchial smooth muscle and mucous glands and stimulation leads to bronchoconstriction and mucus production.[17]

The physiological derangements occurring during severe attacks of asthma include a marked impairment of cardiopulmonary function. These are manifested by reduced airflow rates, air trapping, large changes in intrathoracic pressure, ventilation-perfusion abnormalities resulting in hypoxemia and hypercapnea, increased pulmonary capillary resistance, right ventricular systolic overload, and increased effort of breathing.[18] Additional airflow limitation can result in further hypercapnea, metabolic acidosis, muscle fatigue, exhaustion, and death.[19]

Epidemiology and Natural History. It is estimated that 3-6% of the population of the United States may be affected by asthma.[20] Asthma is more common in children than in adults, with boys being more frequently affected than girls.[21] The prevalence also varies greatly among different countries, and there is evidence that it increases when populations move from rural to urban environments.[22] The prevalence of bronchial hyperactivity far exceeds that of frank asthma.

The mortality from asthma rose in some countries in the 1960s,[23] and there have been sporadic increases in the mortality in the United States, especially among the elderly, in the 1980s.[24] Despite these statistics, rates of death from asthma in the United States remain lower than those in many other countries. The annual mortality from asthma in the United States among persons 5 to 34 years of age is 0.4 per 100,000 population.[19] Mortality for blacks is double that of whites. Inadequate assessment and treatment probably play a role in many deaths from asthma.[19,25] A recent study described four young patients who died unexpectedly and suddenly without apparent cause.[26] Most deaths occur outside the hospital and are most likely the result of inadequately treated airflow obstruction. Whether the background prevalence or severity of asthma have changed in recent years is not clear.

The natural history of asthma has not been extensively delineated. The remission rate appears to be highest in children and adolescents and ranges from 50 to 75%.[27,28] Normal pulmonary function and infrequent symptoms are favorable prognostic factors.[28] Adults age 30-60 have lower remission rates (in the range of 10% over a nine year period) in one study but the remission rate appears to increase somewhat after the age of 60.[28] Relapses after symptom-free periods occur with increasing frequency in the adult asthmatic. A recent study reviewed the clinical features and outcome in 61 asthmatic patients presenting with hypercapnea.[29] In this study: (1) men more commonly presented with hypercapnea than women (50% vs. 18%), (2) patients with hypercapnea had a longer duration of chronic asthma and were more likely to be steroid dependent, (3) hypercapneic patients had greater airway obstruction, respiratory rate, and pulsus paradoxus than did non-hypercapneic patients, (4) findings of a quiet chest on auscultation, inability to talk, and cyanosis suggested the presence of hypercapnea, (5) in nonventilated patients, hypercapnea resolved in a mean time of 5.9 hours; 50% of episodes resolved by 4 hours and all by 16 hours, (6) none of the patients presenting with normocapnea progressed to hypercapnea.[29] They concluded that most patients with hypercapnea from acute asthma have rapid reversibility with appropriate medical therapy and mechanical ventilation can usually be avoided, although close inpatient observation is necessary.[29]

Treatment. There is now considerable evidence that asthma is associated with airway inflammation that leads to contraction of airway smooth muscle, microvascular leakage, and bronchial hyperresponsiveness,[30] which potentially culminates in intermittent wheezing, coughing, and dyspnea. Consequently, pharmacologic treatment strategies are directed at both promoting bronchodilation and reducing the airway inflammation. Initially, supplemental oxygen or mechanical ventilation may also become necessary to support ventilation.

Oxygen and Mechanical Ventilation. Hypoxemia is invariably present in an acute asthmatic attack, and supplemental oxygen administered via nasal cannula or mask may be required. If the PaO_2 drops below 55-60 mm Hg or the oxygen saturation drops below 90%, supplemental oxygen should be given in order to raise the PaO_2 to levels of 80-100 mm Hg. An adequate PO_2 should always be maintained and if hypercapnea, respiratory acidosis, or a decreased level of consciousness develops, strong consideration should be given for endotracheal intubation and mechanical ventilation. However, mechanical ventilation in this setting is associated with a high incidence of complications which the physician should be aware of, such as pneumonia, pneumothorax, mucus plugging, and rarely tracheal stenosis. In order to reduce the risks of barotrauma, the following measures should be taken to reduce both the mean and peak airway pressures: (1) institute pharmacologic treatment for the airflow obstruction as soon as possible, (2) intubate the patient with as large an endotracheal tube as possible (8.0 mm, internal diameter or larger), (3) use a volume-cycled ventilator, (4) attempt to increase the inspiratory-to-expiratory ratio by increasing the inspiratory flow rate, (5) keep the tidal volume and respiratory rate as low as is necessary to maintain adequate ventilation in order to allow complete emptying during expiration, and (6) sedate or, if necessary, paralyze the patient to minimize the patient's efforts to fight the ventilator.

Bronchodilators. β-adrenergic agonist drugs are the most effective and have the most rapid onset of action of the bronchodilating agents currently used. Airway smooth muscle[31] and mast cells[32] have only β2-adrenergic receptors; thus, drugs possessing β1-agonist effects (which are associated with cardiovascular side effects) should be avoided. β2-adrenergic receptor stimulation on airway smooth muscle leads to activation of adenylate cyclase and increased intracellular concentrations of cyclic AMP. This increase subsequently leads to activation of protein kinase A, which inhibits phosphorylation of myosin and lowers intracellular ionic calcium concentrations. The result is airway dilation from the trachea to the terminal bronchioles.[30] β2-adrenergic agonists have also been shown to increase the clearance of mucus, decrease the release of mediators from various cells, and decrease the amount of edema formation.

The preferred method of administration of β2-adrenergic agonists in adults is via inhalation. β2-adrenergic agonists are available for injection but cardiovascular side effects (tachycardia, palpitations, arrhythmias, and hypertension) and cerebral side effects (anxiety, tremor, dizziness, nausea, and nervousness) limit their usefulness. In the young asthmatic patient without cardiac disease who presents with an acute attack, initial therapy can include: (1) epinephrine 0.3 ml of 1:1000 solution subcutaneously every 20 minutes up to three doses or (2) terbutaline 0.25-0.5 mg subcutaneously every four to six hours. It should be stressed that this form of therapy should be avoided in older patients especially those with possible ischemic cardiac disease as the β1 effects could potentially precipitate angina. β2-adrenergic agonists are also available in oral preparations but generally this route of administration offers no advantages over inhaled therapy and is associated with a higher incidence of side effects. The possible exception to this is the use of sustained release β2-adrenoceptor agonists for the treatment of nocturnal asthma.[33]

Inhaled β2-adrenergic agonists have a rapid onset of action (within minutes) and are effective for three to six hours,[34] and are the first line treatment of choice for acute exacerbations of asthma and for the prevention of exercise-induced asthma. Available agents include albuterol, metaproterenol, terbutaline, fenoterol, and bitolterol. They are usually administered on an as needed basis up to two puffs four to six times daily. Side effects to the inhaled agents are uncommon but include palpitations, tachycardia, and tremor. Often, tolerance to the side effects develops with continued use but tolerance to the bronchodilating effects does not occur.[35]

The methylxanthines, including theophylline, are effective bronchodilators, though not as effective as the inhaled β2-adrenergic agonists. Although theophylline has been used for many years, the mechanism by which it produces bronchodilation is unknown. Theories that theophylline promotes bronchodilation by inhibiting phosphodiesterase (and consequently increasing intracellular cyclic AMP) or by antagonizing the effects of adenosine, a known mediator of bronchoconstriction, have been seriously challenged.[36] Other potential modes of action include inhibition of the intracellular release of calcium or stimulation of catecholamine release.[30] In addition to its bronchodilating actions, theophylline may decrease the release of mediators from mast cells, reduce microvascular permeability, and increase the contractility of the diaphragm. Theophylline is available for both oral and intravenous administration. Optimal therapeutic drug levels (10 to 20 mg/ml) should be achieved to avoid adverse and potentially life-threatening reactions which can occur at higher drug levels. Side effects include nausea, vomiting, headache, and restlessness. At higher drug concentrations, cardiac arrhythmias and seizures may occur.

Intravenous aminophylline is often administered as a 5-6 mg/kg loading dose over 20-30 minutes. The maintenance dose (assuming a normal half-life) is 0.5-0.6 mg/kg/hr. Conditions which increase the half-life and may necessitate lower maintenance doses include age greater than 50 years, heart failure, liver disease, and acute viral infections. The use of erythromycin or cimetidine can increase plasma concentrations of theophylline. Cigarette smoking or use of phenobarbital can increase the clearance of theophylline.

Anticholinergic agents achieve bronchodilation by blocking muscarinic receptors in airway smooth muscle and by inhibiting vagal cholinergic tone. They are generally less effective bronchodilators than β2-adrenergic agonists in patients with asthma, but are occasionally useful in combination therapy. Atropine has limited usefulness due to its systemic absorption and anticholinergic side effects (dry mouth, blurred vision, and urinary retention). Synthetic atropine-like drugs have recently been introduced into the United States. Ipratropium bromide is associated with minimal systemic side effects, although it has occasionally precipitated bronchospasm.[37] The usual dose of ipratropium bromide is two puffs four times daily.

Anti-inflammatory Drugs. Anti-inflammatory drugs, in general, do not have immediate bronchodilating effects. They do, however, play an important role in the treatment of status asthmaticus and in the prevention of recurrent asthma.

Corticosteroids can be administered via intravenous, oral, or inhaled routes. Their precise mode of action has not been elucidated but it has been postulated that corticosteroids reduce the inflammatory response in the airways.[38,39] In addition, they have been shown to reduce the formation of relevant inflammatory mediators and cytokines,[40] prevent increased vascular permeability,[41] increase β-adrenergic responsiveness,[42] and reduce the peripheral-blood eosinophilia.[43]

Corticosteroids are an essential component of therapy in the management of acute life-threatening asthma.[44] There is controversy as to the optimum dose, mode of administration, and frequency. Recent studies have shown intravenous methylprednisolone, 125 mg (either one dose in the emergency room or every 6 hours, intravenously) results in considerable improvements in the first 24 hours.[45,46] Another study showed oral prednisolone (45 mg followed by 15 mg every 8 hours) to be as effective as intravenous hydrocortisone.[47] Another recent study found no significant differences between either oral (160 or 325 mg daily) or intravenous (500 or 1000 mg daily) methylprednisolone.[48]

Less severe exacerbations of asthma can be managed with oral administration of corticosteroids. Often, prednisone is given in doses of 40-60 mg with a rapid taper over 10 days to two weeks. Inhaled corticosteroids have greatly enhanced the ability to suppress asthmatic attacks on a chronic basis.[49] Available agents including beclomethasone dipropionate, triamcinolone acetonide, and flunisolide appear to be effective in doses of two puffs two to four times daily.

The side effects associated with prolonged intravenous or oral corticosteroids are well known.[50] These include weight gain, hypertension, diabetes, osteoporosis, cataracts, myopathy, CNS disturbances, skin fragility, and growth inhibition in children. Significant suppression of the adrenal gland can occur after 10-14 days of treatment but is more common after a more prolonged period of corticosteroid therapy. Inhaled corticosteroids are associated with few, if any, systemic side effects. Oral candidiasis can occur as well as dysphonia. There have been instances in which suppression of the adrenal glands has occurred (doses higher than 400 mg per day).[51]

Cromolyn can prevent asthma in some patients. Its mechanism of action is unknown, but it is thought to be anti-inflammatory as it prevents both the early and late asthmatic response and the subsequent hyperresponsiveness. It may stabilize mast cells. Cromolyn protects against various nonspecific bronchoconstrictors such as exercise.[52] It is often used as a prophylactic drug to prevent attacks. In the past, cromolyn was administered as a powder from a Spinhaler, but it is now available in a metered dose inhaler. The drug is relatively safe with few side effects. Occasional throat irritation has been noted when the powder is inhaled.

Other miscellaneous anti-inflammatory agents such as methotrexate have been shown to allow significant reduction in the use of corticosteroids in patients with severe asthma.[53] Some studies have suggested gold therapy can help control the disease.[54]

Other Forms of Treatment. Hyposensitizing injections have been used but evidence of therapeutic efficacy is lacking.[55] Diet has been implicated in some cases of asthma and some children have responded favorably to an elimination diet.[56]

References

1. American Thoracic Society: Definitions and classification of chronic bronchitis, asthma, and pulmonary emphysema. Am Rev Respir Dis. 1962;85:762.
2. Kelsen SG, Kelsen DP, Fleeger BF, et al: Emergency room assessment and treatment of patients with acute asthma: Adequacy of the conventional approach. Am J Med. 1978;64:622.
3. McFadden ER Jr, Lyons HA: Arterial-blood gas tension in asthma. N Engl J Med. 1968;278:1027.
4. Weiss EB, Faling LJ: Clinical significance of PaCO2 during status asthma: The cross-over point. Ann Allergy. 1968;26:545.
5. Houston JC, DeNavasquez S, Trounce JR: A clinical and pathological study of fatal cases of status asthmaticus. Thorax. 1953;8:207-213.
6. Hogg JC: The pathology of asthma. Clin Chest Med. 1984;5:567.
7. Dunnill MS, Massarella GR, Anderson JA: A comparison of the quantitative anatomy of the bronchi in normal subjects, in status asthmaticus, in chronic bronchitis, and in emphysema. Thorax. 1969;24:176.
8. De Monchy JGR, Kauffman HF, Venge P, et al: Bronchoalveolar eosinophilia during alleren-induced late asthmatic reactions. Am Rev Respir Dis. 1985;131:373-376.
9. Tomoika M, Ida S, Shindoh Y, et al: Mast cells in bronchoalveolar lumen of patients with bronchial asthma. Am Rev Respir Dis. 1984;129:1000-1005.
10. Drazen JM: Chemical mediators of immediate hypersensitivity reactions, in Fishman AP, Macklem PT, Mead J (eds): Handbook of Physiology. Bethesda, American Physiological Society, 1985, pp 711-718.
11. Serafin WE, Austin KF: Mediators of immediate hypersensitivity reactions. N Engl J Med. 1987;317:30.
12. Frigas E, Gleich GJ: The eosinophil and the pathophysiology of asthma. J Allergy Clin Immunol. 1986;77:527.
13. Boushey HA, Holzman MJ, Sheller JR, et al: Bronchial hyperreactivity. Am Rev Respir Dis. 1980;121:389-413.
14. Barnes PJ: Adrenergic receptors of normal and asthmatic airways. Eur J Respir Dis. 1984;65(Suppl 135):72-79.
15. Paterson JW, Lulich KM, Goldie RG: The role of B-adrenoceptors in bronchial hyperreactivity, in Morley J (ed): Perspectives in Asthma: Bronchial Hyperreactivity. New York, Academic Press, 1982, pp 19-37.
16. Black JL, Salome CM, Yan K, et al: Comparison between airways response to an alpha-adrenoceptor agonist and histamine in asthmatic and non-asthmatic subjects. Br J Clin Pharmacol. 1982;14:464-466.
17. Partanen M, Laitenen A, Hervonen A, et al: Catecholamine and acetyl cholinesterase containing nerves in human lower respiratory tract. Histochemistry. 1982;76:175-188.
18. Pride NB: Physiology of asthma. In: Clark TJH, Godfrey S (eds):Asthma. London, Chapman and Hall, 1983, 12-56.
19. Benatar SR: Fatal asthma. N Engl J Med. 1986;314:423-429.
20. O'Conner GT, Weiss ST, Speizer FE: The epidemiology of asthma. in Gershwin ME (ed): Bronchial Asthma: Principles of diagnosis and Treatment. Orlando, Grune & Stratton Inc, 1986, p 3.
21. Gregg I: Epidemiological aspects. In: Clark TJH, Godfrey S (eds): Asthma. London, Chapman & Hall, 1983, pp 242-284.
22. Waite DA, Eyles EF, Tonkin SL, et al: Asthma prevalence in Tokelauan children in two environments. Clin Allergy. 1980;10:71-75.

23. Speizer FE, Doll R, Heaf P: Observations on recent increase in mortality from asthma. Br Med J. 1968;1:335-339.

24. Sly RM: Increases in deaths from asthma. Ann Allergy. 1984;53:20-25.

25. Barriot P, Riou B: Prevention of fatal asthma. Chest. 1987;92:460-466.

26. Robin ED, Lewiston N: Unexpected, unexplained sudden death in young asthmatic subjects. Chest. 1989;96:790-793.

27. Rackemann FM, Edwards MC: Asthma in children. N Engl J Med. 1952;246:815-823.

28. Bronnimann S, Burrows B: A prospective study of the natural history of asthma: Remission and relapse rates. Chest. 1986;90:480-484.

29. Mountain RD, Sahn SA: Clinical features and outcome in patients with acute asthma presenting with hypercapnea. Am Rev Respir Dis. 1988;138:535-539.

30. Barnes PJ: A new approach to the treatment of asthma. N Engl J Med. 1989;321:1517-1527.

31. Carstairs JR, Nimmo AJ, Barnes PJ: Autoradiographic visualization of beta-adrenoceptor subtypes in human lung. Am Rev Respir Dis. 1985;132:541-547.

32. Butchers PR, Skidmore IF, Vardey CJ, et al: Characterization of the receptor mediating the antianaphylactic effects of beta-adrenoceptor agonists in human lung tissue in vitro. Br J Pharmacol. 1980;71:663-667.

33. Koeter GH, Postma DS, Keyzer JJ, et al: The effects of oral slow-release terbutaline on early morning dyspnoea. Eur J Clin Pharmacol. 1985;28:159-162.

34. Nelson HS: Adrenergic therapy of bronchial asthma. J Allergy Clin Immunol. 1986; 77:771-785.

35. Tattersfield AE: Tolerance to beta-agonists. Bull Eur Physiopathol Respir. 1985;21:1s-5s.

36. Church MK, Featherstone RL, Cushley MJ, et al: Relationships between adenosine, cyclic nucleotides, and xanthines in asthma. J Allergy Clin Immunol. 1986;78:670-675.

37. Rafferty P, Beasley R, Holgate ST: Comparison of the efficacy of preservative free ipratropium bromide and Atrovent nebuliser solution. Thorax. 1988;43:446-450.

38. Morris HG: Mechanisms of action and therapeutic role of corticosteroids in asthma. J Allergy Clin Immunol. 1985;75:1-13.

39. Pauwels R: Mode of action of corticosteroids in asthma and rhinitis. Clin Allergy. 1986;16:281-288.

40. Blackwell GJ, Carnuccio R, Di Rosa M, et al: Macrocortin: A polypeptide causing the anti-phospholipase effect of glucocorticoids. Nature. 1980;287:147-149.

41. Boschetto P, Rogers DF, Barnes PJ: Inhibition of airway microvascular leakage by corticosteroids. Thorax. 1989;44:320P-321P (abstr).

42. Townley RG, Reeb R, Fitzgibbons T, et al: The effects of corticosteroids on beta-adrenergic receptors in bronchial smooth muscle. J Allergy. 1970;45:118-121 (abstr).

43. Baigelman W, Chodosh S, Pizzuto D, et al: Sputum and blood eosinophils during corticosteroid treatment of acute exacerbations of asthma. Am J Med. 1983;75:929-936.

44. Fanta CH, Rossing TH, McFadden ER: Glucocorticoids in acute asthma: A critical controlled trial. Am J Med. 1983;74:845-851.

45. Haskell RJ, Wong BM, Hansen JE: A double blind randomized clinical trial of methylprednisolone in status asthmaticus. Arch Intern Med. 1983;143:1324-1327.

46. Littenberg B, Gluck EH: A controlled trial of methylprednisolone in the emergency treatment of acute asthma. N Engl J Med. 1986;314:150-152.

47. Harrison BD, Stokes TC, Hart GJ: Need for intravenous hydrocortisone in addition to oral prednisone in patients admitted to hospital with severe asthma without ventilatory failure. Lancet. 1986;1(8474):181-184.

48. Ratto D, Alfaro C, Sipsey J, et al: Are intravenous corticosteroids required in status asthmaticus?. JAMA. 1988;260:527-529.

49. Li JTC, Reed CE: Proper use of aerosol corticosteroids to control asthma. Mayo Clin Proc. 1989;64:205-210.

50. Smyllie HC, Connolly CK: Incidence of serious complications of corticosteroid therapy in respiratory disease. A retrospective survey of patients in the Brompton Hospital. Thorax. 1968;23:571-581.
51. Konig P: Inhaled corticosteroids—their present and future role in the management of asthma. J Allergy Clin Immunol. 1988;82:297-306.
52. Anderson SD, Seale JP, Ferris L, et al: An evaluation of pharmacotherapy for exercise-induced asthma. J Allergy Clin Immunol. 1979;64:612-624.
53. Mullarkey MF, Blumenstein BA, Andrde WP, et al: Methotrexate in the treatment of corticosteroid-dependent asthma. A double-blind crossover study. N Engl J Med. 1988;318:603-607.
54. Bernstein DI, Bernstein IL, Bodenheimer SS, et al: An open study of auranofin in the treatment of steroid-dependent asthma. J Allergy Clin Immunol. 1988;81:6-16.
55. Lichtenstein LM, Valentine MD, Norman PS: A reevaluation of immunotherapy for asthma. Am Rev Respir Dis. 1984;129:657-659.
56. Dannaeus A: Diet and asthma in infancy and childhood. Eur J Respir Dis. 1984;65 (Suppl 136):165-167.

Case 8

Diabetes Mellitus and Hypertension

Daniel Caruso, MD and Kwame Osei, MD

Case Histories

The relationship between diabetes mellitus (DM) and hypertension has been recognized since the 1920's.[1-3] Diabetics are at increased risk for atherosclerotic complications and hypertension increases this risk. It is now becoming evident that complications associated with diabetes, including nephropathy and retinopathy, are related not only to the duration of diabetes and degree of diabetic control but also to the presence, duration and severity of hypertension. Furthermore, the relationship of hypertension to diabetes differs somewhat between type I DM (insulin-dependent [IDDM], juvenile onset, ketosis-prone) and type II DM (non-insulin-dependent [NIDDM], adult onset, nonketotic) and could modulate the prognosis of diabetes in the respective diabetic groups. The case summaries of three diabetic patients discussed below illustrate important differences and similarities in the etiology and natural history of hypertension in diabetic patients.

Case 1. A 26-year-old patient has been treated for type I diabetes for 18 years. His hemoglobin A1C has ranged from 9.5% to 12.5% (normal <8.0%), with the values being under 10% since using a continuous infusion insulin pump. He developed hypertension at the age of 25; the blood pressure normalized with the administration of a calcium channel blocker. After one year his blood pressure was again elevated, requiring the addition of an angiotensin-converting enzyme (ACE) inhibitor to normalize his blood pressure. Urinary total protein and microalbumin have been in the normal range prior to and during antihypertensive therapy. His creatinine clearance is 139 ml/min. His total cholesterol has dropped from 195 mg/dl to 121 mg/dl over the past three years; triglycerides have been consistently under 70, the high-density lipoprotein (HDL) cholesterol 45-50 mg/dl and the calculated low-density lipoprotein (LDL) cholesterol has decreased from 133 mg/dl to 65 mg/dl.

Case 2. A 28-year-old patient with type I diabetes and congenital absence of one kidney developed subclinical proteinuria (326 mg/24 hr, normal <150 mg/24hr). at the age of 25. The following year his 24-hr urinary protein was 494 mg. Six months later he was found to be hypertensive and was started on an ACE inhibitor. His blood pressure responded well, but proteinuria progressed to 1747 mg/24 hr. Recently his blood pressure was again elevated and his ACE inhibitor dose was increased. His creatinine clearance is 116 ml/min. In four years his total cholesterol has increased from 128 mg/dl to 193 mg/dl; the HDL-cholesterol increased from 35 to 51 mg/dl and the triglycerides have ranged from 60 to 120 mg/dl. The corresponding calculated LDL-cholesterol levels increased from 87 mg/dl to 118 mg/dl.

Case 3. A 53-year-old patient was diagnosed with hypertension 11 years ago. Her blood pressure has been difficult to manage despite polytherapy with loop diuretics, clonidine, ACE inhibitors, beta adrenergic blockers and calcium channel blockers. Because of the lability of her hypertension she was evaluated for surgically curable hypertension, but no reversible causes were found. She was diagnosed with DM seven years ago, and her diabetes has been difficult to control while on insulin and oral hypoglycemic agents; her Hb A1C has ranged from 10% to 15%. In the last 20 months her serum creatinine has deteriorated from 2.8 to 7.8 mg/dl. Urinary protein is greater than 5000 mg/24 hr. She has suffered recurrent hypertensive encephalopathy with blood pressures as high as 300/160 mm Hg, accompanied by coma and intracerebral hemorrhage. Because of accelerated proliferative retinopathy she underwent laser photocoagulation therapy. In 1988, when her creatinine was 3.5 mg/dl and urinary protein was 5.33 gm/24 hr, the cholesterol was 356 mg/dl, triglycerides 1143 mg/dl and HDL-cholesterol 31 mg/dl. She is currently on hemodialysis.

Discussion

Epidemiology. Approximately 58 million Americans have hypertension, 12 million have diabetes and 2.5 million are afflicted by both diabetes and hypertension.[4] Hypertension has long been recognized as being more prevalent in diabetics compared to nondiabetics; it tends to occur more frequently in type I DM than type II DM[4] although this is not a consistent finding.[5,6] The etiology of hypertension can be conveniently categorized into essential (case 1), surgically correctable, and secondary to diabetic nephropathy (case 2).[7] Although any of these etiologies may play a role in the development of hypertension, both type I and II diabetics have an incidence of essential hypertension similar to the general population.[5] The causal relationship between diabetes and hypertension is not well-established. Hypertension clearly precedes clinical proteinuria (> 500 mg/day or Albustix positive),[5] but microalbuminuria (Albustix negative but urinary albumin above 30 μg/min) may precede hypertension,[8,9] as evident by case 2. Somewhere between 20% and 45% of type I diabetics and 40% and 70% of type II diabetics have hypertension with normal urinary albumin; however, most will eventually progress to some degree of albuminuria.[10,11] On the other hand, albuminuria without hypertension is present in 30 to 45% of patients with type I DM and 15 to 50% of type II diabetics.[5-10]

Pathophysiology. The etiologies of hypertension in diabetic patients are numerous; Table 1 summarizes the etiolgies and pathophysiology of diabetic hypertension.

The exact pathophysiology of diabetic renal hypertension is unknown, but has been attributed in part to the renin-angiotensin system. Normotensive diabetics (both type I and II) with microalbuminuria have increased exchangeable sodium

Table 1

Pathogenesis of Hypertension in Diabetes Mellitus

- **Essential**
  Cause Unknown

- **Diabetic Hypertension**
  Hyperinsulinemia (Type II DM)
  Increased vascular tone
  Hypersensitivity to catecholamines

- **Renal**
  Associated with microalbuminuria and later
    clinical proteinuria
  Increased exchangeable sodium
  Supressed renin
  Possibly compounded by poor glycemic control,
    family history of hypertension (type IDM)

- **Surgically Correctable**[a]
  Renal artery stenosis
  Cushing's syndrome
  Primary aldosteronism
  Pheochromocytoma
  Obstructive uropathy
  Coarctation of the aorta

---

[a]*These are rare causes of hypertension in diabetic patients and should be suspected in all patients who fail to respond to maximum antihypertensive therapy.*

and decreased plasma renin activity; the sodium-renin product is normal. In the face of macroalbuminuria with hypertension, exchangeable sodium, plasma renin activity and the sodium-renin product are elevated.[6] However, it should be noted that diabetic patients with hyporeninemia can be hypertensive.[12] Thus, the role of the renin-angiotensin system is not universally accepted.

Second, the risk of nephropathy in type I DM has been suggested to be increased by factors commonly recognized as risk factors for essential hypertension: a parental history of hypertension and increased maximal velocity of lithium-sodium countertransport in red cells.[8,13] The parental history, however, has not been found to be significant by Deckert et al.[14] These risk factors appear to be compounded by poor control of glycemia, particularly in the first ten years after the diagnosis of diabetes.[8]

Excluding renal hypertension, hypertension in type II diabetes probably has a different pathophysiology than hypertension in type I diabetes. Because of the high prevalence of hypertension in type II DM, hyperinsulinemia has been postulated to be the underlying factor linking the two conditions. There is an 80% higher fasting serum insulin in type II DM with hypertension compared to normotensive type II diabetes.[15] The latter group had twofold higher fasting serum insulin levels than the nondiabetic hypertensives and nondiabetic controls. The hypertensive diabetics also had higher insulin/glucose and insulin/C-peptide ratios compared to normotensive diabetics. These findings respectively indicate both significant insulin resistance and impaired hepatic extraction of insulin in the diabetic hypertensives. Insulin secretion was not, however, different between normotensive and hypertensive diabetics, based on similar C-peptide levels in both diabetic groups.[15]

Recently, Ferrannini et al,[16] presented further evidence that has strengthened the relationship between hypertension and hyperinsulinemia. Their study showed that nondiabetic hypertensive patients had increased insulin levels in response to a glucose tolerance test and manifested impaired insulin-mediated nonoxidative glucose disposal. This study indicated that essential hypertension is an insulin-resistant state. The causal relationship between insulin and hypertension is not clear from these studies. It should, however, be noted that insulin has been shown to increase renal tubular absorption of sodium.[17]

Hypertension and Diabetic Nephropathy. There are significant complications that diabetic patients may face, and these complications can be aggravated by hypertension. A summary of the relationship of hypertension to diabetic complications is found in Table 2. One of the most prominent consequences of diabetes and hypertension is renal insufficiency and end-stage renal disease requiring dialysis. Indeed, the third patient presented is now on chronic renal dialysis. The extent of diabetic renal failure is significant; approximately 30% of new cases of end-stage renal disease (ESRD) are diabetic.[5,18] Of those diabetics needing dialysis, anywhere from 20% to 80% are type I.[5] The risk of developing ESRD with DM over a 10 year period is 0.5% for type II DM and 5.8% for type I DM. There is a

Table 2

Summary of Deleterious Effects of Hypertension on Diabetic Complications

- **Renal**
  Accelerates nephropathy to end stage renal disease
  Associated with higher morbidity and mortality rates
  Accelerated by hypertension

- **Ophthalmic**
  Higher prevalence of proliferative retinopathy — neovascularization
  Increases severity of background retinopathy — hemorrhage,
    exudates and microaneurysms which are accelerated by
    hypertension

racial difference, with blacks, Hispanics and Pima indians having a 50-600% increase in ESRD with DM compared to whites.[19-21]

Case # 2 with one kidney, proteinuria and normal creatinine is also at risk for renal failure. Microalbuminuria is recognized as the precursor to proteinuria, which in turn precedes frank renal failure.[5,10,22] A prospective study by Hasslacher et al found a 63% incidence of albuminuria in type I DM and a 38% incidence in type II DM over 18 years.[5] In a nine year follow-up of hypertensive type II diabetics by Mogensen[23] 22% advanced from microalbuminuria (30-140 μg/ml, normal < 30 μg/ml) to proteinuria (> 400 mg/24 hr total protein, normal < 150 mg/24 hr. A similar pattern is seen in type I DM,[24] and the likelihood of developing albuminuria is correlated to the duration of type I DM.[10,22]

A possible marker that precedes microalbuminuria has been recently recognized. Plasma prorenin, the inactive precursor to renin, has been observed to be elevated in normotensive type I DM prior to the development of microalbuminuria.[25] The prorenin level continues to rise as albuminuria increases[10] and microvascular complications, including nephropathy, retinopathy and neuropathy, typically develop in the following two years. When hypertension develops the plasma prorenin declines.[25] With the deterioration in renal function, a distinct pattern of hypertension and the complications emerges in the two diabetic subgroups. In type I DM, the incidence of hypertension increases 50% as the patient progresses from normoalbuminuria to microalbuminuria. This figure increases to 200-300% in patients with established macroalbuminuria.[5,22] By the time renal insufficiency is present, as evidenced by elevated serum creatinine, 90-100% of all diabetic patients are hypertensive.[5] Even when not overtly hypertensive, diabetic patients with albuminuria as a group have higher mean blood pressures than those with normoalbuminuria, especially during exercise.[8,9,26] Several studies have demonstrated increased mortality in patients with diabetic nephropathy. In this regard, Mogensen[23] have shown that type II diabetics with urinary albumin of less than 15 μg/min (lower half of the normal range) had a 37% increase in mortality compared to nondiabetics; mortality was increased 76% in those with urinary albumin of 16-29 μg/min, 148% in those with urinary albumin of 30-140 μg/min, and 105% in patients losing more than 140 μg/min of urinary albumin. Of the deaths, uremia was the cause in 20%, myocardial infarction or insufficiency in 30%, stroke in 15%, infection in 20% and 5% in "other".

Despite the poor prognosis associated with hypertension and diabetes, recent investigations have demonstrated that aggressive antihypertensive therapy can delay the course of progression to end-stage renal failure, thus postponing the need for dialysis. We believe in patient #3 that the uncontrolled hypertension might have played a significant role in the progressive deterioration to ESRD. In 1983 a study by Parving et al[27] prospectively evaluated 10 type I diabetics. Following a 27 mo (mean) baseline the patients were treated with metoprolol, hydralazine and furosemide or thiazide for a mean of 39 mo. Mean arterial pressure was reduced from 112 mm Hg to 99 mm Hg. Albuminuria was reduced with therapy from 977 μg/min to 433 μg/min and the rate of decline in glomerular filtration rate dropped from 0.91 ml/min/mo to 0.31 ml/min/mo.

Hypertension and Diabetic Retinopathy. Diabetic retinopathy is the leading cause of newly diagnosed blindness in the United States.[28] Diabetic retinopathy is categorized into two major groups: background retinopathy, which includes microaneurysms, hemorrhages and exudates, and proliferative retinopathy, which manifests as neovascularization of the retina (see also Table 2). Patient 3 had evidence of both types of retinopathy and required laser photocoagulation. The prevalence of diabetic retinopathy is closely correlated with diabetic nephropathy in both type I and II DM; retinopathy is seen in 10-20% of those with normal urinary albumin, 30-60% with microalbuminuria and 60-100% with macroalbuminuria, similar to the rates of hypertension.[22,26] Retinopathy without hypertension correlates to albuminuria in a similar fashion.[10] Therefore, the finding of diabetic retinopathy on funduscopic examination can be used as an indicator that microvascular renal disease is also present. Conversely, the presence of macroproteinemia without angiographically proven retinopathy and/or hypertension virtually excludes diabetes as the cause of the nephropathy.

It has been argued that hypertension without nephropathy does not appear to increase the risk of retinopathy; Krolewski et al[8] found no difference in blood pressure or degree of hyperglycemia between diabetics with no complications and those with isolated retinopathy. However, hypertension does reduce the time interval between the onset of persistent proteinuria and the diagnosis of proliferative retinopathy by as much as 70%.[5] Hypertension has been associated with the severity of diabetic retinopathy and contributes to blood-retinal leakage in background retinopathy of diabetics with proteinuria. This leakage can be reduced by antihypertensive therapy.[29] Thus, the available literature would argue for intensive antihypertensive therapy in diabetic patients with retinopathy as well.

Therapy. A wide variety of interventions have been proven or proposed to modify the course of diabetic complications in the presence of hypertension. Table 3 summarizes therapeutic options for the diabetic hypertensive patient. Essential hypertension in diabetics is defined as an average of two or more diastolic blood pressures of 90 mm Hg or higher, or multiple systolic blood pressures consistently over 140 mm Hg, with normal renal function and in the absence of surgically correctable hypertension and clinical proteinuria.[28] The Working Group on Hypertension in Diabetes[28] has advised first step therapy with a thiazide diuretic,

Table 3

Interventions Which Modify the Course of Diabetic Complications

---

- **Antihypertensive Therapy**
   Reduces rate of loss of renal function and proteinuria
   Reduces blood-retinal leakage
   Decreases incidence of cerebrovascular accidents

- **Choice of Antihypertensive Agents**
   Angiotensin converting enzyme inhibitors – protective effect
      on renal function
   Prazosin hydrochloride – increases HDL-C and reduces LDL-C
   Calcium channel blockers – no adverse effects on lipids
   Thiazide diuretics – may cause electrolyte or lipoprotein
      abnormalities
   Beta-adrenergic blockers – may cause lipid abnormalities
      (when no intrinsic sypathomimetic activity is present) or
      mask symptoms of hypoglycemia
   Hydralazine – may cause reflex tachycardia or peripheral edema

- **Metabolic Control**
   Strict metabolic control may prevent or delay diabetic
      nephropathy

- **Diet**
   Low-protein diet may reduce the degree of albuminuria and
      protect renal function

---

beta-adrenergic blocker, ACE inhibitor, prazosin hydrochloride or a calcium channel blocker. The report acknowledges the risk of hypokalemia and elevation of low-density lipoprotein from thiazide diuretics. The latter was emphasized by Kaplan in his critique[30] of the final report. As seen by case 2 and 3, lipids and lipoproteins could deteriorate due to either progression of renal disease (i.e., nephrotic syndrome), poor glycemic control or as an adverse effect of antihypertensive therapy. Limitations of beta-adrenergic blockers in respect to masking symptoms of hypoglycemia, particularly in type I DM, have been addressed by The Working Group and the Canadian Consensus Conference report on diabetes and hypertension.[31] In addition to effects on lipids and lipoproteins, nonselective beta-adrenergic blockers could also worsen control in type II DM. The current consensus is that calcium-channel blockers, ACE inhibitors or prazosin hydrochloride may be the treatment of choice for hypertensive diabetics. Both the Working Group and the Canadian Consensus Conference advise hydralazine for refractory hypertension, although reflex tachycardia and peripheral edema may necessitate the use of a diuretic and beta-adrenergic blocker. As a general rule, most diabetics can be effectively treated with current agents. However, the discovery of hypertension refractory to maximum antihypertensive therapy warrants investigation into surgically correctable causes such as renal artery stenosis, Cushing's syndrome, primary aldosteronism, pheochromocytoma, obstructive uropathy and coarctation of the aorta.[7]

Treatment of renal hypertension in diabetes differs little from therapy advised for essential hypertension.[28,31] It is evident that conventional therapy, including β-adrenergic blockers, loop diuretics and hydralazine, will lower blood pressure and benefit renal function.[27] Further reduction in proteinuria may be accomplished by adherence to a low-protein diet while on conventional antihypertensive therapy.[32] The ACE inhibitors decrease systemic hypertension, thereby theoretically reducing renal perfusion pressure and subsequent damage; they also have a direct effect of reducing glomerular pressure, further protecting the kidney from damage.[33,34] The measurable effect of lowering the glomerular perfusion pressure is the reduction of proteinuria. Although these benefits associated with the ACE inhibitors have been investigated in only a limited number of patients over a short term, the ACE inhibitors may prove to be the drug of choice for renal hypertension in diabetics.

Ideally, it would be preferable to prevent or delay renal damage prior to the development of renal hypertension. Trials addressing this issue have attempted to reduce or prevent normotensive microalbuminuria by administering antihypertensives, based on the observation that normotensive diabetics with microalbuminuria tend to have higher mean blood pressures than controls.[35] Studies on small groups have demonstrated that metoprolol[36] and clonidine[37] have beneficial effects on microalbuminuria in normotensive diabetics. In 1987, Marre et al[38] reported their comparison of enalapril, an ACE inhibitor, to placebo for six months with 10 patients in each group. Blood pressure was reduced and albuminuria fell in the treated group from 124 mg/day to 37 mg/day (normal < 30 mg/24 hr mg), while in the placebo group blood pressure was unchanged and the urinary albumin climbed from 81 mg/day to 183 mg/day. These preliminary reports deserve further investigation in a large patient population.

A second approach to delaying the onset of albuminuria has been through strict metabolic control. Evidence suggests that chronic hyperglycemia correlates with albuminuria.[8,10,26] However, the effect of strict glycemic control on the development of established diabetic nephropathy, retinopathy and hypertension is debatable. Several studies evaluating strict glycemic control of up to one year's duration have found no beneficial effects on renal function.[39-41] It is believed that two years of tight glycemic control may be the minimum time necessary to detect any benefit; one study demonstrated that the use of an insulin pump led to an arrest in the progression of albuminuria and hypertension, a decrease in serum creatinine and no change in retinopathy over two years.[9] However, another two-year study found no significant difference in renal function when comparing strict glycemic control to average control.[42]

Summary. Diabetes mellitus and hypertension frequently coexist, and this coexistence accelerates the end-organ damage associated with diabetes. Antihypertensive therapy can reduce the rate of progression of diabetic complications. The choice of antihypertensive agents must be individualized because diabetics have an increased risk of suffering from the side effects of these medications, including severe electrolyte and lipoprotein changes that may be detrimental to the patient. It is uncertain if diabetic control prevents or delays diabetic complications, including renal hypertension; studies are in progress to help answer this question. Finally, in established renal disease it may be prudent to restrict total protein intake in diabetic patients.

References

1. Hitzenberger K. Uber den Blutdruck bei Diabetes mellitus. Wien Arch Inn Med. 1921;2:461.
2. Maranon G. Uber hypertonic und Zuckerkrankheit. Zentralbl Med. 1922;43:169-176.
3. Major SG. Blood pressure in diabetes mellitus: A statistical study. Arch Intern Med. 1929;44:781-797.
4. National Diabetes Data Group. Summary. in National Diabetes Data Group (ed): Diabetes in America. US Dept of Health and Human Services; 1985, pp 1-6.
5. Hasslacher C, Ritz E, Tschope W, et al: Hypertension in diabetes mellitus. Kidney Int Suppl. 1988;25:S133-S137.
6. Ferriss JB, O'Hare JA, Cole M, et al: Blood pressure in diabetic patients: relationships with exchangeable sodium and renin activity. Diabetic Nephropathy. 1986;5:27-30.
7. Christlieb AR. Treating hypertension in the patient with diabetes mellitus. Med Clin North Am. 1982;66:1373-1388.
8. Krolewski AS, Canessa M, Warram JH, et al: Predisposition to hypertension and susceptibility to renal disease in insulin-dependent diabetes mellitus. N Engl J Med. 1988;318:140-145.

9. Feldt-Rassmussen B, Mathiesen ER, Deckert T: Effect of two years of strict metabolic control on progression of incipient nephropathy in insulin-dependent diabetes. Lancet. 1986;2:1300-1304.
10. Luetscher JA, Kraemer FB. Microalbuminuria and increased plasma prorenin. Prevalence in diabetics followed up for four years. Arch Intern Med. 1988;148:937-941.
11. Mathiesen ER, Hommel E, Olsen UB, et al: Elevated urinary prostaglandin excretion and the effect of indomethacin on renal function in incipient diabetic nephropathy. Diabetic Med. 1988;5:145-149.
12. Christlieb AR, Kalding A, D'Elia JA. Plasma renin activity and hypertension in diabetes mellitus. Diabetes. 1976;25:969-974.
13. Mangili R, Bending JJ, Scott G, et al: Increased sodium-lithium transport activity in red cells of patients with insulin-dependent diabetes mellitus. N Engl J Med. 1988;313:146-150.
14. Deckert T, Feldt-Rasmussen B, Borch-Johnsen K, et al: Albuminuria reflects widespread vascular damage. The Steno hypothesis. Diabetologia. 1989;32:219-226.
15. Mbanya JC, Thomas TH, Wilkinson R, et al: Hypertension and hyperinsulinaemia: A relation in diabetes but not essential hypertension. Lancet. 1988;1:733-734.
16. Ferrannini E, Buzzigoli G, Bonadonna R, et al: Insulin resistance in essential hypertension. N Engl J Med. 1987;317:350-357.
17. DeFronzo RA: The effect of insulin on renal sodium metabolism. Diabetologia. 1981;21:165-171.
18. Eggers PW: Effect of transplantation on the Medicare End Stage Renal Disease Program. N Engl J Med. 1988;318:223-229.
19. Cowie CC, Port FK, Wolfe RA, et al: Disparities in incidence of diabetic end-stage renal disease according to race and type of diabetes. N Engl J Med. 1989;321:1074-1079.
20. Nelson RG, Pettitt DJ, Carraher MJ, et al: Effect of proteinuria on mortality in NIDDM. Diabetes. 1988;37:1499-1504.
21. Pugh JA, Stern MP, Haffner SM, et al: Excess incidence of treatment of end-stage renal disease in Mexican Americans. Am J Epidemiol. 1988;127:135-144.
22. Parving HH, Hommel E, Mathiesen E, et al: Prevalence of microalbuminuria, arterial hypertension, retinopathy and neuropathy in patients with insulin dependent diabetes. Br Med J Clin Res. 1988;296:156-160.
23. Mogensen CE: Microalbuminuria predicts clinical proteinuria and early mortality in maturity-onset diabetes. N Engl J Med. 1984;310:356-360.
24. Mogensen CE, Christensen CK. Predicting diabetic nephropathy in insulin-dependent diabetes mellitus. N Engl J Med. 1984;311:89-93.
25. Luetscher JA, Kraemer FB, Wilson DM. Prorenin and vascular complications of diabetes. Am J Hypertens. 1989;2:382-386.
26. Barnett AH, Dallinger K, Jennings P, et al: Microalbuminuria and diabetic retinopathy. Lancet. 1985;1:53-54.
27. Parving HH, Smidt UM, Andersen AR, et al: Early aggressive antihypertensive treatment reduces rate of decline in kidney function in diabetic nephropathy. Lancet. 1983;1:1775-1779.
28. The Working Group on Hypertension in Diabetes. Statement on hypertension in diabetes mellitus. Arch Intern Med. 1987;147:830-842.
29. Parving HH, Larsen M, Hommel E, et al: Effect of antihypertensive treatment on blood-retinal barrier permeability to fluorescein in hypertensive type 1 (insulin-dependent) diabetic patients with background retinopathy. Diabetologia. 1989;32:440-444.
30. Kaplan NM. Critique of recommendations from Working Group on Hypertension in Diabetes. Am J Kidney Dis. 1989;13:38-40.

31. Hamet P, Kalant N, Ross SA, et al: Recommendations from the Canadian Hypertension Society Consensus Conference on Hypertension and Diabetes. Can Med Assoc J. 1988; 139:1059-1062.

32. Zucchelli P, Zuccala A, Sturani A. Glomerular dysfunction in diabetic nephropathy. Postgrad Med J. 1988;64(Suppl 3):22-30; discuss.

33. Hommel E, Parving HH, Mathiesen E, et al: Effect of captopril on kidney function in insulin-dependent diabetic patients with nephropathy. British Med J. 1986;293:467-470.

34. Bjorck S, Nyperg G, Mulec H, et al: Beneficial effects of angiotensin converting enzyme inhibition on renal function in patients with diabetic nephropathy. BMJ. 1986;293:471-474.

35. Christensen CK. Abnormal albuminuria and blood pressure rise in incipient diabetic nephropathy induced by exercise. Kidney Int. 1984;25:819-823.

36. Christensen CK, Mogensen CE. Effect of antihypertensive treatment on progression of incipient diabetic nephropathy. Hypertension. 1958;7:9-13.

37. Friedman PJ, Dunn PJ, Jury DR. Metoprolol and albumin excretion in diabetes. Lancet. 1986;2:43.

38. Marre M, Leblanc H, Suarez L, et al: Converting enzyme inhibition and kidney function in normotensive diabetic patients with persistent microalbuminuria. British Med J. 1987;294:1448-1452.

39. Viberti GC, Bilous RW, Mackintosh D, et al: Long-term correction of hyperglycemia and progression of renal failure in insulin-dependent diabetes. British Med J. 1983;286:598-602.

40. Christiansen JS, Parving HH: The effect of short term strict metabolic control on albuminuria in insulin-dependent diabetics with normal kidney function and diabetic neuropathy. Diabetic Nephropathy. 1984;3:127-129.

41. Feldt-Rassmussen B, Mathiesen ER, Hegedus L, et al: Kidney function during 12 months of strict metabolic control instrument insulin-dependent diabetic patients with incipient nephropathy. N Engl J Med. 1986;314:665-670.

42. Deckert T, Lauritzen T, Parving HH, et al: Effect of two years of strict metabolic functions in long term insulin-dependent diabetics. Diabetic Nephropathy. 1984;3:6-10.

Case 9

Hypothyroidism and Chest Pain in an Elderly Woman

Ernest L. Mazzaferri, MD, FACP and Lorraine M. Birskovich, MD

Case History

A 71-year-old woman from West Virginia first presented to The Ohio State University Hospital General Medicine Clinic for preoperative evaluation in preparation for surgical biopsy of a hypopharyngeal tumor that had been found by CT scan after she had experienced hemoptysis. She had suffered a myocardial infarction 11 years previously and shortly thereafter had undergone triple coronary artery bypass grafting. During the past several years she had been experiencing stable angina with 2 or 3 episodes of chest heaviness per week relieved with one sublingual nitroglycerine. Two months prior to consultation she had been admitted to University Hospital for congestive heart failure which responded to captopril, furosemide, and digoxin. During that hospitalization gated cardiac radionuclide angiography showed her left ventricular ejection fraction to be 34%. Recently her exercise tolerance was restricted to walking around the house. She also had long standing type 2 diabetes mellitus with background retinopathy, nephropathy, and peripheral neuropathy as well as severe peripheral vascular disease. About 30 years previously she had been told she had "throat cancer" which had been treated with surgery and external radiation therapy. She had an 80 pack year history of smoking.

Physical Examination. She was an alert and cooperative elderly woman in a wheelchair who weighed 130 pounds, had a regular pulse rate of 80 beats per minute, a respiratory rate of 18, and a blood pressure of 150/70 mm Hg. Her cardiac examination revealed a moderately enlarged and sustained point of maximum impulse, with a grade II/VI systolic ejection murmur along the left sternal border over the left ventricular outflow tract, and a soft S_4 gallop. Her jugular venous pulsation appeared normal. Bilateral bruits were present over both carotid and femoral arteries. Her electrocardiogram was unchanged from previous studies and showed normal sinus rhythm with a right bundle branch block and left anterior fascicular block patterns.

Hospital Course. Shortly thereafter she underwent biopsy and subsequent right radical neck dissection for an invasive squamous cell carcinoma of the hypopharynx. Her surgery included laryngectomy, partial pharyngectomy, right thyroid lobectomy, tracheostomy, and flap reconstruction. She had an uneventful hospital course and was discharged with codeine for pain.

Several weeks later she noted weakness, and 2 months later experienced abdominal discomfort, mild nausea and severe constipation. The only new physical findings were moderate abdominal distension and tympany without tenderness. She did not have a fecal impaction. Abdominal roentgenograms showed a pattern consistent with ileus. Her routine laboratory studies, including serum calcium and potassium concentrations, were normal or unchanged from previous studies. She failed to respond to laxatives, and shortly thereafter was admitted to the hospital because of chest pain. At the time of admission she was alert and oriented. There were no new physical findings. Her skin was dry and wrinkled, and she had some periorbital puffiness, particularly in the lower lids. Her pulse was 74 beats per minute, her respiratory rate 17, and her blood pressure 160/80 mm Hg. Her abdomen remained mildly distended, was tympanic to percussion and showed hypoactive bowel sounds without tenderness to palpation. Her chest pain responded promptly to nitrates and bed rest. Routine laboratory studies were unchanged from her previous hospital admissions over the past year and continued to show fasting hyperglycemia (fasting plasma glucose 130 mg/dl) with mild elevation of her blood urea nitrogen (30 mg/dl) and creatinine (1.7 mg/dl). Her electrocardiogram was unchanged and her cardiac enzymes showed no evidence of an acute myocardial infarction. Thyroid function tests obtained on admission disclosed a T_4 of 2.1 μg/dl (normal 3.5-11), a free T_4 index (FTI) of 2.2 (normal 3.5-11), and a TSH greater than 50 μU/ml (normal 0.2-5).

Discussion

This patient has primary hypothyroidism, a common problem in elderly persons, particularly in aging women. This disorder frequently poses perplexing diagnostic and therapeutic challenges in the aged as occurred in the patient in this case study. Recognition of hypothyroidism in elderly persons is often enigmatic, and replacement therapy with thyroid hormone frequently presents unique problems.

Hypothyroidism is often referred to as being subclinical or overt, terms that do not have standard definitions in the literature on this subject. Subclinical (sometimes termed biochemical) hypothyroidism is often defined as *asymptomatic* disease in which the *only* laboratory abnormality is a clearly elevated serum TSH concentration. However, some attribute subtle symptoms to this stage of the disease. Serum thyrotropin (TSH) elevations between 5 and 10 μU/ml are usually regarded as being uncertain insofar as hypothyroidism is concerned, while levels over 10 μU/ml are clearly abnormally high. Overt hypothyroidism refers to *symptomatic* disease that is apparent from the history and physical examination, which can be confirmed by low serum free thyroxine (FT$_4$) concentrations. Myxedema refers to long standing hypothyroidism which is characterized by widespread tissue infiltration with mucopolysaccharides. Hypothyroidism can be the result of thyroid, pituitary, or hypothalamic disease, sometimes referred to as primary, secondary, and tertiary hypothyroidism. Primary thyroid disease, by far the most common cause of hypothyroidism, accounts for at least 95% of the cases and is distinguished by a low serum FT$_4$.[a]

Prevalence of Primary Hypothyroidism in the Elderly. The prevalence of hypothyroidism in elderly persons is quite high but variable around the world. Worldwide it is between 1 and 2% of the population over age 60 and is highest in women.[2] In the United States even higher figures have been reported. In one study of a group attending a senior citizen's center who were older than 60 years of age, Sawin et al[3] reported a 5.9% prevalence of hypothyroidism defined by serum TSH concentrations higher than 10 μU/ml. The prevalence of subclinical hypothyroidism in this same group, defined as a TSH between 5 and 10 μU/ml, was 14.4%.[3] The same authors, in a more recent study of the elderly population in the city of Framingham, found the prevalence of overt and subclinical hypothyroidism to be 4.4% and 5.9%, respectively.[4] In this study, the frequency of overt hypothyroidism was more than twofold greater in women than men (5.9% versus 2.4%).[4]

Etiology of Hypothyroidism in the Elderly. The causes of hypothyroidism are listed in Table 1.[1] Hypothyroidism in the elderly is most often due to primary thyroid disease, most frequently autoimmune thyroiditis.[5] However, thyroid failure in elderly persons is commonly a late consequence of Graves' disease treated with ^{131}I, surgery, or antithyroid drugs. As many as 75% of patients with Graves' disease treated with ^{131}I eventually develop hypothyroidism.[6] In surgically treated Graves' disease patients, the eventual prevalence of hypothyroidism was 27% in a recent study.[7] In another study,[8] the annual incidence of overt and subclinical hypothyroidism following antithyroid drug therapy for Graves' disease was 0.6% and 2.5%, respectively.[8] Thyroid failure in the elderly is thus frequently caused by Hashimoto's thyroiditis and is common in patients previously treated for Graves' disease.

Autoimmune thyroiditis occurs with increasing frequency in the aged population, and is particularly prevalent in women. It is probably the most frequent cause of hypothyroidism in elderly persons.[9] There is a high prevalence of serum antithyroid antibodies in the aged, which varies somewhat around the world,[1] but is

---

[a]*The FT$_4$ is usually estimated from the FTI or by RIA. The FTI is calculated from the total T$_4$ and the thyroid hormone binding ratio (THBR) which is measured by various methods such as the T$_3$ resin uptake. This calculated estimate of FT$_4$ is valid in most cases, but can be misleading in patients with severe nonthyroidal illness.*

Table 1

Causes of Hypothyroidism

- **Primary (Thyroidal) Hypothyroidism**
  Thyroid agenesis
  Destruction of the thyroid gland
  - surgical removal
  - therapeutic irradiation ^{131}I or external radiation
  - autoimmune disease (Hashimoto's thyroiditis)
  - replacement by cancer or other disease
  - postthyroiditis (acute or subacute)
  - following allogeneic bone marrow transplantation
  - treatment with interleukin-2 and lymphokine-activated killer cells
  Idiopathic atrophy (following autoimmune disease)
  Inhibition of synthesis of thyroid hormones
  - iodine deficiency
  - excess iodine in susceptible patients
  - antithyroid drugs
  - inherited enzyme defects
  Transient
  - after surgery or ^{131}I therapy
  - postpartum
  - during the course of thyroiditis

- **Secondary (Pituitary) Hypothyroidism**
  Tumors
  - pituitary adenomas, intrasellar (functioning and nonfunctioning)
  - craniopharyngioma
  - metastatic tumors (to pituitary gland)
  Ischemic necrosis
  - postpartum (Sheehan's syndrome)
  - severe shock, coma, diabetes mellitus, vasculitis
  Iatrogenic — radiation or surgery
  Chronic autoimmune lymphocytic hypophysitis
  Infectious diseases — tuberculosis, pyogenic, syphilis
  Sarcoidosis

Table 1 (Continued)

Causes of Hypothyroidism

- **Secondary (Pituitary) Hypothyroidism (Continued)**
  Histiocytosis (Hand-Schuller-Christian disease)
  Hemochromatosis
  Pituitary aplasia or hypoplasia
  Idiopathic hypopituitarism
  Lymphocytic hypophysitis

- **Tertiary (Hypothalamic) Hypothyroidism**
  Tumors
  - suprasellar extension of pituitary adenomas
  - craniopharyngiomas
  - meningioma, glioma, other primary brain tumors
  - metastatic tumors (especially breast, lung cancers)
  Traumatic
  Ischemic necrosis
  Iatrogenic
  - surgery, irradiation
  Sarcoidosis
  Histiocytosis
  Congenital malformations
  Idiopathic

- **Peripheral Tissue Resistance to Thyroid Hormones**
  Inherited or acquired

quite high in the United States. In a group of women aged 60 years and older residing in Worcester, MA, the prevalence of thyroglobulin and/or antimicrosomal antibodies at titers $\geq$ 1:400 was 25% while in a group of 243 women residing in Reggio Emilia, Italy, only 2 subjects had positive antibodies.[2] In another study by Rosentahl et al[10] TSH levels were elevated above 4.0μ U/ml in 13.2% of 258 healthy elderly subjects. Of the 26 subjects with elevated serum TSH concentrations, one third developed biochemical hypothyroidism (serum T_4 levels less than 58 nmole/liter (4.5 μg/dl) over a 4 year period. Overt hypothyroidism occurred in all subjects with initial TSH levels above 20 μU/ml, and 80% of those with high-titer antimicrosomal antibodies (> 1:1,600).

There are other important causes of hypothyroidism. Recently, hypothyroidism was reported in 21% of 34 patients treated with interleukin-2 and lymphokine activated killer cells, possibly as a result of exacerbating preexisting autoimmune thyroiditis.[11] Hypothyroidism also occurs following allogeneic bone marrow transplantation, possibly as the result of direct damage to follicular cells or to pituitary thyrotropic cells caused by irradiation.[12] Hypothyroidism may be induced in elderly subjects by administration of drugs with antithyroid activity, including thionamides, iodides, lithium, and other less commonly used preparations.[2] Excess iodine ingestion is an important cause of hypothyroidism, particularly in elderly subjects with Hashimoto's thyroiditis or previously treated Graves' disease.[2] Amiodarone, an antiarrhythmic agent that causes hypothyroidism, not only contains large amounts of iodine, but also impairs T_4 to T_3 conversion. The prevalence of hypothyroidism in patients treated with this drug ranges from 4% to 20% and is especially common in subjects with Hashimoto's thyroiditis.[1,2]

The patient under discussion developed hypothyroidism following laryngectomy for squamous carcinoma of the hypopharynx. After treating nodal metastases from squamous carcinoma of the head and neck, the incidence of occult hypothyroidism (manifested by elevated TSH levels) has been estimated to be as high as 25% following either surgery or radiation therapy alone, and 70% after combinations of the two. Of 261 patients who underwent total laryngectomy, Biel et al[13] found hypothyroidism had developed in 70% treated with radiotherapy and hemithyroidectomy, in 38% treated with radiotherapy alone, in 23% who had undergone hemithyroidectomy alone, and in 20% who had not received hemithyroidectomy or radiotherapy. Adding chemotherapy, however, does not appear to increase the incidence or severity of thyroid dysfunction. Posner et al[12] prospectively evaluated 43 previously untreated patients who were managed with aggressive chemotherapy in addition to standard surgery with or without radiotherapy. Thyroid abnormalities appeared within the first four months after therapy and were slowly progressive. Occult hypothyroidism appeared in 37% of patients a median of 9 months after chemotherapy and subsequent surgery and/or radiotherapy. Although elevated TSH levels occurred in 30% of patients given radiotherapy alone and in 43% of patients receiving surgery and radiotherapy, only one developed clinical symptoms while the others were asymptomatic despite persistently elevated TSH levels. In another study of 100 successive patients treated for tumors of the head and neck, none developed hypothyroidism after radiation therapy alone.[15] However, 10 to 17 (59%) patients developed occult hypothyroidism more than a year after irradiation combined with surgery, all but one of whom had been treated with hemithyroidectomy. The interval between hemithyroidectomy and postoperative irradiation was shorter in those developing hypothyroidism than those who remained euthyroid (31 versus 49 days). In view of the extended survival of patients treated with surgery and irradiation for head and neck squamous cell carcinomas, all patients receiving irradiation to the neck — particularly those undergoing neck dissections or total laryngectomies — should have routine thyroid function studies performed every 3 to 6 months the first year after treatment. Thereafter, it seems prudent to perform thyroid function tests at yearly intervals.

Clinical Presentation of Hypothyroidism in the Elderly. The classic signs and symptoms of hypothyroidism, listed in Table 2, are observed in as few as 25% of hypothyroid patients, making the diagnosis difficult to recognize in many patients.[2]

Table 2

Symptoms and Signs of Hypothyroidism

● General Symptoms		● Central Nervous System	
Dry thick skin and/or hair	89%	Mental/physical slowness	57%
Fatigue	70	Sleepiness	25
Edema-puffy hands, face, eyes	67	Headaches	22
Pallor	59	Dizziness	16
Cold intolerance	58	Nervousness	16
Hoarseness	48	Insomnia	13
Weight gain > 15 pounds	48	Psychological disturbance	5
Alopecia, loss/thinning hair	32	Stroke	2
Weakness	26	● Gastrointestinal System	
Lethargy	25	Constipation	37
Enlarged tongue	19	Anorexia	14
Neuropathy	17	Nausea and vomiting	13
Loss of sweating	11	Abdominal pain	12
Weight loss	6	Dysphagia	9
● Musculoskeletal System		Bloating or indigestion	8
Arthritis	15	Ascites	4
Muscle cramps	10	● Cardiovascular System	
Backache	9	Short of breath (subjective)	9
Stiff muscles or joints	8	Hypertension	18
Myopathy (weak muscles)	1	Bradycardia	14
● Genitourinary System		Dyspnea (objective)	11
Menstrual disorders	17	Heart failure	8
Polyuria and nocturia	11	Angina	4
Impotence and infertility	1	Pleural effusion	4
● Special Senses		Myocardial infarction	1
Blurred vision	7	Pericardial effusion	1
Tinnitus	7	Peripheral vascular insufficiency	1
Decreased hearing	6		
Diplopia	5		
Deafness	3		

From Watanakunakorn et al: Arch Intern Med. 1965;116:183.

The paucity of clear symptoms in many patients may be due to the characteristically insidious onset and slow progression of the disease over many years. In some cases, hypothyroidism may be manifested by only one dominant symptom. In others it may present with puzzling or atypical symptoms such as intestinal pseudo-obstruction, a von Willebrand-like bleeding disorder, an enlarged pituitary gland, seizures and neurologic dysfunction, and behavioral abnormalities such as psychosis, dementia, delirium, paranoia, and perseveration.[16] In the elderly, hypothyroidism is even more difficult to diagnose. Lloyd and Goldberg[17] screened 3417 patients for hypothyroidism admitted to a geriatric institution and found only 10% with laboratory confirmation of hypothyroidism were diagnosed by clinical examination. The others were thought to have a variety of other diagnoses such as chronic bronchitis, anemia, cardiac failure, and cerebral vascular disease. In some patients the symptoms of hypothyroidism were attributed to the aging process *per se*. Similar observations were made by Bahemuka and Hodkinson[18] who screened 2,000 geriatric inpatients and found only 28% (13 of 46) hypothyroid patients had clinically recognizable signs or symptoms of hypothyroidism, while a similar number (28%) had virtually no clinical evidence of hypothyroidism. Another 22% of unrecognized hypothyroid patients demonstrated symptoms of psychiatric disease. Sawin et al[4] found that although 95 of 2139 subjects screened had distinctly elevated serum TSH concentrations, none were clinically suspected of having hypothyroidism.

Because of its high frequency in the aging population, and the paucity of clear symptoms to readily identify its presence, some have suggested screening all asymptomatic persons for hypothyroidism. A recent report of the U.S. Preventive Services Task Force[19] recommended against routine thyroid function testing for asymptomatic adults, but noted that thyroid screening in the absence of symptoms may be clinically prudent for populations at increased risk, such as older persons, especially women. Elderly patients with vague symptoms, or unexplained neuromuscular, central nervous system, pulmonary, gastrointestinal, or genitourinary symptoms, or with impaired hearing, should be tested for hypothyroidism.

Laboratory Diagnosis of Hypothyroidism. The laboratory diagnosis of hypothyroidism is summarized in Table 3.[1] Decreased serum total and free T_4 and T_3 concentrations are consistent with but not diagnostic of hypothyroidism. Low thyroid hormone values, especially serum T_3 concentrations can be seen with a number of nonthyroidal illnesses. A wide variety of nonthyroidal illnesses lower serum total T_3 concentrations. In addition, many apparently normal elderly persons have lower than normal serum T_3 concentrations. In physically vigorous elderly persons who maintain a normal diet, this may not be the case. Nonetheless, the serum T_3 is basically useless in the diagnosis of hypothyroidism. In contrast, the T_4 does not change significantly with age and is not altered by most acute or chronic nonthyroidal illnesses. Even the serum T_4 concentration may fall dramatically, however, in patients who are critically ill;[1,2] however TSH usually remains

Table 3

Thyroid Function Tests in Hypothyroidism and Other Low-T₄ Syndromes

Diagnosis	T_4	T_3RU	FT_4I	T_3	TSH	TRH
Hypothyroid						
Thyroidal (primary)						
Overt hypo-						
thyroidism	low	low	low	low	high	excessive
Preclinical						
hypothyroidism	nl	nl	nl	nl	high	excessive
Pituitary (secondary)	low	low	low	low	low	blunted
Hypothalamic						
(tertiary)	low	low	low	low	low	nl/hi/ delayed
Euthyroid						
Low TBG	low	high	nl	low	nl	normal
Nonthyroidal Illness						
Low T_3 syndrome						
(mild NTI)	nl	nl	nl	low	nl	normal
Severe NTI	low	low/nl	low	low	nl	normal/ delayed

normal in these patients, thus clearly excluding primary hypothyroidism. In a few critically ill patients the serum TSH may rise, closely mimicking primary hypothyroidism. Unless there is clear evidence of myxedema in a critically ill patient with this combination of tests, it is prudent to withhold levothyroxine therapy and to repeat the tests several weeks after the patient has recovered from the acute illness. However, a very low serum T_4 is an ominous prognostic sign for survival in patients with nonthyroidal illness.

Measurement of the serum TSH concentrations is the most reliable and accurate test of hypothyroidism. In patients with primary hypothyroidism the serum TSH rises long before abnormalities in the serum FT_4I are appreciated. Patients suspected of having hypothyroidism who have normal TSH concentrations either have pituitary or hypothalamic disease (which is usually accompanied by deficiencies of other trophic hormones) or the diagnosis of hypothyroidism is incorrect. The latter is usually the case.

Treatment of Hypothyroidism in the Elderly. Synthetic levothyroxine is the treatment of choice for hypothyroidism. However, there are important differences in the bioavailability of currently available preparations. Over the past 10 years reformulation of a form of levothyroxine (Synthroid) raised considerable concern about the tablet strength and bioavailability of currently available preparations.[20] With current preparations of this drug the mean replacement dose in a group of carefully studied hypothyroid patients was found to be 112 ± 19 (SD) $\mu g/day$ (1.63 $\mu g/kg/day$) which is significantly less than the dose of an earlier formulation.[20] The median replacement dose in this study was 125 $\mu g/day$, and all patients required between 75 and 150 μg of levothyroxine/day.

In elderly patients, the average dose required to return the serum TSH concentrations to normal ranges is at least 10% less than in younger patients, and there is no difference between men and women.[2] It is prudent to begin therapy of hypothyroidism in the elderly with small daily dosages of levothyroxine in the range of 25 μg. The daily dosage is increased by 12.5 to 25 μg increments every 2 to 4 weeks until the calculated total daily dosage is reached or until adverse reactions occur.

The most serious adverse reactions are cardiac arrhythmias, angina, and myocardial infarction. Other rare but serious adverse reactions include manic behavior, sometimes so severe as to require hospitalization, pseudotumor cerebri, and cardiac tamponade in patients with myxedematous pericardial effusion. Ordinarily, slowly increasing the daily dosage will avoid serious complications in the elderly patient. However, concurrent coronary artery disease and hypothyroidism pose a particularly serious therapeutic problem which is discussed in greater detail below.

With adequate therapy, the serum TSH will return to the normal range about 6 weeks after achieving the full replacement dose, although occasionally much longer periods elapse before the TSH returns to normal. With adequate therapy, the serum FT4I should be in the normal range, but may be substantially higher in treated subjects than normal individuals.[20] In the study by Fish et al,[20] suppression of serum TSH concentrations was more clearly related to the serum T3 level than the serum T4 concentration. The serum TSH is thus the key test to follow in patients on replacement levothyroxine therapy. It should be in the normal range, along with serum T3 concentrations, while serum FT4I may be at the higher end of normal or slightly above normal in euthyroid patients on replacemnt levothyroxine therapy. One should not suppress serum TSH below the normal range since this is, in effect, subclinical thyrotoxicosis which should be avioded because of its association with osteoporosis. This is of particular concern since many treated hypothyroid patients are postmenopausal women.

The Problem of Concurrent Hypothyroidism and Arteriosclerotic Heart Disease. Many patients with hypothyroidism have severe concurrent coronary artery disease. An excellent review by Becker[21] on this relationship concluded that despite a large body of data linking the two disorders, the precise relationship between them remains obscure. The pathogenetic mechanisms involved in the progression of coronary artery disease in patients with hypothyroidism remain complex and poorly understood.[21]

Patients presenting with untreated hypothyroidism and severe angina pose a serious challenge for the clinician. Such patients usually have extensive underlying coronary artery disease, and the potential for exacerbating the angina or precipitating an acute myocardial infarction by thyroid hormone replacement is great. In an older retrospective study of 1503 patients seen at the Mayo Clinic, 90 patients had angina and hypothyroidism.[22] Of these, 49% had new onset or worsening of the angina, and 15% had an acute myocardial infarction during the first year after initiating thyroid hormone therapy. Subsequent studies have shown similar results.[21] Thyroid hormone treatment of hypothyroid patients who have angina requires hospitalization, at least during the initial phases of treatment. Patients should have their cardiovascular status closely monitored during the initial phases of therapy when they are particularly susceptible to cardiac arrhythmias. Since levothyroxine has a slower onset of action, and results in more stable serum and tissue levels of thyroid hormone, it is the drug of choice in this situation. The dose is decreased at the first sign of any cardiac problems. The patient under study had levothyroxine therapy started in the hospital where she was closely monitored. After several weeks, when a daily dosage of 25 μg was achieved, she was discharged and followed closely as an outpatient. The dose of levothyroxine was slowly increased over several months to 75 μg daily without worsening of her angina. Medical management of angina may be difficult in the hypothyroid patient because nitrates may precipitate hypotension or syncope, and β-blockers may be poorly tolerated. Until recently, however, no other form of therapy was available and surgical intervention was considered contraindicated.

Newer studies indicate that surgical intervention for coronary artery disease should be considered in hypothyroid patients whenever medical management of either the angina or hypothyroidism cannot be achieved.[21] Until recently it was felt that hypothyroid patients could not be taken to surgery until replacement levothyroxine had been given. Several studies have shown that this is not true. In a case control study comparing 59 hypothyroid patients with 59 controls, Weinberg et al[23] concluded that it is safe to send mild to moderate hypothyroid patients to surgery without preoperative thyroid hormone therapy. This study has been criticized as probably generalizing beyond the limits of a small sample size.[21] A second retrospective case control study[24] of 40 hypothyroid patients concluded that this group had significantly higher frequencies of perioperative hypotension, gastrointestinal hypomotility, and central nervous system disturbances compared with controls. More serious complications were encountered among 17 patients undergoing cardiac surgery, including impaired hemostasis, delayed recovery from anesthesia, marked friability of the aortic root, and a significantly higher prevalence of perioperative heart failure among hypothyroid patients as compared with controls. However, none of these complications had serious or lasting sequelae for the patients. The authors concluded that complications in hypothyroid patients can occur and should be anticipated, but that necessary surgery should not be postponed simply to replete thyroid hormone. This is not true for patients with severe myxedema who should be given preoperative thyroid hormone except in the most urgent of surgical emergencies or uncontrollable ischemic heart disease. In a review of this subject, Becker[21] concluded that the overall consensus in the literature is that cardiac catheterization and coronary artery bypass surgery can be done safely in hypothyroid patients with or without preoperative thyroid hormone replacement. Hypothyroid patients who have undergone coronary artery bypass surgery are relieved of their angina and are stable even after several years of follow-up.[21]

References

1. Mazzaferri EL: Adult hypothyroidism. Postgrad Med. 1986;79:64-85.
2. Robuschi G, Safran M, Braverman L, et al: Hypothyroidism in the elderly. Endo Rev. 1987;8:142-153.
3. Sawin CT, Chopra D, Azizi F, et al: The aging thyroid: Increased prevalence of elevated serum thyrotropin levels in elderly. J Am Med Assoc. 1979;242:247-254.
4. Sawin CT, Castelli WP, Hershman JM, et al: The aging throid. Thyroid deficiency in the Framingham study. Arch Intern Med. 1985;145:1386-1394.
5. Hurley JR: Thyroid disease in the elderly. Med Clin North Am. 1983;67:497-512.
6. Srudana V, McCormic M, Kaplan EL, et al: Long-term follow-up study of compensated low-dose 131I therapy for Graves' disease. N Engl J Med. 1984;311:426-431.
7. Max MH, Scherm M, Bland KI: Early and late complications after thyroid operations. South Med J. 1983;76:977-983.
8. Lamberg BA, Salmi J, Wagar G, et al: Spontaneous hypothyroidism after antithyroid treatment of hyperthyroid Graves' disease. J Endocrinol Invest. 1981;4:299-308.
9. Riniker M, Tieche M, Lupi GA, et al: Prevalence of various degrees of hypothyroidism among patients of a general medical department. Clin Endocrinol (Oxford). 1981;14:69-77.
10. Rosenthal MJ, Hunt WC, Garry PJ, et al: Thyroid failure in the elderly. Microsomal antibodies as a discriminant for therapy. J Am Med Assoc. 1987;258:209-213.
11. Atkins MB, Mier JW, Parkinson DR, et al: Hypothyroidism after treatment with interleukin-2 and lymphokine-activated killer cells. N Engl J Med. 1988;318:1557-1563.
12. Lio S, Arcese W, Papa G, et al: Thyroid and pituitary function following allogeneic bone marrow transplantation. Arch Intern Med. 1988;148:1066-1071.
13. Biel MA, Maisel RA: Indications for performing hemithyroidectomy for tumors requiring total laryngectomy. Am J Surg. 1985;150:435-439.
14. Posner MR, Ervin TJ, Miller D, et al: Incidence of hypothyroidism following multimodality treatment for advanced squamous cell cancer of the head and neck. Laryngoscope. 1984;94:451-454.
15. de Jong JM, van Daal WA, Elte JW, et al: Primary hypothyroidism as a complication after treatment of tumours of the head and neck. Acta Radiol [Oncol]. 1982;21:299-303.
16. Tachman ML, Guthrie GP Jr. Hypothyroidism: Diversity of presentation. Endo Rev. 1984;5:456-465.

17. Lloyd WA, Goldberg IJL: Incidence of hypothyroidism in the elderly. Br Med J. 1961;2: 1256-1259.

18. Bahemuka M, Hodkinson HM: Screening for hypothyroidism in elderly inpatients. Br Med J. 1975;1:601-605.

19. Guide to Clinical Preventive Services. Report of the U.S. Preventive Services Task Force. Washington, D C, U S Public Health Service, 1989, p 71.

20. Fish LH, Schwartz HL, Cavanaugh J, et al: Replacement dose, metabolism, and bioavailability of levothyroxine in the treatment of hypothyroidism. N Engl J Med. 1987;316:764-770.

21. Becker C: Hypothyroidism and arteriosclerotic heart disease: Pathogenesis, medical management, and the role of coronary artery bypass surgery. Endo Rev. 1985;6:432-440.

22. Keating FR Jr, Parkin TW, Selby JB, et al: Treatment of heart disease associated with myxedema. Prog Cardiovasc Dis. 1961;3:364-385

23. Weinberg AD, Brennan MD, Gorman CA, et al: Outcome of anesthesia and surgery in hypothyroid patients. Arch Intern Med. 1983;143:893-899.

24. Ladenson PW, Leven AA, Ridgway EC, et al: Complications of surgery in hypothyroid patients. Am J Med. 1984;77:261-269.

Case 10

Skin Lesions and Pulmonary Infiltrates in Acute Myelogenous Leukemia

Loretta S. Davis, MD

Case History

A 27-year-old white woman with ovarian dysgerminoma underwent surgical resection and chemotherapy with adriamycin, cyclophosphamide and methotrexate. Two years later, she developed acute myelogenous leukemia, which was thought to have been induced by the chemotherapeutic regimen. She then received high dose cytarabine and daunorubicin and responded with a partial remission. Follow-up bone marrow examination revealed increased blast forms, and she was treated with low-dose cytarabine. This therapy was discontinued secondary to cytarabine-induced hepatitis. Subsequently, the patient did reasonably well, but required regular platelet and red blood cell transfusions. Several months later, she developed symptoms of recurrent sinusitis and complained of painful red lesions on her thighs and lower legs. These skin lesions steadily increased in size and number and became increasingly tender. Fever as high as 102°F developed. She was admitted for further evaluation and therapy.

Physical Examination. The patient was an overweight woman in no acute distress. Temperature was 100.7°F, pulse 118, respirations 18, and blood pressure 130/80 mm Hg. Skin examination was remarkable for multiple erythematous plaques and nodules scattered over the lower extremities and abdomen. These lesions were exquisitely tender to palpation. Head and neck examination was unremarkable except for a healing labial herpes lesion. No lymphadenopathy was appreciated. Cardiothoracic examination was unremarkable. The liver percussed to 11 cm, and the spleen was palpable 7 cm below the left costal margin. Neurologic examination was normal.

Laboratory Data. The white cell count was 13,800/mm^3 with a mildly left shifted differential. The hemoglobin was 13.2 gm/dl and the hematocrit was 38.4%.

Electrolytes, BUN and creatinine were all normal. The glucose was elevated at 181 mg/dl. Liver function tests included an elevated aspartate aminotransferase of 96 U/liter (normal < 60), alanine aminotransferase of 49 U/liter (normal < 40), and alkaline phosphatase of 221 U/liter (normal < 85). Total bilirubin was elevated at 3.2 mg/dl (normal < 1.5) with a direct fraction of 1.2 mg/dl. Electrocardiogram showed sinus tachycardia but was otherwise within normal limits. The chest roentgenogram showed normal heart size and no acute cardiopulmonary disease.

Hospital Course. Work-up was initiated for a presumed infectious disease. Multiple cultures of blood and an aspirate from one of the typical skin lesions were negative for bacteria and fungus. Empiric antibiotic therapy was initiated with vancomycin. Despite this therapy, the patient remained febrile and many other antibiotics were instituted during her hospitalization.

Subsequently, several skin lesions developed bullae while others became studded with small pustules. Dermatology consultation was sought and skin biopsies were performed. Histopathologic examination revealed collections of mature neutrophils within the fat globules and surrounding blood vessels. A sparse superficial and perivascular mixed inflammatory cell infiltrate was present in the dermis. PAS, AFB and tissue Gram stains were negative for organisms. Tissue cultures were also negative for bacteria, fungi, and atypical mycobacteria.

Given the patient's persistent fever, previous history of sinusitis and current left maxillary sinus pain, sinus films were obtained, which confirmed bilateral maxillary and ethmoid sinusitis. The left maxillary sinus was aspirated. Cultures from this aspirate also remained negative.

Over the hospital course, the patient developed bilateral pulmonary infiltrates. Bronchoscopy revealed heavy purulence in the bronchoalveolar lavage fluid, with 47% mature neutrophils, 17% lymphocytes, and 36% alveolar pneumocytes. Special stains for fungi, AFB, parasites and viral inclusions were negative. Cultures of lavage fluid and transbronchial biopsy material were likewise negative except for a light growth of *Candida albicans*.

Despite aggressive antibiotic therapy, the patient's clinical status began to deteriorate. The skin lesions progressed in size and number, fever was persistent, and pulmonary infiltrates enlarged. Increased edema and renal insufficiency developed, with a rise in creatinine from 0.8 mg/dl to 1.4 mg/dl. The urinalysis, however, remained unremarkable.

Given the prominent neutrophilic infiltrate on skin biopsy, in the setting of fever with negative cultures, the diagnosis of acute febrile neutrophilic dermatosis, or Sweet's syndrome, was strongly entertained. Prednisone, the therapy of choice for Sweet's syndrome, was instituted at a dose of 30 mg twice a day. Dramatic improvement promptly occurred. There was a marked diuresis with recovery of baseline renal function, and the pulmonary infiltrates and cutaneous lesions rapidly resolved. She became afebrile, and antibiotics were stopped. With continued clinical improvement, she was discharged from the hospital. Within two weeks of discharge, however, the patient's leukemia fulminantly relapsed, and she expired shortly thereafter.

Discussion

The "neutrophilic dermatoses" represent a spectrum of noninfectious, nonvasculitic, skin lesions which have frequently been reported in patients with myeloproliferative diseases. This cutaneous spectrum ranges from typical lesions of acute febrile neutrophilic dermatosis, also known as Sweet's syndrome, to typical forms of pyoderma gangrenosum. Histologically, such diseases share polymorphonuclear infiltrates as their predominant finding. These infiltrates are neither neoplastic nor infectious but rather sterile collections of mature neutrophils.

Clinically, our case is quite typical of the entity first described by Sweet in 1964.[1] The hallmarks of Sweet's syndrome are fever, leukocytosis, tender erythematous plaques, a neutrophilic infiltrate on skin biopsy and rapid response to steroids. In 1973, Matte et al[2] reported two cases of Sweet's syndrome which occurred in patients with leukemia. Perry and Winkelmann reported[3] cases from the other end of the spectrum, i.e. superficial pyoderma gangrenosum lesions in association with myeloproliferative diseases. The lesions they described share the histologic hallmark of neutrophilic infiltrates but with clinical findings of superficial pyoderma gangrenosum. Subsequently, the literature has been filled with the spectrum of Sweet's syndrome (acute febrile neutrophilic dermatosis) and atypical pyoderma gangrenosum presenting in patients with underlying hematologic malignancies.

Epidemiology. Roughly 10-15% of reported Sweet's syndrome cases have been associated with malignancy, with acute myelogenous leukemia accounting for nearly half of these. The other associated neoplastic diseases include myeloproliferative and myelodysplastic disorders, B and T cell lymphoproliferative disorders, and rarely solid tumors.[4] The reason for these associations remains obscure. For simplicity, these typical skin lesions in a setting of leukemia are probably best thought of as one of the many "leukemids"; an entity associated with leukemia but without direct leukemic cell infiltration of involved skin sites.[5] The remaining 85-90% of reported cases have occurred in otherwise healthy individuals, typically middle-aged women. The etiology is not clear. Most of these cases have occurred one to two weeks after an upper respiratory infection. In such cases a hypersensitivity phenomenon has been postulated.

Clinical Presentation. The typical skin lesion of Sweet's syndrome is a tender, red to bluish-red, indurated plaque. Papules and nodules have been described. The lesions are usually well-marginated, often with central clearing leading to arcuate or annular patterns. The marked inflammatory edema may give the "illusion of vesiculation" or actual blistering. Tiny pustules may stud the lesion's surface. While uncommon, severe vesiculobullous and ulcerative lesions as well as mucosal lesions have been reported and are more likely to occur in cases associated with underlying malignancy. The lesions of Sweet's syndrome are usually asymmetrically distributed on the extremities, although the face and neck are also frequently involved. Typical lesions occurring in sites of trauma, specifically intravenous catheter sites, have been noted in the leukemia-associated variety.[4,6]

Histopathology. Skin biopsy is usually quite diagnostic. The epidermis is typically normal, although rarely microscopic intraepidermal abscesses form. The dermis is edematous with a dense infiltrate of polymorphonuclear leukocytes. Early on, this neutrophilic infiltrate surrounds blood vessels. In time, however, neutrophils are seen in perivascular nodules and among collagen bundles. Nuclear dust may be seen and blood vessels appear dilated, but there is typically no fibrin deposition to suggest vasculitis.[7] The process may extend into the subcutaneous tissue.[6] Our case is unusual in that the subcutaneous tissue was the primary area of involvement, while the dermis was relatively spared. Such localization of findings to the subcutaneous fat has not previously been reported in Sweet's syndrome. A repeat biopsy may have provided more classic histology as clinically both pustular and bullous lesions were present.

Systemic Manifestations. Our patient demonstrated the leukocytosis which is a cardinal feature of this entity. A leukocytosis is routinely expected in the non-leukemia-associated cases (idiopathic Sweet's syndrome). Cooper et al,[6] however, observed that cases which eventuate into the leukemia-associated variety may in fact lack this leukocytosis and are much more likely to have lower hemoglobin values than their truly idiopathic counterparts. They suggest that anemia in the setting of what appears to be the idiopathic variety should be viewed as a "red flag," possibly heralding a preleukemic state. The absence of a neutrophilia has also been observed in a number of patients with preexisting leukemia. This finding is likely due to the natural history of leukemia or bone marrow suppression resulting from chemotherapy.[4] As in our patient's case, an elevated erythrocyte sedimentation rate is a typical laboratory abnormality in Sweet's syndrome.

The noninfectious nature of this process is well documented in our case, as well as throughout the literature. Numerous blood cultures were negative. PAS, AFB, and tissue Gram stains performed on the skin biopsy were likewise negative. Deep fungal and hepatitis serologies were negative. Cultures of the maxillary sinus aspirate were negative for aerobic and anaerobic bacteria as well as AFB. Bronchoalveolar lavage fluid was cultured for bacteria, fungi, AFB, legionella, and virus, and CMV immunofluorescence was performed. All results were entirely negative except for a light growth of *Candida albicans*. Such compulsive sampling and culturing is typical in Sweet's syndrome where every clinical sign is easily interpreted as infectious in nature. As in our case, compulsive culturing and empiric antibiotic therapy is unrewarding. Broad-spectrum antibiotics fail to halt disease progression. All too often, the appropriate therapy is delayed as clinicians "assume infection until proven otherwise."

The typical patient with Sweet's syndrome is not only febrile but appears systemically ill. Myalgias and articular complaints are common. Polyarthralgia and nondestructive polyarthritis involving large and small joints of the extremities have been described. Eye involvement, typically conjunctivitis and episcleritis, have frequently been reported.[4] Proteinuria and renal insufficiency have also been documented. Matta et al reported five cases in which four had some degree of proteinuria.[2] One patient underwent kidney biopsy which revealed a lymphocytic infiltration of the renal interstitium and hypercellularity of the mesangium with focal basement membrane thickening. Following prednisone therapy, this patient's urinalysis, creatinine clearance and renal biopsy returned to normal. One of their five cases underwent diagnostic liver biopsy which revealed a mild neutrophilic invasion of the portal triad as well as foci of fatty change in the liver cells. From their findings, Matta et al contend that the lesions of Sweet's syndrome may not be limited to the skin but involve other organ systems.

Our patient clearly had pulmonary involvement. Several recent reports of Sweet's syndrome have identified the lungs as a neutrophilic target. Lazarus et al[8] reported a patient with preleukemia and classic Sweet's syndrome who presented with pulmonary infiltrates. Extensive cultures of blood, sputum and bronchoscopic washings were negative. During the patient's hospital course, bilateral lung biopsies were performed. The pulmonary histology paralleled that of the skin: sterile neutrophilic infiltrates and small areas of fibrosis. Numerous negative cultures, failure to respond to antibiotics, neutrophilic histology on lung biopsy and dramatic improvement with prednisone therapy strongly suggested that Sweet's syndrome had involved both lungs and the skin. Gibson, et al[9] and Soderstrom[10] have also reported cases of Sweet's syndrome presenting with sterile pulmonary infiltration. Our patient's case is likewise noteworthy for this paralleling of skin and lung pathology. In both organs, sterile infiltrates of mature neutrophils simultaneously progressed despite broad- spectrum antibiotic coverage and promptly improved with prednisone therapy.

Differential Diagnosis. Clearly, an infectious etiology must be diligently sought when abscesses appear on skin biopsy. The neutrophilic histology of Sweet's syndrome mandates special stains and cultures. Early on, however, the classic clinical presentation should trigger the differential diagnosis of Sweet's syndrome and appropriate management should not be unduly delayed.

Clinically, lesions of Sweet's syndrome have been called atypical erythema nodosum or erythema multiforme. However, the classic primary lesions of these three entities are actually quite diagnostic. Characteristic distribution and histology further serve to differentiate them. Erythema elevatum diutinum may have similar-appearing skin lesions but tends to be chronic with variable response to steroids and shows vasculitis on biopsy.[11] Sweet's syndrome, as previously noted, is not a vasculitic process. Leukemic infiltrates can present as erythematous plaques and nodules, but once again, the histology should be diagnostic revealing heavy infiltrates of immature cells.

Notably, pyoderma gangrenosum shares several characteristics with Sweet's syndrome: both entities exhibit dermal neutrophilic infiltrates, without vasculitis; both have been well described in the setting of myeloproliferative diseases; both exhibit pathergy, i.e. new lesion development at sites of trauma; both respond to immunosuppressive therapy. The classic lesions, however, are not easily confused. Pyoderma gangrenosum flaunts ulceration with an indurated, purple, undermined border while Sweet's syndrome remains a well-marginated red plaque occasionally studded with pustules or exhibiting vesiculation. Atypical forms of pyoderma gangrenosum, however, have been described and indeed may cause more confusion with Sweet's syndrome. This atypical variety is more superficial with bullous borders and a subdued blue-gray halo. It would also appear that the superficial bullous variety compared to classic pyoderma gangrenosum is more likely to be associated with myeloproliferative diseases.[12] Thus, many authors contend that these neutrophilic eruptions associated with myeloproliferative diseases represent a continuum ranging from classic Sweet's syndrome to atypical and classic pyoderma gangrenosum. The term "neutrophilic dermatosis of myeloproliferative disorders" has been suggested to reflect this spectrum of clinical disease.[11]

Natural History and Management. In 1983, Cooper et al[6] reviewed the literature on Sweet's syndrome with specific attention given to the differences between the idiopathic and leukemia-associated varieties. Patients with the idiopathic variety who received no specific therapy experienced spontaneous resolution within two weeks to four months with an average of five weeks.

With prednisone therapy, patients with both the idiopathic and leukemia-associated varieties had similar, impressive, responses. At prednisone doses of 30 to 80 mg/day, dramatic clinical improvement predictably ensued within 24 to 48 hrs. Complaints of tenderness, fever and malaise rapidly responded, and cutaneous lesions began to wane with complete resolution within one to four weeks. Prednisone remains the treatment of choice, with much support for the contention that steroid responsiveness is mandatory for confirming the diagnosis. It has been noted that recurrences are more common with the leukemia-associated variety and often develop during tapering of the steroid dosage.[6] Other authors have noted that the disease may be more easily controlled while patients are receiving effective antileukemic therapy.[8] Single or multiple recurrences of Sweet's syndrome have been observed in about two-thirds of patients with underlying hematologic malignancies. Recurrence has coincided with or immediately preceded a hematologic relapse in more than half of these cases.[4]

Since Sweet's syndrome is known to occur not only with preexisting leukemia but to herald leukemia-to-come, the clinician should attempt to identify patients at highest risk for the development of leukemia. The current literature suggests that both the absence of leukocytosis as well as a profound leukocytosis (greater than 25,000/mm^3) should alert the clinician to the possibility of concurrent or imminent myeloproliferative abnormalities. An immature differential count in the peripheral blood, marked anemia, and thrombocytosis may also be indicators of myeloproliferative disease.[4,6,10] In this subset of patients with abnormal hematologic screening, initial bone marrow aspirates and biopsies may be inconclusive, demonstrating a myeloproliferative disorder, but not frank leukemia. Unfortunately, fairly rapid conversion to leukemia has often been the case. In this same setting, a relapse of Sweet's syndrome appears to be even more telling with regard to leukemic conversion. The conclusion may be drawn that in such patients with screening bone marrow abnormalities, Sweet's syndrome may indeed forewarn of imminent leukemic disease.

References

1. Sweet RD: An acute febrile neutrophilic dermatosis. Br J Dermatol. 1964;76:349-356.
2. Matta M, Malak J, Tabet E, et al: Sweet's syndrome: Systemic association. Cutis. 1973;12:561-565.
3. Perry HO, Winkelmann RK: Bullous pyoderma gangrenosum and leukemia. Arch Dermatol. 1972;106:901-905.
4. Cohen PR, Kurzrock R: Sweet's syndrome and malignancy. Am J Med. 1987;82:1220-1226.
5. Spector JI, Zimbler H, Levine R, et al: Sweet's syndrome: Association with acute leukemia. JAMA. 1980;244:1131-1132.
6. Cooper PH, Innes DJ Jr, Greer KE: Acute febrile neutrophilic dermatosis (Sweet's syndrome) and myeloproliferative disorders. Cancer. 1983;51:1518-1526.
7. Ackerman AB: Histologic Diagnosis of Inflammatory Skin Diseases. Philadelphia, Lea and Febiger, 1978.
8. Lazarus AA, McMillan M, Miramadi A: Pulmonary involvement in Sweet's syndrome (acute febrile neutrophilic dermatosis). Chest. 1986;90:922-924.
9. Gibson LE, Dicken CH, Flach DB: Neutrophilic dermatoses and myeloproliferative disease: Report of two cases. Mayo Clin Proc. 1985;60:735-740.
10. Soderstrom RM: Sweet's syndrome and acute myelogenous leukemia: A case report and review of the literature. Cutis. 1981;28:255-260.
11. Chmel H, Armstrong D: Acute febrile neutrophilic dermatosis: Sweet's syndrome. South Med J. 1978;71:1350-1352.
12. Caughman W, Stern R, Haynes H: Neutrophilic dermatosis of myeloproliferative disorders. J Am Acad Dermatol. 1983;9:751-758.

Case 11

Diagnosis and Management of Thyrotoxicosis

Edith T. de los Santos, MD and Ernest L. Mazzaferri, MD, FACP

Case History

A 54-year-old housewife was seen in consultation at the Ohio State University Thyroid Clinic because of weight loss. Twelve years previously, she had experienced substantial weight loss and other symptoms that had been attributed to Graves' disease which was treated with ^{131}I resulting in prompt resolution of her symptoms. She remained well until four months prior to her present consultation when she was hospitalized for pneumonia from which she recovered quickly; nonetheless, since having pneumonia she had lost 25 pounds despite having a good appetite. In addition, she had recently been developing symptoms of easy fatigability, palpitations, nervousness, heat intolerance, muscle weakness, and hair loss.

She had undergone a hysterectomy and oophorectomy in 1972 for dysfunctional uterine bleeding, and since then had been taking estrogen replacement therapy. There was no history of hepatitis or blood transfusion. She smoked 2 packs of cigarettes per day for 35 years. She denied alcohol intake. Her family history was unremarkable.

Physical Examination. Her blood pressure was 130/50 mm Hg, and her pulse rate was 130 beats per minute and regular. She weighed 100 pounds and was 67 inches tall. The skin was smooth, warm, and moist, and her scalp hair was fine and thinning. The thyroid, which was firm and diffusely enlarged, was estimated by palpation to be 80 grams (normal 15 to 20 gm). Neither cervical lymphadenopathy nor thyroid bruit was present. She had lid lag on downward gaze, but proptosis and other signs of Graves' ophthalmopathy were not present. The cardiovascular exam demonstrated a hyperdynamic precordium, tachycardia and a grade 3/6 ejection murmur loudest over the second intercostal space. The deep tendon reflexes were brisk and hyperactive. She had temporal muscle wasting and a fine finger tremor. She was unable to stand unassisted from a squatting position and could not rise easily from the sitting position without using her arms for support. The remainder of her physical examination was unremarkable.

Laboratory Data. The complete blood count and routine serum chemistry values were normal. The thyroid function tests showed: serum thyroxine (T4) 21.8 μg/dl (normal 3.5-11) and free thyroxine index (FT4I) 23.2 (normal 3.5-11), thyroid hormone binding ratio (THBR) 0.94 mg/dl (normal 0.7-1.25), thyrotropin (TSH) μU/ml (normal 0.2-5). The thyroid ^{123}I scan showed diffuse radionuclide concentration in both lobes with an elevated 24 hour uptake (60%). The electrocardiogram was normal except for sinus tachycardia. Her chest roentgenogram had changes consistent with chronic obstructive pulmonary disease.

Subsequent Course. After starting therapy with 300 mg of propylthiouracil daily and atenolol 50 mg twice daily, she began regaining weight and experiencing improved strength. However, within four weeks of starting this therapy, she developed a pruritic maculopapular rash over the trunk and extremities, her stools became pale, her urine darkened, and her sclerae became icteric. The rash spared only her face and soles of the feet. Her liver was enlarged and tender. Propylthiouracil was immediately discontinued and she was admitted to the hospital. A complete blood count was within normal limits. Total bilirubin was 3.7 mg/dl (normal 0.2-1.2), direct bilirubin 1.8 mg/dl (normal up to 0.5), alanine aminotransferase (ALT) 399 U/liter (normal 0-40), aspartate aminotransferase (AST) 478 U/liter (normal 0-60), lactic dehydrogenase (LDH) 348 U/liter (normal 60-220), gamma glutamyltransferase (GGT) 324 U/liter (normal 5-85), and alkaline phosphatase 655 U/liter (normal 0-100). The hepatitis A and B profiles were negative. Skin biopsy showed vacuolar interface dermatitis and deep perivascular inflammation consistent with a severe drug reaction.

Discussion

This patient, who had recurrent thyrotoxicosis due to Graves' disease, developed a severe reaction to propylthiouracil. Several major questions immediately should come to mind. Why did the thyrotoxicosis recur so many years after her initial therapy? What type of reaction did she have in response to propylthiouracil and will it resolve? This discussion will focus on the diagnosis, treatment, and complications of Graves' disease, and will attempt to answer some of these questions.

Definitions. The terms thyrotoxicosis and hyperthyroidism, although commonly used interchangeably, are distinctly different with important diagnostic and therapeutic implications. Thyrotoxicosis is a clinical syndrome resulting from the peripheral tissue responses to thyroid hormone excess, while hyperthyroidism simply refers to an overactive thyroid gland which is manifested by a high thyroidal radioiodine uptake (RAIU).[1,2] The distinction between the two can be appreciated by considering the problems of factitial thyrotoxicosis and Graves' disease. In the former, the patient is thyrotoxic but the thyroid gland is quiescent and has a low ^{123}I uptake. With thyrotoxic Graves' disease the thyroid gland becomes overactive which is reflected in its high ^{123}I uptake. This idea is well illustrated in Table 1 which is modified from Ingbar's classification of thyrotoxicosis according to the presence or absence of hyperthyroidism.[1] A high RAIU is the key to hyperthyroidism and the opposite is true in thyrotoxicosis without hyperthyroidism as occurs with thyroiditis or excessive exogenous thyroid hormone intake.[2]

Clinical Features

Table 2 lists the frequency of various clinical manifestations of thyrotoxicosis based on a study of 880 thyrotoxic subjects.[3] Older patients frequently have less typical features. Many of the usual signs and symptoms of thyrotoxicosis are often

Table 1

Classification of Thyrotoxicosis

Thyrotoxicosis with hyperthyroidism (High RAIU)
    Inappropriate TSH (TSH excess)[a]
        Neoplastic
        Nonneoplastic (Thyroid hormone resistance)
    Abnormal thyroid stimulator
        Graves' disease
        Trophoblastic tumors (i.e. H-mole, choriocarcinoma)
    Autonomously functioning thyroid nodule
        Solitary
        Multiple

Thyrotoxicosis without hyperthyroidism (Low RAIU)
    Thyroiditis
        Subacute
        Chronic
    Extrathyroidal thyroid hormone source
        Hormone ingestion
        Ectopic thyroid hormone production
            Struma ovarii
            Functioning thyroid cancer metastasis

Adapted from Ingbar.[1]
[a]*TSH is inappropriately normal or elevated, all the others have suppressed TSH.*

absent in the older age groups. Manifestations of thyrotoxicosis that are particularly prevalent in the elderly are weight loss and atrial fibrillation, while increased appetite and weight gain are more likely to occur in younger patients. The patient under discussion had overwhelming clinical evidence of thyrotoxicosis.

Often recognized on initial handshake, the characteristic warm, moist skin of the thyrotoxic person is so different from the cold, clammy feel of an anxious

Table 2

	Frequency of Manifestations of Thyrotoxicosis*		
	Frequency (%)		
	Age < 60 yr **N = 827**	**Age > 60 yr** **N = 50**	**Patient[a]**
Symptoms			
Palpitations	66	51	+
↑ sweating	45	29	−
Heat intolerance	56	32	+
Weight loss	59	79	+
Weight gain	13	0	−
↑ appetite	43	15	+
↓ appetite	11	22	−
↑ bowel movements	22	15	−
Fatigue	69	72	+
Irritability	46	32	−
Nervousness	69	56	+
Signs			
Finger tremors	69	68	+
Warm moist skin	34	22	+
Atrial fibrillation	1	14	−
Pulse 90/min	80	75	+
Goiter	94	81	+
Lid retraction	30	28	−
Lid lag	12	14	+
Shortened Achilles reflex time	39	49	+

Adapted from Nordyke et al.[3]
[a]*Patient under discussion.*

person's hand that it can distinguish the two despite many similar complaints that often exist in the two disorders.[4,5] Significant weight loss in the face of an increased food intake is another hallmark of thyrotoxicosis seen in only a few other conditions such as malabsorption and uncontrolled diabetes mellitus.[5] However, in severe instances of thyrotoxicosis, particularly in elderly patients, anorexia may supervene. Young patients with mild thyrotoxicosis who compensate for their hypermetabolic state by increasing food intake may gain weight.[3,5] Nervousness, excitability, and lack of concentration, typical thyrotoxicosis symptoms, are readily recognized during the interview. Examination of the outstretched hands demonstrates the characteristic fine finger tremor, which usually results in handwriting changes and clumsiness in fine tasks. Tachycardia, a hyperdynamic precordium, and murmur over the left sternal border are typical cardiovascular changes.[4] A widened pulse pressure is characteristic of thyrotoxicosis and is the result of an increased rate and force of cardiac ejection that increases systolic pressure and thyroid hormone-induced vasodilatation that decreases diastolic pressures. Easy fatigability with prominent weakness of the proximal muscles is also typical of thyrotoxicosis and is noted on climbing stairs and when rising from a squatting position. Loss of hair seen prior to treatment persists until the patient becomes euthyroid.[4,5]

The presence of diffuse goiter and thyrotoxicosis is not itself diagnostic of Graves' disease. Both diffuse goiter and thyrotoxicosis may result from thyroiditis. Pituitary TSH hypersecretion and trophoblastic diseases cannot be differentiated from Graves' disease merely on clinical grounds. On the other hand, goiter may be absent in about 20 to 25% of Graves' disease cases, particularly in the elderly.[3] Aside from a diffuse hyperfunctioning goiter, the other manifestations distinctly associated with Graves' disease are ophthalmopathy and dermopathy. These major manifestations can appear singly or in various combinations and may appear to be independent of each other.[4,5]

It is essential to differentiate the eye signs resulting from thyrotoxicosis from the infiltrative ophthalmopathy of Graves' disease. Thyrotoxicosis, regardless of its etiology, may produce ocular manifestations including stare, lid retraction and lid lag which subside when the thyrotoxicosis abates. Infiltrative ophthalmopathy includes proptosis, extraocular muscle palsy, and congestive oculopathy characterized by chemosis, conjunctival congestion and periorbital edema (Fig. 1). Although only about 3% of patients with Graves' disease have clinically apparent ophthalmopathy, a majority have either elevated intraocular pressure, increased retrobulbar tissue or enlarged extraocular muscles as seen on ultrasound or CT scan of the globes (Fig. 2).[6] An unusual feature of Graves' disease is pretibial myxedema which is seen in about 4% of cases.[4,5] It is characterized by thickening and hyperpigmentation of the skin usually over the dorsum of the legs and feet (Fig. 3). Clubbing of the fingers and toes, termed thyroid acropachy, is an unusual and late manifestation of Graves' disease that may accompany the other dermal changes.

Diagnostic Tests

When thyrotoxicosis is clinically apparent, laboratory tests are merely confirmatory. We have previously reported that the FT4I is the most cost-effective initial thyroid test when there is a low clinical suspicion of thyrotoxicosis.[7] However, when there is a high clinical probability of thyrotoxicosis, as in the patient under discussion, it is appropriate to perform a combination of thyroid tests including FT4I and serum TSH, not only to determine the metabolic state but also to establish the etiology of thyrotoxicosis.[2]

Estrogen use, as in the patient under discussion, stimulates hepatic thyroid binding globulin (TBG) synthesis which elevates the total T_4 but not the free T_4.[8] The free T_4 concentration can be estimated from the free T_4 index (FT4I) which is calculated from the total T_4 and the THBR (a test of thyroid hormone binding such as the T_3 resin uptake). The FT4I is more cost-effective than other more cumbersome and expensive methods of estimating free T_4 such as equilibrium dialysis.[7,8,9,10] The latter is almost never necessary to distinguish thyrotoxicosis from thyroid hormone binding abnormalities, particularly since more sensitive tests for measuring thyrotropin (TSH) have become widely available.

Thyroid hormones exert a negative feedback inhibition on pituitary thyrotrophic cells which lowers the serum TSH concentration.[8,10,11] Among the disorders causing thyrotoxicosis (Table 1), only two fairly uncommon conditions — pituitary thyrotroph tumors and pituitary resistance to T_4 — cause thyrotoxicosis without suppressing TSH. In the past, this was most commonly demonstrated by a thyrotropin-releasing hormone (TRH) stimulation test during which the serum TSH failed to rise. This test is now usually unnecessary. New immunometric TSH assays, which are at least 10-fold more sensitive than the older TSH radioimmunoassay, can reliably distinguish between normal and suppressed serum TSH concentrations (i.e. serum TSH concentrations are below the lower detection limit of the assay in thyrotoxicosis).[7,8,10,11]

Triiodothyronine (T_3) or free T_3 index (FT3I) is done when FT4I is normal but thyrotoxicosis is still strongly suspected on clinical grounds. This may occur in patients with overt symptoms of thyrotoxicosis, or with a nodular goiter, or elderly persons with unexplained symptoms (i.e. atrial fibrillation or unexplained weight loss) that may be due to thyrotoxicosis. This is usually termed T_3 toxicosis, a condition wherein only serum T_3 concentration is elevated.[7,8]

Once a diagnosis of thyrotoxicosis has been established on clinical and laboratory grounds, an RAIU is essential to classify the causes of thyrotoxicosis (Table 1).[1,2,8,10] In the patient under discussion, a diagnosis of thyrotoxicosis was strongly suspected on clinical grounds and proven with an elevated FTI and suppressed serum TSH concentration. Her diffuse goiter, elevated RAIU and diffuse pattern on thyroid scan confirmed the diagnosis of Graves' disease.

Thyroid-stimulating immunoglobulin (TSI) is an abnormal gamma globulin that can stimulate thyroid gland activity. TSI is present in most patients with Graves' disease. In one study, TSI was detectable in 95% of untreated patients with hyperthyroid Graves' disease, in only 4% of nongoitrous euthyroid controls and 5% of patients with Hashimoto's disease.[10] An elevated TSI in a pregnant woman increases the likelihood of thyrotoxicosis in the neonate.[12,13] The absence of TSI in a patient on antithyroid drugs seems associated with an increased chance of long-term remission following discontinuation of the drugs.[14] In most cases, however, it is not necessary to determine TSI concentrations, although it may be helpful in confusing cases of hyperthyroidism whose clinical signs are not adequate to make a diagnosis of Graves' disease.[10] Its measurement during pregnancy in women with Graves' disease, regardless of whether they are thyrotoxic or not, is good practice.

Autoimmune thyroid antibodies against thyroglobulin and thyroid microsomal membranes are frequently present in autoimmune thyroid diseases. Antimicrosomal antibody is present in about 95% of patients with Hashimoto's thyroiditis and 85% of those with Graves' disease while antithyroglobulin antibody is detectable in 60% and 30% of cases, respectively.[15] However, from 2% to 17% of asymptomatic euthyroid individuals are positive when screened for thyroid antibodies, particularly older women.[10] Other autoimmune diseases such as pernicious anemia, myasthenia gravis, lupus erythematosus and rheumatoid arthritis may also have detectable antithyroid antibodies, particularly antimicrosomal antibodies, which are not specific for Hashimoto's thyroiditis.[10] Determination of antithyroid antibodies may be helpful in evaluating patients with atypical manifestations of autoimmune thyroid diseases.

The natural history of Graves' disease is unpredictable. The disease — and its attendant thyrotoxicosis — may wax and wane in severity, it may remain subclinical for years, or it may be relentlessly progressive. It is not unusual for thyrotoxicosis to occur many years after the initial manifestations of the disease, particularly ophthalmopathy, are first recognized. In a small number of cases Graves' disease spontaneously results in hypothyroidism. Rarely, autoimmune hypothyroidism precedes Graves' disease. In the patient under discussion, Graves' disease was initially treated with an unknown amount of ^{131}I, presumably at a dose small enough to have left enough thyroid tissue viable to ultimately respond to ongoing TSI stimulation, thus accounting for her late recurrence of thyrotoxicosis.

Therapy

The main choices for treating Graves' disease are antithyroid drugs, radioactive iodine therapy (^{131}I) and surgery. Choice of therapy for a particular patient is influenced by a number of factors, including the treatment's efficacy and risk, the patient's age and goiter size, severity and complications of the thyrotoxicosis, and concurrent disorders.[2] Due to the severity of thyrotoxicosis in the patient under discussion, an antithyroid drug (propylthiouracil) and a β-blocker (atenolol) were selected for initial therapy. Unfortunately, she developed a severe adverse reaction to propylthiouracil.

Antithyroid Drugs. Antithyroid drugs block thyroid hormone production by inhibiting tyrosine iodination.[16] The antithyroid drugs are themselves iodinated, thereby diverting iodine from thyroid hormone synthesis. They do not affect thyroid hormone release and thus are not fully effective until stored hormone in the gland is depleted. Their effect is therefore a function not only of drug dosage and timing, and severity of the underlying disease, but also of thyroid gland size which reflects the amount of stored thyroid hormones. Other reported extrathyroidal effects of antithyroid drugs include immunosuppression and inhibition of peripheral T_4 to T_3 conversion which is true only for propylthiouracil.[16] Although the intrinsic immunosuppressive action of antithyroid drugs is controversial, several studies have shown a reduction of TSI levels during propylthiouracil treatment of Graves' disease which is unchanged with placebo or β-blocker therapy.[17,18] The added effect of propylthiouracil on inhibition of peripheral T_4 to T_3 conversion is only a theoretical advantage over methimazole, since no studies have actually compared the two drugs in this situation.

Side effects of antithyroid drugs are listed in Table 3.[2,16] Jaundice may be cholestatic which is typically associated with methimazole, or cytotoxic (hepatitis) which occurs almost exclusively with propylthiouracil, or mixed cytotoxic-cholestatic injury.[19] The pathogenesis of liver injury is unknown but is theorized to be an

Table 3

Side Effects Associated With Antithyroid Drugs

Minor
Fever, rash
Arthralgia, arthritis
Transient leukopenia
Major
Agranulocytosis
Toxic hepatitis
Others (rare)
Cholestatic jaundice, Alopecia
Hypoprothrombinemia, Thrombocytopenia
Aplastic anemia, Nephrotic syndrome
Vasculitis, Lupus-like syndrome
Autoantibody induction (insulin, glucagon)
Loss of taste

Adapted from de los Santos et al.[2]

allergic host reaction.[19,20] Manifestations of propylthiouracil-induced hepatitis are jaundice, nausea, vomiting, malaise and liver tenderness. There is no age predilection, and onset of symptoms may occur two weeks to six months after initiating propylthiouracil intake.[19] The patient under discussion developed a combined hepatocellular-cholestatic hepatitis one month after propylthiouracil therapy was started. Propylthiouracil-induced hepatitis usually improves with prompt drug withdrawal as in the patient presented, but may be fatal in some cases.[19,20]

Another important adverse reaction to antithyroid drugs is agranulocytosis. It usually occurs within the first three months of therapy, is more frequent in older patients, and is dose related only for methimazole at daily dosages over 30 mg.[16] Methimazole may be a somewhat safer drug since agranulocytosis is predictably less common at lower doses. Agranulocytosis is characterized by fever and infection mostly in the oropharynx and a white blood cell count of less than 250/mm.[3,16] Serial white blood cell counts are not done. They are not very useful because agranulocytosis typically occurs with explosive abruptness, and it may give both patient and physician an unwarranted sense of security.[2,16]

Although there is no way of predicting a severe reaction to antithyroid drugs, this possibility should not discourage their use, considering the infrequent occurrence of severe reactions. The frequency of side effects from antithyroid drugs is 1% to 5%, a rate comparable to other commonly used drugs, and severe reactions occur much less frequently.[16] Prolonged use of antithyroid drugs is suitable for Graves' disease in children, pregnant women and patients who are compliant and whose disease is easily controlled. Otherwise, antithyroid drugs are used for preparation of severely thyrotoxic patients for permanent thyroid ablation either by radioactive iodine therapy or surgery. It is essential to carefully educate patients about the possible side effects of antithyroid drugs and to reiterate the problem every time they are seen. Should any untoward effects such as fever, sore throat, mouth sores, skin lesions, or jaundice occur, the medication should be immediately stopped and the physician promptly informed. If a major reaction to one drug occurs, the use of the other is discouraged because of common cross-reactions.[16] With less severe drug reactions such as arthralgia, one may choose to switch from one to another antithyroid drug.

The remission rate of thyrotoxicosis due to Graves' disease with antithyroid drugs averages about 50%.[21] Remissions were thought to follow the natural history of Graves' disease, but it is unclear whether other factors such as the drug's immunosuppressive effects, iodine depletion, or concomitant thyroiditis may also influence outcome.[26]

The patient under discussion had a decreased chance of achieving spontaneous remission because of the severity of her hyperthyroidism, presence of a large goiter and history of relapse after previous radioactive iodine therapy, so we chose to treat her with β-blockers and to permanently ablate her thyroid. Three days after propylthiouracil was stopped, 20 mCi of ^{131}I was given. Atenolol was continued, and other medications given were 60 mg of terfenadine twice daily and prednisone 30 mg once daily.

β-blockers. These drugs can ameliorate the symptoms of thyrotoxicosis but do not alter the underlying disease. This class of drugs serve as adjunctive but not as primary therapy. β-blockers are helpful for short-term symptomatic management and when other drugs are contraindicated.[22,23]

Although propranolol is the most extensively studied β-blocker for thyrotoxicosis, there are only minor differences between it and the other β-blockers regarding symptom relief.[2,22] Cardioselective drugs without intrinsic sympathomimetic activity (ISA) are as efficient as propranolol in heart rate reduction. The effect of propranolol on peripheral inhibition of T_4 to T_3 conversion is also shared by the other β-blockers.[23] Tremors which are most likely mediated via $β_2$-receptors are better controlled with propranolol than cardioselective blockers.[23] Atenolol, a cardioselective β-blocker without ISA, was chosen for our patient to avoid aggravating her chronic obstructive pulmonary disease.

Iodides. About 100 μg/day of iodine is needed for thyroid hormone synthesis, but much larger doses of iodine inhibit thyroid hormone production and release.[2] The effect of iodine-containing radiocontrast agents such as sodium ipodate (Oragrafin™) and iopanoic acid (Telepaque™) is hastened by their additional action of inhibiting peripheral T_4 to T_3 conversion.[24] Although sodium ipodate is highly effective in reducing the serum concentrations of both T_4 and T_3 when used for short periods of time, many patients experience exacerbations of thyrotoxicosis when it is continued for more than a month.[24] In addition, withdrawal of ipodate when used alone for the treatment of thyrotoxicosis may cause worsening of thyrotoxicosis.[25] Iodides, like β-blockers, are suitable supplementary therapy for thyrotoxicosis.

Radioactive Iodine Therapy. This therapy (^{131}I) causes permanent thyroid ablation by acutely producing follicular cell necrosis and later causing vascular and stromal fibrosis.[26] It does not ameliorate thyrotoxicosis at once but usually takes full effect over 3 to 6 months. During the first week after radioactive iodine therapy, radiation thyroiditis with release of stored thyroid hormone may ensue, consequently exacerbating thyrotoxicosis. Although thyrotoxicosis seen after radioactive iodine therapy is often mild and commonly controlled by β-blockers, thyroid storm is a possibility especially in severely thyrotoxic patients who are not rendered euthyroid prior to ^{131}I administration.[26] This is why ^{131}I therapy was postponed for several days in the patient under discussion. However, three days after she was given ^{131}I therapy she developed congestive heart failure which responded to diuresis. This was undoubtedly in part precipitated by ^{131}I exacerbation of thyrotoxicosis.

Although radioactive iodine therapy is very effective in ablating the thyroid, it has the main disadvantage of being associated with a high frequency of hypothyroidism. In a study of 261 hyperthyroid patients treated with graded doses of ^{131}I, 54% became euthyroid while an additional 29% needed supplementary antithyroid medications.[27] However, the incidence of hypothyroidism was at least 10% in the first year of follow-up and increased by 3% to 5% per year for several years thereafter.[27] The incidence of hypothyroidism 10 years after radioactive iodine therapy ranges from 40% to 70%.[26] Therefore, patients who undergo radioactive iodine therapy should be able to accept the strong possibility of becoming permanently hypothyroid later and should be educated about the importance of lifelong continuous follow-up. The risks of leukemia and other malignancies are not increased in hyperthyroid patients treated with [131]I.[26,28]

Role of Surgery. Subtotal thyroidectomy has the advantage over radioactive iodine therapy of ameliorating thyroid hormone overproduction immediately. Postoperative hypothyroidism occurs in about 2% to 40%, while persistent or recurrent hyperthyroidism ranges from 6% to 12%.[26] Even in the most experienced hands, surgery is associated with some complications, particularly permanent hypoparathyroidism which occurs in about 1% to 2%, and recurrent laryngeal nerve paralysis which is seen in 3% to 5%.[26] The patient under discussion was certainly not a good surgical candidate because of her hepatitis, concomitant chronic lung disease and heart failure. Surgery may have a special role in treating extremely large goiters (80 gm) causing obstruction or if co-occurrence of malignancy is being considered.

The patient under discussion gradually experienced an improvement in her condition following ^{131}I therapy. Her liver function tests returned to normal, and her rash disappeared. She was clinically and biochemically euthyroid three months after ^{131}I therapy but became mildly hypothyroid three months later. She was doing well as of the last follow-up while being treated with an appropriate replacement dosage of levothyroxine that maintained her FTI and TSH in normal ranges.

References

1. Ingbar SH: Thyrotoxicosis: Classification and manifestations, in Ingbar SH, Braverman LE (eds): Werner's The Thyroid: A Fundamental and Clinical Text, ed 5. Philadelphia, JB Lippincott Co., 1986, pp 809-810.
2. de los Santos ET, Mazzaferri EL: Thyrotoxicosis. Results and risks of current therapy. Postgrad Med. 1990 Apr;87(5):277-278,281-286,288,291-294..
3. Nordyke RA, Gilbert FI, Harada AS: Graves' disease. Influence of ages on clinical findings. Arch Intern Med. 1988 Mar;148:626-631.
4. McKenzie JM, Zakarija M: Hyperthyroidism, in: DeGroot LJ (ed): Endocrinology, ed 2. Philadelphia, WB Saunders Co, 1989, pp 846-682.
5. Mazzaferri EL: The thyroid, Mazzaferri EL (ed): Textbook of Endocrinology ed 3. New York, Medical Examination Publishing, 1986, pp 89-350.
6. Bahn RS, Garrity JA, Bartley GB, et al: Diagnostic evaluation of Graves' ophthalmopathy. Endocrinol Metab Clin North Am. 1988;17:527-545.
7. de los Santos ET, Starich GH, Mazzaferri EL. Sensitivity, specificity and cost-effectiveness of sensitive thyrotropin assay in the diagnosis of thyroid disease in ambulatory patients. Arch Intern Med. 1989;149:526-532.

8. de los Santos ET, Mazzaferri EL: Thyroid function tests. Guidelines for interpretation in common clinical disorders. Postgrad Med. 1989;85:333-352.

9. Larsen PR, Alexander NM, Chopra IJ, et al: Revised nomenclature for tests of thyroid hormone and thyroid related protein in serum. J Clin Endocrinol Metab. 1987;64:1089-1094.

10. Hay ID, Klee GG. Thyroid dysfunction. Endocrinol Clin North Am. 1988;17:473-509.

11. de los Santos ET, Mazzaferri EL: Sensitive thyroid stimulating hormone assays: Clinical applications and limitations. Compr Ther. 1988;14(9):26-33.

12. Zakarija M, McKenzie JM. Pregnancy-associated changes in the thyroid stimulating antibody of Graves' disease and the relationship with neonatal hyperthyroidism. J Clin Endocrinol Metab. 1983;57:1036-1040.

13. Tamaki H, Amino N, Aozasa M, et al. Universal predictive criteria for neonatal overt thyrotoxicosis requiring treatment. Am J Perinatol. 1988 Apr;5:152-158.

14. Orgiazzi J, Madec AM, Genetet N, et al: Immunological parameters in Graves' disease: Are they useful for indication and monitoring of antithyroid drug treatment? Horm Res. 1987;26:131-136.

15. Refetoff S: Thyroid function tests and effects of drugs on thyroid function, in DeGroot LJ (ed): Endocrinology, ed 2. Philadelphia, WB Saunders Co, 1989 pp 590-639.

16. Cooper DS. Antithyroid drugs. Engl J Med. 1984;311:1353-1362.

17. Fenzi G, Hashizume K, Roudebush CP, et al: Changes in thyroid stimulating immunoglobulins during antithyroid therapy. J Clin Endocrinol Metab 1979;48:572-576.

18. Teng CS, Yeung RTT: Change in thyroid-stimulating antibody activity in Graves' disease treated with anti-thyroid drugs and its relationship to relapse: A prospective study. J Clin Endocrinol Metab. 1980;50:144-147.

19. Hanson JS: Propylthiouracil and hepatitis. Two cases and a review of literature. Arch Intern Med. 1984;144:994-996.

20. Limaye A, Ruffolo PR: Propylthiouracil-induced fatal hepatic necrosis. Am J Gastroenterol. 1987;82:152-154.

21. Leclere J: Anti-thyroid drugs - A rational treatment for Graves' disease? Horm. Res. 1987;26:125-130.

22. Mazzaferri EL, Reynolds JC, Young RL, et al: Propranolol as primary therapy for thyrotoxicosis. Result of a long-term prospective study. Arch Intern Med. 1976;136:50-56.

23. Feely J, Peden N: Use of beta-adrenoceptor blocking drugs in hyperthyroidism. Drugs. 1984;27:425-446.

24. Kamel N, Upsala AR, Kologlu S, et al: Sodium ipodate in the treatment of toxic diffuse goiter. Short-term or long-term effects on thyrotoxicosis. Rom J Med. 1988;26:99-105.

25. Roti E, Robuschi G, Manfredi A, et al. Comparative effect of sodium ipodate and iodide on serum thyroid hormone concentrations in patients with Graves' disease. Clin Endocrinol. 1985;22:489-496.

26. Orgiazzi J: Management of Graves' hyperthyroidism. Endocrinol Clin North Am. 1987;16:365-389.

27. Goolden AWG, Stewart JSW: Long-term results from graded low-dose radioactive iodine therapy for thyrotoxicosis. Clin Endocrinol. 1986;24:217-222.

28. Graham GD, Burman KD. Radioiodine treatment of Graves' disease. An assessment of its possible risks. Ann Intern Med. 1986;105:900-905.

Case 12

Rapidly Progressive Rosacea in an Adult Male With Flushing Attacks, Pruritus, and "Freckles"

Jonathan K. Wilkin, MD, FACP, FAAD

Case History

A 58-year-old man had a 12-month history of facial flushing and a progressively deteriorating facial "complexion." He was a salesman who traveled frequently by automobile, and he had flushing attacks when traveling on hot days in his non-air-conditioned vehicle. Over the past year, the flushing had become more severe and was associated with a burning sensation of the face and copious rhinorrhea. He also described abundant "freckles" on his chest and back which appeared approximately one year before this presentation. Over the past few months he had noted an increase in pruritus and urticaria localized to these "freckles," especially after ingestion of alcoholic beverages, after hot showers, and following aspirin ingestion. He described having one episode of explosive diarrhea weekly, almost always after ingestion of 3-5 cans of beer. Persistent rhinitis, epigastric discomfort, and watery, burning eyes had been problems over recent months. The pruritus and substernal burning sensation occurred during and shortly after the flushing reactions. There had been no localized skeletal pain, fainting spells, or bleeding problems.

Physical Examination. Examination of the skin disclosed many 2-3 mm brown-tan macules which were scattered over the thorax. They were particularly abundant over the medial aspect of the upper arms and in the axillae. The lesions urticated with stroking, developing substantial pseudopodia over a 3-5 minute period with a peripheral flare. A less intense, but definite, urticarial response was obtained by stroking apparently uninvolved skin. He also had an intense, blanchable facial erythema. This was most prominent over the malar areas, the glabella, nose, and the chin. Both fine and coarse telangiectasias were present over the nose and the malar areas. The conjunctivae were moderately, diffusely injected.

Diagnostic Studies. A cutaneous biopsy specimen of one of the tan macules demonstrated an infiltrate consisting predominantly of mast cells around dilated blood vessels of the superficial dermal plexus. The peripheral blood smear showed no basophils or mast cells. The white cell count of the peripheral blood was 8,300/mm^3, with 8% eosinophils. The hemoglobin value was 15.7 g/dl, and the hematocrit was 46.3%. The urinary histamine concentration was 366 μg/24 hr (normal 17-68 μg/24 hr). No abnormalities were identified in the following studies: stool guaiac test, technetium liver-spleen scan, histopathology of bone marrow biopsy obtained from right iliac crest, upper GI series with small bowel follow through, chest x-ray, and radionuclide bone scan.

Ophthalmologic examination disclosed extremely profuse telangiectasia on the margins of the lids. There was also a moderate, diffuse injection of the conjunctivae. Further, there was plugging of the Meibomian glands and excessive discharge.

At the follow-up visit the patient had a flushing reaction which persisted longer than 30 min. The blush distribution was a bright pink throughout, with no patches of pallor or cyanotic hues. There was no eccrine sweating associated with the flushing.

The flushing, rhinorrhea, facial erythema and telangiectasia, and eye manifestations improved considerably during treatment with tetracycline HCl 250 mg, qid; ranitidine HCl 300 mg, bid; and, terfenadine 120 mg, bid. Fluocinonide ointment 0.05% applied to the cutaneous macules provided no apparent benefit beyond that obtained by the systemic medications and was discontinued.

Discussion

The presentation of this patient raises several important points. When patients have an explosive onset of rosacea and are flushing, the physician must consider the differential diagnosis of flushing reactions. The explosive onset of the facial stigmata of rosacea can be seen in the carcinoid syndrome. This and other observations underscore the role of flushing reactions in the progression of rosacea.[1] Several clues are helpful in focusing on mast cell-mediated flushing, and these are especially relevant in considering this patient's condition, systemic mastocytosis. In addition to the clinical evidence pointing to the diagnosis of systemic mastocytosis in this patient, the histamine assay provides a critical piece of evidence supporting the diagnosis of mastocytosis. Recent views on the variety of assays and biological materials tested will be reviewed.

Rosacea. Rosacea is not a disease but a cutaneous syndrome.[2] It is the sequential or simultaneous presence of some or all of a fixed combination of disease indicants. Patients with classical rosacea have a fairly persistent erythema or cyanosis of the blush distribution, as well as telangiectasia, facial edema, papules, pustules, ocular lesions, and rhinophyma. Most patients with rosacea have only a few of these stigmata at any one time.

The telangiectasias may be coarse or fine. In many patients fine telangiectasias are limited to the forehead, malar areas, and ears. Coarse telangiectasias, when found, are more frequent along the nasal and malar areas. Telangiectasia is also frequent on the pinnae. Both fine and coarse telangiectasias were present over the nose and the malar areas in the patient reported here.

Ocular rosacea is common but frequently undiagnosed. Among the most common signs and symptoms are foreign body sensation, burning, superficial punctate erosions, chalazia, and blepharitis. Less common, but ophthalmologically more important, are corneal thinning, vascularization, and infiltrates. The most common ocular signs are vascular or have a vascular basis. There is also a strong correlation between the degree of eye involvement and tendency to flushing.[3] The patient reported here had extremely profuse telangiectasia on the margins of the lids and also a moderate, diffuse injection of the conjunctivae. He also had plugging and excessive discharge of the Meibomian glands.

Papules and pustules may be present over the forehead, malar areas, nose, and chin. The papules are nontender, nonscarring, and nonfollicular. They do not leave any residual fibrous nodule, nor are they preceded by a comedo as in acne vulgaris. Pustules appear much less frequently than papules. Papules and pustules often appear in crops. Occasionally, the discrete papules will appear as yellowish-brown nodules upon diascopy and as noncaseating granulomas histologically. Quite a few patients may have the vascular components of rosacea without any trace of papules or pustules; conversely, there are also individuals with papules and pustules and few vascular changes. The patient reported here is of the former category, having no inflammatory lesions (papules or pustules), but having only the vascular components of rosacea, persistent erythema and telangiectasia.

Rhinophyma, the cosmetically important disfigurement which afflicted W.C. Fields, is due to soft tissue hypertrophy of the nose. Some "phymatous" changes may also be seen in the malar areas, forehead, chin, and edges of the pinnae. The first perceptible change is the presence of patulous follicles. The patient presented here had neither rhinophyma nor patulous follicles, although rhinophyma has been associated with intense flushing reactions due to carcinoidosis[4].

In fact, patients with severe flushing due to carcinoid syndrome develop all of the various rosacea stigmata, including ocular rosacea, facial telangiectasia, and severe connective tissue hypertrophy.[1,2] These findings suggest that intense flushing reactions play a role in the pathogenesis of rosacea and, given the present report of a patient, that mastocytosis with intense flushing can lead to a vascular variety of rosacea, as well. The earliest findings are the ocular rosacea, the facial telangiectasia, and the erythema localized to the "blush distribution." In fact, a pronounced injection of the bulbar conjunctiva has been regarded as the earliest and most reliable sign of the carcinoid flush.[5] Further, in this same series of 16 patients, the authors frequently observed during the flushing episodes moderate to marked lacrimation. Additionally, when flushing was intense and frequent, the periorbital tissues and the lids became edematous. The severe connective tissue hypertrophy is a later development. While there were no signs of connective tissue hypertrophy, all of the other rosacea stigmata associated with carcinoid syndrome were found in the patient reported here.

There are several other lines of evidence that support a role for flushing in the pathogenesis of rosacea. There is an increased frequency of flushing in patients with rosacea.[6] There is a correlation between severity of ocular rosacea and tendency to flushing. Mild rosacea is more common in women and usually appears after age 35 when the frequency of "hot flashes" and flushing increases.[7] Flushing is invariably the earliest component of rosacea to be apparent. Rosacea can be exacerbated during vasodilator therapy accompanied by flushing.[8] Finally, there is an extensive clinical literature that has broadly incriminated flushing in the genesis and exacerbation of rosacea.[2]

Since rosacea is a syndrome, much as jaundice is, the physician should look for a specific diagnosis beyond the accurate, but trivial, statement that the patient has rosacea and flushing. Rosacea does not cause flushing, but rather results from it. Therefore, the specific diagnosis is based on the nature of the flushing reaction which leads to the vascular variety of rosacea.

Mechanism of Flushing. Because flushing is a phenomenon of transient vasodilation, flushing mechanisms may be broadly classified into two categories: those flushing reactions resulting from direct smooth-muscle effects of circulating agents and those reactions mediated by nerves. Autonomic nerves also control the eccrine sweat glands; whenever vasodilation is mediated by autonomic nerves, an accompanying eccrine sweating (e.g., menopausal flushing) also occurs. On the other hand, agents that act directly on the vascular smooth muscle cause flushing reactions in which there is no increase in eccrine sweating (e.g., niacin-provoked flushing).

Therefore, two mechanisms of flushing can be distinguished at the bedside or in the office: neural-mediated flushing, which includes eccrine sweating ("wet flush"), and flushing from agents that act directly on vascular smooth muscle ("dry flush"). The first step in the diagnosis of a flushing reaction is to decide whether the flushing reaction is caused by events at some level in the neural control of vascular smooth muscle or by a circulating, direct-acting vasodilator.

Clinical Approach. The physician should also consider four clinical characteristics in an initial evaluation of the patient with flushing: (1) provocative and palliative factors, (2) morphology of the flushing reaction, (3) associated features, and (4) temporal characteristics, i.e., the timing of the specific features during each flushing reaction and also the frequency of the flushing reactions. Data of much better quality than a simple history can be obtained from a two-week diary in which the patient records qualitative and quantitative aspects of the flushing reaction and lists exposure to all exogenous agents, such as drugs, physical exertion, alcoholic beverages, and occupational chemicals.

Although this initial information may be sufficient for diagnosis of the type of flushing reaction, occasionally the patient is found to have one of the less common varieties of flushing reactions which are catalogued elsewhere.[1,9] In this report I will consider both common and important flushing reactions in the differential diagnosis.

The three most important flushing reactions to rule out in a patient with severe flushing are the carcinoid syndrome, pheochromocytoma, and mastocytosis. Although the clinical characteristics of each condition are distinctive, the diagnosis of each ultimately depends on a biochemical assay or demonstration of increased numbers of mast cells.

The Carcinoid Syndrome. The carcinoid syndrome comprises two subtypes based on clinical characteristics that correlate with the site of origin of the carcinoid tumor. Although tumors from foregut and midgut origin both produce serotonin, the foregut carcinoid tumors also produce histamine, which may explain their association with peptic ulcer disease. Compared with that of midgut carcinoid tumors, the flushing reaction seen with foregut tumors is bright, appearing salmon-pink to red, more persistent, with a geographic pattern, and more intense, with prominent associated findings that include lacrimation, sweating (with pallor), vomiting, and asthma. In contrast with this "maiden flush" of the foregut tumors, the midgut tumors are associated with a cyanotic flush of mixed cyanosis, erythema, and pallor. The single most important diagnostic criterion of carcinoid flushing is biochemical evidence of the overproduction of serotonin. This is usually documented by an elevated urinary 5-HIAA level.

Pheochromocytoma. The most common symptoms of pheochromocytoma include a severe, throbbing headache with excessive perspiration, palpitations, and hypotension. A flushed face, if it occurs, is seen after such a paroxysm of hypotension, tachycardia, and chest pain; pallor is typically present during the attack. The diagnosis of pheochromocytoma depends on the biochemical confirmation of excessive catecholamine release. The best current recommendation is to measure 24-hour urinary levels of free norepinephrine and, if the assay becomes generally available, its metabolite, 3,4-dihydroxyphenylglycol.[10]

Systemic Mastocytosis. Findings in mastocytosis include severe throbbing headache, bronchospasm, rhinorrhea, hypotension, lacrimation, tachycardia, dyspnea, syncope, flushing, and intense pruritus. Dermatographism can frequently be elicited in clinically involved skin. Provocative factors include the various drugs, foods, and physical agents that provoke mast cell degranulation, e.g., opiates, aspirin, alcohol, physical exertion, hot baths, cold exposure, and anxiety. The presence of skin lesions demonstrating the infiltration by large numbers of mast cells is extremely helpful in making the diagnosis. The absence of skin lesions would not rule out the possibility of systemic mast cell disease.[11,12] Even in the absence of cutaneous lesions, pruritus is an extremely common complaint.

The patient reported here became more symptomatic after ingestion of alcoholic beverages, hot showers, and infrequent ingestion of aspirin. All of these stimuli are known to provoke mast cell degranulation. The flushing reaction in this patient lacked eccrine sweating, indicating that his flushing resulted from a circulating vasodilator substance. The association with pruritus made histamine a likely candidate. Finally, his "freckles," which were actually cutaneous mastocytomas, urticated with stroking (Darier's sign), strongly suggesting the diagnosis of mastocytosis. The elevation of the urinary histamine was confirmatory.

Alcohol and Flushing. The frequent association with alcohol and symptoms in the present patient also raised the possibility of an alcohol-provoked flushing reaction. The relationship between alcohol ingestion and flushing is complex for several reasons.[1] First, other vasoactive pharmacologic agents found in alcoholic beverages may be important. These include tyramine, histamine, sulfites, and higher-chained alcohols and aldehydes. Second, the sensitivity to ethanol-induced flushing varies among people of different ethnic backgrounds.[13-16] Increased sensitivity is frequently seen in a variety of Mongoloid populations, although a few Caucasoids will also express this biochemical intolerance. Third, various drugs (e.g., disulfiram) and occupational exposures will predispose otherwise normal individuals to the alcohol-provoked flushing reaction.[1] Importantly, in the present case the patient had tolerated alcohol for many years before developing the flushing reactions over the past year.

Pathophysiology of Mastocytosis. Mastocytosis is accompanied by a variety of signs and symptoms caused by the tissue infiltration by large numbers of mast cells and by the release from these cells of a variety of biologically active substances. Many of the mediators from mast cells are preformed and stored and released at the time of degranulation. Others are synthesized at the time of degranulation. The latter include prostaglandin D_2 and a variety of leukotrienes. It is likely that these substances are also important, since the biosynthesis of PGD_2 can be reduced with nonsteroidal antiinflammatory agents, and the addition of these agents to combined antihistamine therapy leads to greater control of these flushing reactions.[17] The metabolite of prostaglandin D_2 may serve as an important biochemical indicant of mastocytosis.[17] Another potential biochemical indicant is a metabolite of histamine, 1-methyl-4-imidazoleacetic acid, which may actually provide a more quantitative correlation with total body histamine stores than histamine itself.[18]

Visceral and Systemic Involovement. Probably 10% of all patients with mastocytosis have systemic involvement.[19] The GI tract and the skeletal system seem to be the most common extracutaneous sites involved. Bone involvement may be manifested as discrete lytic, cystic, or sclerotic lesions, as well as generalized osteoporosis or osteosclerosis. In adults with systemic mastocytosis, technetium scanning of bone appears to be a more sensitive diagnostic test for detection of bone involvement than a radiographic skeletal survey.

Mastocytosis may affect the GI system by direct mast cell infiltration and corresponding high tissue levels of histamine, or the GI symptoms may be simply an effect of high circulating histamine levels.

Hepatomegaly or splenomegaly occurs in over 10% of cases. An infiltration of lymph nodes may lead to palpable adenopathy. Eosinophilia is found in about 15% of cases and, occasionally, leukemia occurs with mastocytosis.

Histamine Assay. A final comment must be made on the assay for histamine which is the mainstay in the diagnosis of systemic mastocytosis. Most physicians rely on elevations of urinary histamine coupled with the clinical picture and, if cutaneous lesions are present, evidence of increased numbers of mast cells infiltrating the skin. Today, if a physician wants to measure histamine in a biological specimen, he can choose from a multitude of techniques. Further, the biological material can be a variety of fluids and tissues. Recently, the European and American Histamine Research Societies conducted a consensus development conference considering the usefulness of the different types of histamine assay. Urinary histamine by radioimmunoassay, enzymeimmunoassay, gas chromatography-mass spectroscopy, high performance liquid chromatography, and bioassay are all acceptable. The radioimmunoassay/enzymeimmunoassay are probably the most reliable for routine clinical use.[22]

Treatment of Mastocytosis. The usual goal in the treatment of mastocytosis is the amelioration of symptoms. Best pharmacologic regulation is thought to occur with a combination of H_1 and H_2 antihistamines along with a non-steroidal antiinflammatory agent to inhibit the production of PGD_2. Since non-steroidal antiinflammatory agents are potent mast cell degranulators, the addition of a non-steroidal antiinflammatory agent to the regimen in a patient with mastocytosis should be undertaken in an appropriate clinical environment. When the majority of the mast cell infiltrations appear to be cutaneous, the combination of oral psoralen with ultraviolet A therapy can lead to improvement.[20] Also, topical corticosteroid preparations have appeared to hasten the resolution of cutaneous infiltrates of mastocytosis.[21] Recently, cromolyn sodium has been found useful in controlling the symptoms.

Since no therapeutic regimen is completely successful, patients should be instructed at each follow-up visit to avoid anything that precipitates symptoms, such as opiates, alcohol, aspirin, hot and cold stimuli, and overexertion. They should also be instructed to let every physician who provides care for them know that they have mastocytosis. Drugs which may exacerbate flushing reactions should be avoided (Table 1).

While the prognosis of childhood mastocytosis is favorable, the occurrence of mastocytosis in adulthood is typically associated with persistence. Serious systemic involvement appears to correlate with a later age of onset and with extensive cutaneous disease. Accordingly, the patient presented in this report will need to

Table 1

Flushing Reactions: A Classification

I. Flushing reactions related to alcohol:
   Increased susceptibility in mongoloid populations
   Occupational "degreasers" flush occurs in women drinking beer after
     exposure to industrial solvents:
           trichloroethylene vapor
           N, N-dimethylformamide
           N-butyraldoxime
           carbon disulfide
           xylene
   Fermented alcoholic beverages (beer, sherry) may contain tyramine or
     histamine, which induce flushing
   Drugs
       disulfiram
       chlorpropamide
       calcium carbamide
       phentolamine
       griseofulvin
       metronidazole
       ketoconazole
       chloramphenicol
       quinacrine
   B-lactams with methyltetrazolethiol side chain (cephalosporin
     antiobiotics)
       cefamanadole
       cefoperazone
       moxalactam
   Eating Coprinus mushrooms
   Carcinoid flushing
   Mastocytosis flushing

II. Flushing related to food additives:
     Monosodium glutamate (MSG) putatively provokes flushing, but this
       is not verified
     Sodium nitrite in cured meats (frankfurters, bacon, salami, ham)
       may cause headache and flushing
     Sulfites (potassium metabisulfite) may cause wheezing and flushing

Table 1

Flushing Reactions: A Classification (Continued)

III.   Flushing associated with eating:
Hot beverages cause flushing through countercurrent heat
    exchange into blood vessels leading to the anterior hypothalamus
Auriculotemporal flushing (especially after chewing a chili pepper)
Dumping syndrome (especially after a meal or ingestion of hot
    liquids or hypertonic glucose)

IV.   Neurologic flushing:
anxiety
simple blushing
brain tumors
spinal cord lesions (autonomic hyperreflexia)
migraine headaches
Parkinson's disease
climacteric (menopausal) flushing = "hot flashes"
cholinergic erythema

V.   Flushing due to drugs:
all vasodilators (e.g., nitroglycerin, prostaglandins, synthetic
    calcitonin-gene-related peptide)
all calcium channel blockers (nifedipine, verapamil, diltiazem)
nicotinic acid (not nicotinamide)
morphine and other opiates
amyl nitrite and butyl nitrite (recreational drugs)
cholinergic drugs (e.g., metrifonate, an anthelminthic)
bromocriptine used in Parkinson's disease
thyrotropin-releasing hormone (TRH)
tamoxifen
cyproterone acetate
oral triamcinolone used with psoriatic arthritis
cyclosporin A

VI.   Flushing due to systemic diseases:
carcinoid syndrome
mastocytosis
basophilic chronic granulocytic leukomia
pheochromocytoma
medullary carcinoma of thyroid
pancreatic tumors (e.g., VIPoma)
renal cell carcinoma
horseshoe kidneys (Rovsing's syndrome)

be reevaluated at intervals in the future, despite success in the clinical suppression of symptoms.

In summary, this patient developed an explosive onset of vascular rosacea. The association of severe flushing with the rapid onset of rosacea is also seen in the carcinoid syndrome and is associated with a variety of other flushing reactions. Both the rosacea and the flushing are syndromic taxa, and they both require a more definitive diagnosis by the physician. The differential diagnosis of flushing reactions is briefly reviewed, with emphasis on systemic mastocytosis, which this patient had. The management of patients with systemic mastocytosis includes symptomatic therapy, evaluation for systemic involvement, and continuing patient education.

References

1. Wilkin JK: Flushing reactions, Rook AJ, Maibach H (eds): in Recent Advances in Dermatology, vol 6. Edinburgh, Churchill Livingstone, 1983, pp 157-187.
2. Wilkin JK: Rosacea. Int J Dermatol. 22:393-400.
3. Starr PAJ, MacDonald A: Oculocutaneous aspects of rosacea. Proc. R Soc Med. 1969;62:9-10.
4. Findlay GH, Simson IW: Leonine hypertrophic rosacea associated with a benign bronchial carcinoid tumor. Clin Exp Dermatol. 1977;2:175.
5. Wong VG, Melmon KL: Ophthalmic manifestations of the carcinoid flush. N Engl J Med. 1967;277:406-409.
6. Marks R, Beard RJ, Clark ML, et al: Gastrointestinal observations in rosacea. Lancet 1967;1:379.
7. Domonkos AN: Andrews' Diseases of the Skin, ed 6. Philadelphia, WB Saunders Co, 1971, p 261.
8. Wilkin JK: Vasodilator rosacea. Arch Dermatol. 1980;116:598.
9. Wilkin JK: Flushing reactions: Consequences and mechanisms. Ann Intern Med. 1981;95:468-476.
10. Duncan MW, Compton P, Lazarus L, et al: Measurement of norepinephrine. Measurement of norepinephrine and 3,4-dihydroxyphenylglycol in urine and plasma for the diagnosis of pheochromocytoma. N Engl J Med 1988;319:136-142.
11. Roberts LJ II, Fields JP, Oates JA: Mastocytosis without urticaria pigmentosa. A frequently unrecognized cause of recurrent syncope. Trans Assoc Am Physicians 1982;95:36-41.
12. Webb TA, Li CY, Yam LT: Systemic mast cell disease: A clinical and hematopathologic study of 26 cases. Cancer. 1982;49:927-938.
13. Wilkin JK: Ethnic contact urticarial reaction to alcohol. Contact Dermatitis 1985;12:118-120.
14. Wilkin JK, Fortner G: Cutaneous vascular sensitivity to lower aliphatic alcohols and aldehydes in Orientals. Alcoholism: Clin Exp Res. 1985;9:522-525.
15. Wilkin JK, Stewart JH: Substrate specificity of human cutaneous alcohol dehydrogenase and erythema provoked by lower aliphatic alcohols. J Invest Dermatol. 1987;88:452-454.
16. Wilkin JK: 4-Methylpyrazole and the cutaneous vascular sensitivity to alcohol in Orientals. J Invest Dermatol. 1988;91:117-119.
17. Roberts LJ, Sweetman BJ, Lewis RA, et al: Increased production of prostaglandin D2 in patients with systemic mastocytosis. New Engl J Med. 1980;303:1400-1404.
18. Granerus G, Wass U: Urinary excretion of histamines, methylhistamine (1-MeHi) and methylimidazoleacetic acid (MeImAA) as an indicator of systemic mastocytosis. Agents and Actions. 1984;14:341-345.

19. Sagher F, Even-Paz Z: Mastocytosis and the mast cell. Chicago, 1967, Year Book Medical Publishers, Inc., pp. 4-242.
20. Granerus G, Roupe G, Swanbeck G: Decreased urinary histamine metabolite after successful PUVA treatment of urticaria pigmentosa. J Invest Dermatol. 1981;76:1-3.
21. Barton J, Lavker RM, Schechter NM, et al: Treatment of urticaria pigmentosa with corticosteroids. Arch Dermatol 1985;121:1516-1523.
22. Lorenz W, Uvnas B. Histamine assays: chapter-writing by consensus. Lancet. 1989;1:1278.

Case 13

Refractory Ventricular Tachycardia

Charles Love, MD

Case History

P.W. is a 57-year-old white man who was in good health until 1972, when he suffered an acute anterior myocardial infarction. His immediate postinfarction course was uncomplicated. He did well for the next two years, when he then began to have symptoms of progressive dyspnea and fatigue. Subsequent physical examination revealed a systolic murmur, and further evaluation proved this to be severe calcific aortic stenosis. He underwent aortic valve replacement in March of 1978 with a Starr-Edwards prosthesis. At this time he developed intraoperative and postoperative runs of ventricular tachycardia (VT). He was treated with propranolol and quinidine with resolution of the arrhythmia. The medications were discontinued after discharge as the rhythm disturbance was felt to be related to the stress of the operative procedure.

In November of 1983 he was undergoing supine bicycle ergometry with multigated radioisotope ventriculography at which time he developed sustained VT. He was on no antiarrhythmia medications at the time. He was admitted to the hospital and underwent cardiac catheterization with coronary angiography. This revealed a resting ejection fraction of 31%, with an anterio-apical aneurysm as well as high-grade stenosis of both the left anterior descending and obtuse marginal coronary arteries. An electrophysiologic study with programmed electrical stimulation was then performed at which time sustained monomorphic VT was induced (Fig. 1). The patient was treated with quinidine gluconate; however, he had a febrile reaction which resolved upon withdrawal of the medication. He was then treated with procainamide, but developed intolerable gastrointestinal upset. Propranolol was given, but he devloped profound bradycardia at doses needed to prevent the arrhythmia from occurring. He was then started on amiodarone, with resolution of his symptoms.

He did well until August of 1986, when he presented to his local hospital's emergency room with a wide-complex tachycardia, hypotension and dyspnea.

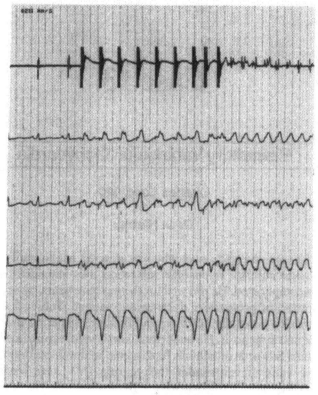

Figure 1
Induction of sustained monomorphic ventricular tachycardia by programmed stimulation. Top to bottom: intraventricular electrogram, lead I, lead II, lead III and lead V.

Attempts to treat the rhythm with intravenous verapamil, propranolol and bretylium were not successful. He was subsequently converted to sinus rhythm with DC cardioversion. While in the coronary care unit, he had frequent ventricular ectopy which responded to the addition of oral mexiletine to the amiodarone.

In January 1987 he suffered a cardiac arrest, but was promptly and successfully resuscitated. Further evaluation at his local hospital revealed no evidence of myocardial infarction by serial cardiac isoenzyme assay. The patient was subsequently discharged, but continued to have periodic episodes of tachycardia.

In August 1987 he again presented with sustained VT resistant to medical therapy and requiring DC cardioversion. He underwent repeat electrophysiologic study, and programmed stimulation using single premature ventricular depolarizations induced sustained monomorphic VT. This was able to be terminated by rapid ventricular pacing in all cases. Though each episode was monomorphic, the episodes were of separate morphologies and cycle lengths (500, 440, and 420 msec). The patient was returned to the coronary care unit and encainide was added to the amiodarone. He underwent repeat programmed stimulation 6 days later, with the finding of easily inducible VT which was of a shorter cycle length (higher rate) degenerating to ventricular fibrillation. The patient was defibrillated successfully, returned to the CCU, and the encainide was discontinued.

The following week an automatic implantable cardioverter defibrillator and an antitachycardia pacemaker were implanted. The patient was maintained on amiodarone and mexiletine. He was discharged and did well with consistent termination of his tachycardia by the pacemaker, but in December 1987, three episodes of accelerated tachycardia over a 2-week period were terminated by discharge of the automatic implantable cardioverter. He was admitted to the CCU and the antitachycardia pacemaker was reprogrammed. The reprogramming was necessary because the antitachycardia pacemaker appeared to have accelerated the VT instead of terminating it as it was supposed to have done.

The following month he had repeated episodes of VT, and was admitted again for further medical therapy. The mexiletine was discontinued, and tocainide was added to the amiodarone, but spontaneous nonsustained VT continued. Procainamide was started at 500 mg every 6 hr. This abolished the spontaneous VT, and was tolerated this time by the patient. He did well for 2 months, and then presented again with VT, which was controlled by increasing the procainamide dose to 750 mg. The following month he became increasingly fatigued, and was found to have marked elevation of his liver enzymes. This was felt to be due to the amiodarone, and amiodarone was stopped. In addition, the antinuclear antibodies were found at a titer of 1:320. Despite the development of antinuclear antibodies, procainamide was continued because of its efficacy and because the patient did not have disabling symptoms of drug-induced lupus. He has remained stable since that time.

Discussion

The treatment of refractory VT remains one of the most difficult therapeutic problems facing the clinician. Though there have been many recent advances in drug, surgical, and device therapy, many patients continue to experience recurrences of VT or sudden death. This case demonstrates many of the concepts and modes of therapy involved in the approach to a patient with VT. Changing patient substrate and intolerance to drugs play a continuing role in the therapy of this patient's rhythm disturbance.

Etiology. The majority of patients with sustained or hemodynamically significant VT have ischemic cardiac disease and infarcted myocardium.[1] Other groups that are at risk include those with dilated cardiomyopathy, congenital heart disease (i.e., tetralogy of Fallot), asymmetric septal hypertrophy (idiopathic hypertrophic subaortic stenosis/hypertrophic obstructive cardiomyopathy), arrhythmogenic right ventricular dysplasia, mitral valve prolapse, long QT syndrome, and familial cardiomyopathy.

All arrhythmias are caused by abnormalities of either impulse formation, impulse conduction, or a combination of both. This holds true for VT, in that there appear to be two mechanisms that are responsible for the initiation and maintenance of VT. The first and most common mechanism is reentry.[1,2] This is the same mechanism as in accessory-pathway tachycardia (i.e., Wolff-Parkinson-White). In VT, the pathway involves slowed conduction through the peri-infarction tissue (Fig. 2). Unidirectional block may also be present. The impulse may then reenter into tissue that is no longer refractory. This provides the loop necessary to maintain the rhythm. Patients with idiopathic dilated cardiomyopathy may also have reentry as the basis for VT. This can occur via excitation from a physiologic circuit rather than from an anatomic circuit as noted above (Fig. 3). In this example, the impulse propagates in a circular manner around a "core" that remains refractory due to constant stimulation.

The cycle length of the tachycardia is related to the length of the "circuit" and the refractory period of the tissue. In order to be able to sustain and propagate a tachycardia, the proper milieu must be present in the ventricular myocardium. Reentry is favored by slow conduction and short refractory times. Conduction is influenced by sodium flux during phase 0 of the action potential (fast sodium channels), abnormalities of cell-to-cell coupling, autonomic changes, drug therapy, cellular excitability, tissue geometry, and electronic interactions. Refractory time is influenced by metabolic factors, ischemia, hypoxemia, heart rate, neural influences, and drugs. It is the proper combination of these factors that makes VT possible.

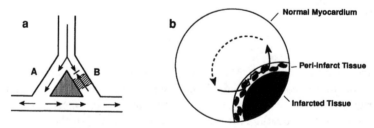

Figure 2
a) Classic reentry. With unidirectional block the impulse cannot travel down pathway B, but reenters B from below then loops from A to B. b) Reentry through a region of slowed conduction. The impulse enters the peri-infarction tissue where "islands" of viable myocardium conduct the impulse to a distal point of exit. If the myocardium at the point of exit is no longer refractory, it is depolarized and the loop begins.

Figure 3

Reentry around a physiologic obstacle. The tissue in the center of the loop remains constantly depolarized.

Conversely, it is the modification of one or several factors that allows us to treat rhythm disturbances.

The second mechanism involves abnormal impulse formation. This can be caused by either abnormal automaticity or by triggered activity.[3] Abnormal automaticity allows impulses to occur de novo and without dependence on the previous impulse. This is usually the result of an abnormal resting potential. Triggered activity is due to the presence of afterdepolarizations which represent abnormal depolarization of cardiac tissue occurring just after the previous depolarization (Fig. 4). This results in repeated depolarization of a cell or group of cells resulting in an increased firing rate and thus tachycardia. Afterdepolarizations are subclassified as early or delayed, depending on whether they occur when repolarization is in process (early) or completed (delayed). Early afterdepolarizations can be produced by hypoxia, hypercarbia, increased catecholamine levels, injury, fiber stretch, and drugs prolonging the action potential. The clinical significance of early afterdepolarizations is uncertain. Delayed afterdepolarizations are made possible

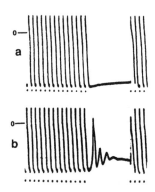

Figure 4

a) Normal response to repeated stimulation. b) Response after digitalis glycoside given demonstrating triggered afterdepolarizations.

by factors causing abnormally high or low resting potentials, digitalis, and catecholamine excess. Unlike reentry where the length and characteristics of the circuit determine the cycle length of the tachycardia, triggered tachycardias are dependent upon the stimulation rate that initiates the process.

Natural History. The one-year survival for patients with untreated refractory VT is poor, and for some groups of patients (dilated cardiomyopathy) may be as low as 50%. If treated effectively the prognosis may improve to higher than 95% survival at one year.[4] Obviously, the effect of treatment and thus the prognosis will vary with the underlying substrate.

The most common presentations for a patient with sustained VT are palpitations, near-syncope, syncope, and sudden death. The diagnosis of VT can be made by a number of methods. The current electrophysiologic definition of sustained VT is the finding of VT lasting a minimum of 20 sec, or VT that causes hemodynamic collapse requiring CPR and/or cardioversion.

The approach to diagnosing the presence and etiology of VT may involve the use of a number of standard and newer diagnostic modalities. These include the following:

1) *Standard 12-lead electrocardiogram:* The presence of frequent or complex ventricular ectopy may provide a clue that VT is present. In addition, Q-waves can show the presence of myocardial scar tissue providing the substrate for VT.

2) *24-48 hour continuous ECG (Holter) monitoring:* Frequent, complex, or sustained ventricular ectopy found during monitoring provides very valuable information. This modality has become one of the keystones of diagnosis and therapy. The major weakness of this modality is that patients having infrequent symptoms may not have a diagnosis confirmed when the arrhythmia does not occur during the monitoring period. There are now restrictions on the frequency and number of recordings allowed on a patient by third-party payers, making documentation of the rhythm more difficult using this technique.

3) *Real-time ECG transtelephonic transmission:* Patients who have symptoms infrequently and who remain functional while symptomatic can use a hand-held transmitter placed on the chest to transmit a continuous, real-time rhythm strip by telephone to a receiving station. This type of device will work from any telephone and can be carried in a pocket or purse. Patients for whom this technique should not be used are those who have short runs of tachycardia, are unable to be near a telephone when symptomatic, or are too symptomatic and thus unable to operate the transmitter or telephone.

4) *Stored real-time ECG transtelephonic transmission:* This is similar to the former device in operation except it has the capability of storing the recorded rhythm strip. The ECG may then be transmitted through any telephone minutes or hours later when the patient is able to do so. This may be an alternative to the real-time devices if the patient is not frequently near a telephone, is relatively compromised during symptoms, or has shorter runs of tachycardia.

5) *Looping memory recorders:* These recorders are worn similar to 24-hr recorders. They can be worn for days to weeks, and store the ECG continuously in an electronic memory. When symptoms occur, either the patient or observer presses an "event" button which freezes the previous 30 sec of ECG in memory and then continues to record the next minute of ECG into the memory (these time periods vary by manufacturer). The stored information may then be transmitted over the telephone to a receiving station. This type of device represents one of the major diagnostic advances in the past 10 years.

6) *Exercise testing:* Treadmill or bicycle testing can be used to provoke arrhythmias and thus provide a diagnosis. Exercise may result in many changes (ischemia, catecholamine increase, hypoxemia, electrolyte shifts, autonomic imbalance) that favor the initiation and propagation of VT. This type of study should only be performed when adequate personnel are present and measures assuring patient safety have been taken.

7) *Signal-averaged electrocardiogram:* This is the newest diagnostic tool to predict the presence of inducible sustained VT in patients with previous myocardial infarction.[5] This technique involves recording several hundred QRS complexes and averaging the complexes together. As a result, electrical noise (a random event) is averaged out, and one is able to amplify the resultant QRS to a degree 1,000 times greater than is possible using standard techniques. The presence of delayed electrical activity (late potentials) represents slowed conduction through peri-infarction tissue (Fig. 5). This bears a very high sensitivity and specificity in patients with syncope and previous myocardial infarction. Unfortunately, this type of study cannot be used to predict efficacy of drug therapy, though it can confirm successful surgical ablation.

8) *Electrophysiologic testing using programmed electrical stimulation:* Electrophysiologic testing utilizing programmed stimulation represents the current "gold standard" in the diagnosis of VT. This type of testing involves the placement of a temporary pacing catheter into the heart and delivering one, two or three premature ventricular depolarizations (VPDs) at progressively shorter coupling intervals during sinus and paced rhythms (Figure 1). Usually, the right ventricular apex or outflow tract is used as the primary site of stimulation. However, left ventricular stimulation may be used in patients who cannot be induced from the right ventricle. The protocol is made more aggressive by utilizing faster pacing rates or by delivering a greater number of stimuli (up to 3 VPDs). As with most diagnostic tests, the more aggressive protocols have a higher sensitivity but a lower specificity. Electrophysiologic testing is of greatest value in patients who are post myocardial infarction, and have monomorphic (versus polymorphic) VT.[6]

Treatment. Once the diagnosis of sustained VT is made, the most difficult task then awaits the clinician: selection of therapy. We now have more therapeutic drugs and modalities available than ever before: however, our ability to suppress VT without causing significant morbidity and mortality remains poor. If possible, the

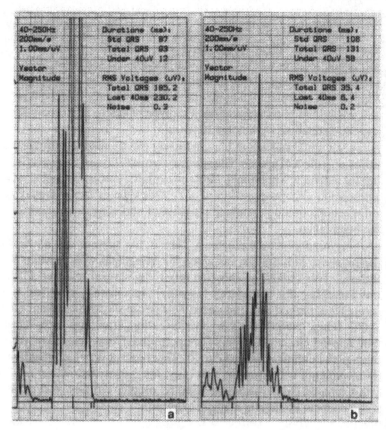

Figure 5

a) Normal SAECG showing abrupt termination of ventricular activity. b) Abnormal SAECG showing late/delayed activity which represents conduction through diseased and arrhythmogenic substrate.

etiology of the arrhythmia should be elucidated prior to the initiation of therapy. Unless a clearly defined cause is present, a thorough cardiac evaluation should be pursued. This should include complete cardiac catheterization with coronary angiography to define both anatomy and function of the heart. Other studies that may be useful include echocardiography and endomyocardial biopsy. Following the institution of therapy, the patient should be reevaluated to establish the effectiveness of the treatment. This preferably involves repeat electrophysiolic study, but may also include exercise testing or Holter monitoring. If electrophysiologic study is to be used to follow the effectiveness of therapy (by noninducibility of the rhythm), then it is preferable that a baseline electrophysiologic study be performed to establish inducibility. There is no question that patients treated by electrophysiologic guided therapy have a better prognosis than those treated by an empiric method.

The following is a summary of currently available therapy:

1) *Correction of underlying or causal metabolic factors*: Ischemia is a frequent cause of VT initiation. Correction via the use of antianginal medication, percutaneous transluminal coronary angioplasty, and coronary artery bypass grafting can relieve ischemia and prevent the initiation and maintenance of the milieu necessary to produce or sustain VT. Cardiac ischemia caused by systemic hypoxemia should be corrected.

Electrolyte disturbances, most notably hypokalemia and hypomagnesemia, alone and in combination with other factors should be noted at the time of recognition of VT and corrected as needed. Obviously, it is preferable to anticipate these types of electrolyte deficiencies when altering drug therapy, especially diuretics.

Inappropriate drug levels of potentially arrhythmogenic drugs (i.e., digitalis glycosides, theophylline, antidepressants, beta agonists) especially when combined with electrolyte disturbances should be addressed. These agents should be discontinued if possible. Antiarrhythmia drugs are potentially proarrhythmic at inappropriately high serum levels of the drug or its active metabolites. Dosage reduction or change in medical therapy should be considered for the latter.

2) *Drug therapy:* The use of antiarrhythmia medications for patients with sustained VT remains the cornerstone of therapy. Drug therapy should always be initiated in an inpatient setting. All of these drugs are potentially proarrhythmic, leading to the possibility of more frequent, faster, or new types of rhythm disturbances. In addition, patients with compromise of their cardiac conduction system can experience SA and/or AV nodal depression as well as infra-Hisian block causing clinically significant bradycardia and heart block.

There is now a consensus that drug therapy for VT should be guided by electrophysiologic studies.[7] Patients on drug therapy who no longer have inducible VT during provocation by programmed stimulation are far less likely to experience a recurrence of VT than those who are treated using an empirical approach. One must keep in mind that the patient's next occurrence of VT could present as sudden death, and that a "second chance" at drug therapy using the empirical approach may never be possible.

Before discussion of initial choice in drug therapy it will be useful to review the classification scheme most commonly used,[8] that of Vaughan Williams (Table 1). Though this is a somewhat useful method of classification, the introduction of newer drugs possessing characteristics of two or more classes has made it more difficult to keep the classification "pure." Moreover, failure of a drug in one class to effectively prevent VT does not mean that other drugs of that class will not be useful. For example, failure of procainamide − a class IA drug − does not

Table 1

Vaughan Williams Classification of Antiarrhythmia Drugs

IA **(Depress phase 0, prolong repolarization)**	II **Beta Blockers**
disopyramide	propranolol
phenytoin	esmolol
procainamide	labetalol
quinidine	atenolol
	nadolol
IB **(Accelerate repolarization)**	sotalol (III)*
lidocaine	metoprolol
aprindine*	timolol
mexiletine	acebutalol
tocainide	pindolol
	III **(Prolongation of repolarization)**
IC **(Little effect on repolarization)**	amiodarone
encainide	bretylium
flecainide	
propafenone (II/IV)	IV **Calcium channel blockers**
moricizine	**(slow inward current)**
	bepridil
I	diltiazem
cibenzoline (III/IV)*	nicardipine
pirmenol (IA/IB)*	nifedipine
lorcainide*	verapamil

* FDA approval pending.

necessarily predict the failure of quinidine which is of the same class. This may be due to active metabolites of the drugs, as well as different effects on a cellular level.

The classical choice for initial treatment of VT has been drugs of group IA, most commonly quinidine or procainamide. It is important to note that failure of one agent does not accurately predict the failure of other drugs in the same class. Thus, if the therapeutic level of one IA drug is adequate but does not achieve effective results, switching to another IA is reasonable. If single agent therapy with a IA is insufficient, addition of a IB (usually mexiletine) to the IA may be tried. The IB drugs are usually well tolerated and have an additive therapeutic effect with other drugs. The use of a IB alone in the treatment of serious ventricular rhythm disturbances is probably not appropriate.

Patients failing the latter therapy should be considered for treatment with amiodarone. Though this drug has many side effects (some of which are potentially fatal), it is the single most effective antiarrhythmia agent available. Indeed, it is the most widely used drug of its type in Europe.[9] Amiodarone may also be used in combination with both IA and IB drugs. Use of amiodarone is difficult since patients need to be monitored closely for pulmonary, thyroid, and hepatic changes.

The issue of the IC drug use has been controversial since the preliminary report of the Cardiac Arrhythmia Suppression Trial (CAST) was made public.[10] The findings of this study indicated that patients who were status post myocardial infarction and treated with IC drugs for asymptomatic premature ventricular contractions (PVCs) and nonsustained VT were at higher risk of sudden cardiac death than those treated with placebo. The current IC drugs have been relabeled for use only in patients with life-threatening arrhythmias that are not responsive to other medical therapy. Due to the fear of potential liability from the use of these drugs, they are only rarely prescribed. They do, however, remain a part of our limited therapeutic arsenal.

The use of beta-blockers for the treatment of VT is limited. There is evidence to suggest that at least one of these agents is as effective as quinidine in the suppression of PVCs. They are quite useful in treating VT that is catecholamine dependent (i.e., exercise induced VT). Though effective, their use at adequate therapeutic levels may be prevented by their negative inotropic effects in patients with poor ventricular function.

The calcium channel blocking drugs (class IV) agents are only rarely useful in the treatment of VT. Their use is limited to VT caused by triggered mechanisms or by increased automaticity. In the real world of clinical practice, this is uncommon.

3) *Antitachycardia pacing:* Devices are available that can recognize the onset of tachycardia by a number of criteria (high rate, sudden onset, rate stability, sustained high rate). The device is implanted in an identical manner as that of a permanent transvenous pacemaker. When the device recognizes an arrhythmia as defined by the physician programming the device, it can deliver single or multiple stimuli to overdrive pace the rhythm. This technique works well only in those with a relatively slow and stable VT rate. It also carries the possibility of accelerating the tachycardia to a less hemodynamically stable rate. These devices are extremely complex and require a great deal of training and experience to use properly. Most physicians experienced in their use are reluctant to use this modality alone for VT.

4) *Automatic Implantable Cardioverter Defibrillator (AICD):* The development of a practical device for recognizing and delivering therapy for sustained VT or VF by delivering an electrical shock to the heart has been a pivotal point in our ability to ensure the survival of patients with VT/VF. Once a tachycardia is recognized by either rate or morphology criteria, the device charges and delivers a shock to the heart. If the rhythm has not been corrected, multiple shocks may be delivered. The

effectiveness of this form of therapy is unsurpassed. Survival rate in high-risk populations can exceed 95% at one year.[4]

The current devices are somewhat large weighing 215 grams (the average pacemaker now weighs 35 grams). They are large in volume, and thus must be placed above the rectus sheath in the abdominal region. Patches are placed directly on the epicardial surface by either a lateral thoracotomy or median sternotomy approach. One lead system allows a single patch on the heart with a transvenous electrode placed into the superior vena cava. Newer configurations will permit totally transvenous systems utilizing superior vena cava, right ventricular and coronary sinus placement. Subcutaneous patch systems are also under investigation This in combination with smaller devices being developed will allow implantation in much the same way as a permanent pacemaker is implanted today. In addition, backup pacing for resultant bradycardia, antitachycardia pacing, telemetered playback of stored ECG acquired during arrhythmia recognition and treatment, and staged therapy allowing combinations of antitachycardia pacing therapy and different levels of energy delivered for different rates of tachycardia are all present in devices currently undergoing clinical trials. The current cost of implantation can exceed $25,000.

5) *Surgical ablation:* Some patients, specifically those with discrete ventricular aneurysm formation, may be curable by a surgical approach. Since the area of reentry is virtually always located in the tissue surrounding the aneurysm, an operative approach combining the skills of the cardiologist/electrophysiologist and the cardiac surgeon can be utilized. The patient has the heart exposed in the operating room, after which VT is induced by programmed stimulation. The epicardial surface is mapped using an electrical probe or a computer-generated map. Once the area of reentry is localized, subendocardial resection or cryo-ablation is performed. Alternatively an encircling incision is made. The patient is then rechecked for inducibility. While the morbidity and mortality of this procedure is around 10%, it represents a possible "cure" for the patient. Even if the rhythm is not totally abolished, the substrate may be modified in such a way to permit effective drug therapy that may not have been possible prior to the operation.

6) *Catheter ablation:* For some patients with refractory VT, it may be possible to modify or totally abolish the tachycardia using this technique. The patient is taken to the electrophysiology lab and a temporary pacing catheter is placed into the appropriate ventricle. The endomyocardium is then mapped utilizing various techniques to localize the site of reentry. The patient is then anesthetized and several 100 joule shocks are delivered through the catheter to the endomyocardial surface. Unfortunately, complications are not rare and success is not common. Investigators are currently working with radio-frequency energy as well as Laser energy as alternatives to this technique.

Thus, the treatment of VT has become increasingly complex as our therapeutic options and our understanding of the mechanisms involved have evolved. The older empirical approach to treatment is no longer justified in most patients with serious ventricular rhythm disturbances. Therapy guided by programmed stimulation has been shown to be significantly safer and more effective. However, even with the many drugs available, finding one that is both well tolerated and effective can be extremely difficult. The most effective form of therapy to ensure patient survival seems to be the AICD. However, the cost of this form of therapy remains very high at this time.

References

1. Josepheson ME, et al: Recurrent sustained ventricular tachycardia: I. Mechanisms. Circulation. 1976;57:431.
2. Josepheson ME, et al: Sustained ventricular tachycardia in coronary artery disease: Evidence for a reentrant mechanism, in Zipes DP, Jalife J (eds): Cardiac Electrophysiology and Arrhythmias, Orlando, Grune and Stratton, 1985, pp 409-418.
3. Brugada P, Wellens JHH: The role of triggered activity in clinical ventricular arrhythmias. PACE. 1984;7:260.
4. Fogoros RN, et al: The automatic implantable cardioverter defibrillator in drug refractory ventricular tachycardia. Ann Intern Med. 1987;107:635-641.
5. Hall PAX, et al: The signal averaged surface electrocardiogram and the identification of late potentials. Prog Cardiovasc Dis. 1989;31:295-317.
6. Fisher JD: Role of electrophysiologic testing in the diagnosis and treatment of patients with known and suspected bradycardias and tachycardias. Prog Cardiovasc Dis. 1981;24:25.
7. MKSAP, Medical Knowledge Self-Assessment Program VIII, 1988, pp 830-831.
8. Vaughan-Williams EM: Classification of antiarrhythmic drugs in Sandow E, Flenstedt-Jensen E, Olesen KH (eds): Sweden, Sodertalje, Cardiac Arrhythmias. 1970.
9. Naccarelli GV, et al. Amiodarone: Pharmacology and antiarrhythmic and adverse effects. Pharmacotherapy. 1985;5:298-313.
10. Preliminary Report: Effect of encainide and flecainide on mortality in a randomized trial of arrhythmia suppression after myocardial infarction. CAST investigators. N Engl J Med. 1989;321:406-412.

Case 14

Temporal Arteritis

Seth M. Kantor, M.D.

Case History

An 83-year-old woman was seen in consultation for evaluation of jaw pain and intermittent diplopia.

The patient was first seen by her internist with a several month history of progressive fatigue and lack of energy. She also noted weight loss and painless anorexia. She complained of generalized weakness without specific muscle dysfunction or myalgia. She felt many of her problems were due to despondency since the death of her husband eight months ago.

She had been generally well in the past. She had osteoarthritis of the fingers, neck, hips and knees symptomatically controlled by acetaminophen. She was doing well on medical therapy for obstructive lung disease, ischemic heart disease, and primary hypothyroidism. Her medications included thyroxine, 0.125 mg daily, and isosorbide dinitrate, 10 mg. t.i.d.

Physical Examination. The weight was 156 lb and the blood pressure was 142/82 mm. Hg. The heart and lung examination was normal. There was some fullness in the epigastrium suggestive of a ventral abdominal wall hernia. There was no lymphadenopathy. Examination of the extremities demonstrated Heberden's nodes and marked crepitation of the knees. The neurologic exam was normal for her age.

Clinical Course. The patient declined a suggested upper GI series. Amitriptyline, 10 mg at bedtime was started, and a follow-up appointment was planned for two months later.

The patient returned in one month for further evaluation. She could not tolerate the amitriptyline so she discontinued it after one week. She complained of continued fatigue and further weight loss. In addition, she noted intermittent diplopia over the preceding week. She had also experienced a mild sensation of vertigo. Further questioning revealed difficulty chewing. She experienced pain in her jaw and fatigue shortly after beginning her meals. There was no dysphagia, and she had not had headache, visual loss or fever. There was no history of myalgia or muscle stiffness.

On repeat physical examination the BP was 158/84 and the weight 153 lb. The fundi were normal and there was no detectable loss of visual field. She had bilateral cataracts. The temporal arteries were prominent and the temporal pulse was present but diminished. The temporal arteries were not nodular nor tender to palpation.

Laboratory tests were obtained at that visit and subsequently reported back as: Hct 33.1, Hb 10.5 gm/dl., MCV 86.5, WBC 9.400/mm3. The Westergren sedimentation rate was 97 mm/hr. The patient was asked to take dipyridamole 25 mg b.i.d., and was referred for rheumatologic consultation.

The patient was seen three weeks later in consultation. Her symptoms had persisted but not worsened. She described jaw claudication and intermittent diplopia. She continued to deny headache, scalp tenderness or myalgia. The temporal arteries were as previously noted. The patient was immediately begun on prednisone 40 mg daily. Arrangements were made for a temporal artery biopsy. Five days later, a 1.5 cm section of the left temporal artery was obtained. Multiple-level histologic study described a prominent vasculitis with evidence of subintimal fibrosis and inflammation. Fragmentation of the elastica was identified. No multinucleated giant cells were seen. The biopsy diagnosis was chronic vasculitis without giant cells.

The patient was seen back one month after beginning prednisone. Her weight had increased to 155 lb. She complained of emotional lability and crying spells. Her jaw claudication and visual difficulties had cleared completely. The hematocrit was now 37.9 and the hemoglobin value had increased to 12.5 g/dl. The Westergren sedimentation rate was 9 mm/hr. The prednisone dose was reduced to 30 mg daily and arrangements were made for further tapering of prednisone depending upon her symptoms and sedimentation rate.

Discussion

Temporal arteritis is a vasculitis of unknown etiology which affects large vessels in older adults. The major morbidity of unrecognized and untreated arteritis is blindness. Corticosteroid therapy is very effective in preventing this complication and in providing symptomatic relief. However, in large dosages, particularly in the elderly, corticosteroid treatment is not without complications. It is therefore imperative to make an accurate and timely diagnosis.

Temporal arteritis and polymyalgia rheumatica are often discussed together, though it is still not clear whether they are two distinct entities or two expressions of one disease. The two disorders have elements in common, including a predilection for those over 50 and the presence of a high sedimentation rate. It is estimated that between 15 and 40% of patients with polymyalgia rheumatica will have positive temporal artery biopsies, even in the absence of symptoms suggestive of vasculitis. Between 20 and 50% of patients with biopsy-proven temporal arteritis will manifest symptoms of polymyalgia rheumatica.[1,2] Nonetheless, since the morbidity and suggested treatment regimens are so different, it is best to think of them as distinct entities for the purpose of diagnosis.

Epidemiology. Temporal arteritis is a disease exclusively of those over 50, with most cases occurring over the age of 60. The incidence and prevalence appear to increase directly with age. If present demographic trends continue, it is likely that clinicians will make this diagnosis with greater frequency.

A three-year study in Sweden estimated the clinical incidence of temporal arteritis in the age group over 50 as 28.6 per 100,000 and 16.8 for biopsy-proven cases.[3] A study from the Mayo Clinic in Olmsted County, Minnesota, estimated the prevalence to be 133 per 100,000 population aged 50 and over. The incidence in this population was estimated at 17.4 cases per year, ranging from 1.4 cases in the group 50-59 years old to 30 cases per year in those 70-79 years old.[4] The two estimates for biopsy-proven cases are quite similar. It is clear that the incidence increases dramatically with age.

Clinical Manifestations. The diagnosis of temporal arteritis should be obvious if an elderly patient presents with headache, visual disturbance, fever and a palpably tender temporal artery. Most cases, however, have a less distinctive presentation. The occurrence of clinical symptoms in temporal arteritis is outlined in Table 1.

Table 1

Symptom	At Initial Presentation (%)	Occurrence During Disease Course (%)
Headache	32	60
Polymyalgia rheumatica	25	45
Fever	15	45
Visual symptoms	7	22
Weakness/malaise	5	35
Jaw claudication	2	40
Weight loss/anorexia	2	45
Visual loss	1	25
Limb claudication	—	21
Depression	—	25

Sensitivity of Symptoms for Temporal Arteritis

Data from Calamia and Hunder,[1] Huston et al,[4] Goodman,[5] Bengtsson,[6] Fernandez-Herlihy.[9]

The onset of the illness is abrupt in about one third of patients. In most patients, the more gradual development of symptoms leads to delayed or missed diagnoses until significant morbidity has occurred. In the case discussed, the onset of her illness was probably gradually manifested by fatigue, weight loss and depression. However, the onset of visual disturbance and jaw claudication was fairly abrupt, causing her to seek medical attention within a week of the development of symptoms.

Headache as a symptom of temporal arteritis is generally different than any type of headache experienced previously by a patient. The location is often unilateral and temporal, leading to a prompt diagnosis. Often, however, the headache can be frontal, global or poorly localized. It is important to emphasize that headache is a very nonspecific symptom. The majority of elderly patients with headache will not have temporal arteritis. More importantly, as indicated in Table 1, the majority of patients with temporal arteritis will not have headache as the presenting symptom.[11]

Polymyalgia Rheumatica. Polymyalgia rheumatica is a clinical syndrome defined by myalgia in a proximal shoulder and hip girdle distribution. Morning stiffness is often present. Many patients will have an associated subdeltoid bursitis. Patients may become considerably disabled, with difficulty abducting the shoulders and flexing and externally rotating the hips. Their functional limitations will include difficulty reaching for objects, getting dressed, and rising from a chair or toilet. If unrecognized, it can cause considerable disability in the elderly, forcing some patients to consider a change in their home setting. A careful physical examination may establish that the functional limitation is from muscle pain and stiffness, and not from loss of motor strength.

Polymyalgia rheumatica is important to recognize because the disability can be completely reversed with low-doses of corticosteroids. It is important to recognize that polymyalgia rheumatica may be the presenting complaint in about one-fourth of patients with temporal arteritis. The majority of the time, however, polymyalgia rheumatica will occur as an isolated syndrome.

Fever in Temporal Arteritis. Fever is a common complaint in patients with temporal arteritis and may be seen in up to 50% of cases. In general, the fever is low-grade and accompanied by more typical symptoms such as headache or visual abnormality. In some patients, the fever is accompanied solely by constitutional symptoms such as fatigue or weight loss. Rather than occurring in a characteristic pattern, fever may be intermittent, recurring or sustained, and as high as 103.6°F.[1]

In one reported series of 100 biopsy-proven cases, fever was present in 42% of patients. Fifteen patients met the classic criteria for fever of unknown origin. In four of these patients, temporal artery biopsy was performed after a thorough clinical evaluation failed to identify symptoms or signs suggestive of temporal arteritis.[12]

In another series of 74 biopsy-proven cases, 12 patients presented with fever of unknown origin, and another 7 patients presented with low-grade fever, anorexia, malaise and weight loss. In the group of 12 patients who lacked major constitutional symptoms other than fever, the fevers were intermittent, and as high as 103°F. In one patient, the fever was persistent and lasted 5 months before diagnosis and initiation of proper therapy.[13] It is clear from these reports that fever may be an underappreciated symptom of temporal arteritis. Unexplained fever in an elderly patient should lead to consideration of temporal arteritis even if other features of the disorder are lacking.

Loss of Vision in Temporal Arteritis. Visual symptoms can occur in up to 30% of patients with temporal arteritis. Typically, patients complain of blurring, diplopia or amaurosis fugax. In one series, unilateral loss of vision had occurred in 7% of patients at the time of diagnosis.[14] In general, visual loss is not the first manifestation of arteritis, and other symptoms of temporal arteritis precede loss of vision by one to several months. In the majority of patients with irreversible visual loss, transient visual symptoms such as diplopia or amaurosis fugax precede the loss by one to several days. In patients with unilateral loss of vision, subsequent involvement of the other side can occur within a few hours or days of the initial loss. In patients with temporal arteritis, visual symptoms are best considered medical emergencies.

Systemic Symptoms is Temporal Arteritis. Constitutional symptoms occur quite frequently in temporal arteritis. Weakness, malaise, weight loss, anorexia and depression occur singly or in combination in virtually all patients. These symptoms can occur in the absence of polymyalgia rheumatica. In general, they are sufficiently nonspecific so that the diagnosis of temporal arteritis is not considered in the absence of a more definitive symptom. In the case presented, the patient complained of malaise, weight loss, fatigue and depression for several months prior to the onset of jaw claudication and visual disturbance. In all likelihood, temporal arteritis was present during that period of time.

Jaw Claudication. Intermittent claudication occurs as a result of narrowing of muscle nutrient arteries. Most often, it involves the muscles of mastication, resulting in jaw claudication. This symptom is pathognomonic for temporal arteritis and is the symptom that most likely will precede blindness. Jaw claudication, though present in up to 40% of patients, may be overlooked if the patient is not directly questioned about the presence of jaw pain or fatigue while chewing. Jaw claudication must be carefully differentiated from pain in the temporomandibular joint that might be experienced by opening and closing the mouth.

Claudication occurring during repeated swallowing may occur in the muscles of deglutition, and tongue claudication may occur with protracted talking. Limb claudication may occur if large arteries such as the subclavian, brachial or femoral arteries are involved. Patients with extremity involvement may develop symptoms suggestive of thoracic outlet syndrome or aortoiliac atherosclerosis.[18]

Table 2

Sensitivity of Physical Examination for Temporal Arteritis

Symptom	At Initial Presentation (%)	Occurrence During Disease Course (%)
Tender artery	3	37
Decreased pulse	–	50
Nodular artery	–	29
Scalp tenderness	–	50

Data from Calamia and Hunder,[1] Huston et al,[4] Goodman,[5] Bengtsson,[6] Fernandez-Herlihy.[9]

Physical Examination. In general, the physical examination in patients with temporal arteritis is not as helpful in making the diagnosis as the history or laboratory evaluation. The most common physical abnormalities are summarized in Table 2. Scalp tenderness to palpation and a tender or nodular artery are the most commonly reported findings. The pulse may be diminished, but in the elderly that may be a finding even in the absence of temporal arteritis.

Ophthalmologic examination is generally normal in the absence of visual loss, and may be normal even in the presence of a visual deficit. Pallor of the disc or other signs of optic neuritis may be present if there has been ischemia to the retina. The arterioles generally are normal since the vasculitis does not affect such small-caliber vessels.

The musculoskeletal examination may be abnormal if polymyalgia rheumatica is present. Typical findings include reduced range of motion in the shoulders. Shoulder abduction is particularly difficult. Patients with polymyalgia also have difficulty rising from a chair because of hip girdle stiffness. If carefully examined, however, the strength of isolated muscle groups can be shown to be intact.

Pathophysiology. When present, the histopathological findings of temporal arteritis are quite typical and indicative of a granulomatous vasculitis. A positive biopsy will usually show intimal fibrosis and thickening, disruption of the internal elastic membrane, and mononuclear cell infiltration of the media of the arterial wall. Granulomas composed of monocytes, lymphocytes and plasma cells are seen associated with the characteristic multinucleated giant cells.[15] The giant cells are often seen in association with fragments of the internal elastic membrane. There is some suggestion that the giant cells actually phagocytose elastic tissue.

A recent study suggests that infiltrating cells in the arterial wall consist predominantly of macrophages which express HLA-DR and T lymphocytes of the CD4 subset. B cells are quite rare and K cells are not present. Interleukin-2 receptor expression was observed in 87.5% of biopsy specimens. In specimens obtained after therapy with steroids, only 14% of specimens contained such receptors.[28] This suggests that steroids do not initially modify cellular distribution, but rather interrupt certain immunologic functions.

Some changes seen in atherosclerosis or normal aged arteries can superficially resemble arteritis. Intimal thickening, fragmentation and calcification of elastic tissue, and patchy adventitial inflammation can be seen in arteries of normal older adults. It is therefore important that the specimens be carefully and thoroughly evaluated. Giant cells, though quite characteristic, may not always be present. Some authors label as "probable" specimens that show transmural lymphohistiocytic infiltrates without giant cells.[8]

One study reports finding evidence of inflammation in only 24% of temporal artery specimens from patients who were felt on clinical grounds to have temporal arteritis, and whose symptoms responded to steroid therapy.[16] Other authors, however, have attributed such findings to the presence of "skip lesions".[17] Such lesions are defined as being present when one or more sections of the artery appear normal, while other sections of the same artery have features characteristic of arteritis. The size of the specimen and the handling of the sections are probably of great importance if false- negative interpretations are to be avoided. A minimum specimen of 1 cm is recommended, and specimens up to 3 cm are preferred.

Specific clinical symptoms of temporal arteritis correlate with the anatomic distribution of the vasculitis. The vessel inflammation leads to compromised blood flow. Often thrombosis may be found at the site of ongoing inflammation.

Blood flow to the optic nerve or retina can be compromised by vasculitic lesions in the arteries supplying the eye. The main blood supply to the eye is the ophthalmic artery, which arises from the internal carotid artery.[14] The central retinal artery supplies the retina and the posterior ciliary arteries supply the optic nerve head. Any or all of these branches of the ophthalmic artery can be involved resulting in infarction of the optic nerve head. If all three posterior ciliary arteries are involved, then loss of vision will be complete. If only one artery is involved, there will be partial defects. Involvement of the central retinal artery will cause ischemic retinopathy with visual loss dependent upon the extent of damage.

Infarction of other tissues of the head and neck can occur. Lingual artery involvement can produce tongue infarction. Interestingly, there is no greater incidence of stroke, since the vasculitis generally spares the intracranial arteries. One series reported involvement of the aorta or its major branches in 15% of patients. Such lesions led to aortic rupture or dissection, myocardial infarction and involvement of the renal arteries.[18] Such complications are generally unusual.

Laboratory Diagnosis. The best screening test for temporal arteritis is the erythrocyte sedimentation rate. The Westergren method is preferred, since most of the published literature is based on this method.[19] It also has the advantage of a greater range, which is useful since some patients with temporal arteritis have an

ESR over 100 mm/hr. The upper limit of normal is generally considered to be 20 mm/hr. In the elderly, however, the sedimentation rate may normally be as high as 40 mm/hr.[20] In general, 30 mm/hr can be considered abnormal, and most patients with temporal arteritis will have values over 50 mm/hr.

In general, the sedimentation rate is an excellent screening test for temporal arteritis, with a sensitivity approaching 100%. Rarely, biopsy-proven cases with visual loss and a normal ESR have been reported.[7] Nonetheless, if the ESR rate is normal, then the likelihood of temporal arteritis is very low.

As might be expected, the ESR is not very specific for the diagnosis of temporal arteritis. Many different conditions can produce elevation of the ESR. These include infectious, inflammatory, and rheumatic disorders. Many of these conditions may mimic temporal arteritis. In clinical practice, a normal ESR, effectively rules out the presence of temporal arteritis. An intermediate elevation is nonspecific and the diagnosis may need to be pursued with further testing. It is the marked elevation (over 50 mm/hr) in ESR, that most strongly indicates the presence of temporal arteritis in the appropriate clinical setting. As discussed below, temporal artery biopsy is the confirmatory diagnostic test that is usually considered when the screening sedimentation rate is either moderately or markedly increased.

Temporal Artery Biopsy. A temporal artery biopsy is a relatively simple outpatient procedure. A sampling of the superficial temporal artery can readily be obtained under local anesthesia. A 2-4 cm sample should be obtained with ligation of the remaining artery. There are no clinical consequences to the procedure, and even elderly patients with chronic medical problems should tolerate it well.

The sensitivity and specificity of the temporal artery biopsy for the diagnosis of temporal arteritis may be overstated since it is the "gold standard" and most clinical series are predicated on the finding of a positive biopsy. As previously mentioned, certain findings, such as inflammation of the arterial wall, and disruption of the internal elastic membrane, are very suggestive. The presence of multinucleated giant cells is pathognomonic, but not always present. If all three findings are present, the specificity of biopsy diagnosis should be 99% and there should not be any false positives.

The sensitivity of the biopsy is quite variable in the literature, ranging from 50 to 90%, probably as a result of variations in surgical technique and pathologic interpretation.[21-24] The utility of the biopsy is therefore not perfect, and in most hospitals there will be false negatives. In part this may also be due to the previously mentioned skip areas of normal artery in pathologic specimens. In approximately 30% of specimens, characteristic pathologic findings are seen only after examination of multiple transverse or longitudinal sections. Thus, biopsy length and the number of sections examined may influence the result. About 5% of patients are felt to have unilateral arteritis and the wrong artery may have been sampled. With all of these considerations, in most hospitals, the sensitivity of the procedure will be about 70%. Adherence to strict clinical and research protocols and biopsy of the contralateral artery could increase this to approximately 95%.

Angiography has been used to try to make the diagnosis or identify specific areas of artery to be biopsied. In general, however, it is more uncomfortable than temporal artery biopsy. It probably does not add much beyond a careful physical examination.

Other laboratory tests have been found to be abnormal in a majority of patients with temporal arteritis. These include the hematocrit, platelet count, serum protein electrophoresis, and alkaline phosphatase. In general, however, these tests lack sufficient sensitivity or specificity to be clinically useful in establishing or excluding the diagnosis. Hypochromic or microcytic anemia is particularly common, suggesting many other possible diagnoses in the elderly. It is critical, therefore, that the history first establish temporal arteritis as a diagnostic possibility.

Diagnostic Strategies. Temporal arteritis is a diagnosis that must be made as early as possible given the possible severe morbidity and the fact that blindness is completely preventable with timely and proper treatment. However, temporal arteritis is a challenging disorder to diagnose clinically. Headache, is the symptom usually associated with the disorder, but is a very nonspecific complaint. In fact, recent onset of headache was no more prevalent in biopsy- positive cases than in those whose biopsy was negative.[9]

Certain symptoms when found in clusters would seem to more strongly support the possibility of temporal arteritis. Jaw claudication in particular is quite specific for temporal arteritis and also often precedes actual visual loss. Polymyalgia rheumatica, a tender or swollen temporal artery and visual loss are also symptoms that are highly correlated with a positive biopsy. Unless several specific findings are present, most often the clinical situation is uncertain and in an elderly patient the differential diagnosis is quite broad.

If temporal arteritis is a reasonable diagnostic possibility at all, the sedimentation rate is the first step in laboratory diagnosis. Selection of patients for biopsy can then be done as discussed previously.

Though there is some debate over the sensitivity of the temporal artery biopsy, it is the test of choice following the ESR.[21,22] Even when the diagnosis seems assured on clinical grounds alone, biopsy is still useful for confirmation so that both the physician and the patient will be comfortable continuing therapy if treatment complications ensue. The biopsy is a simple and safe procedure and should be performed if temporal arteritis is suspected. In a patient over 50 with an ESR over 50 mm/hr and any suggestive symptom such as recent onset of headache, jaw claudication, visual change, scalp tenderness, unexplained fever or anemia or a tender temporal artery, the biopsy should be pursued. If the biopsy is done well and is negative then the diagnosis should be reconsidered. With a negative biopsy there is still a 5-10% chance of establishing the diagnosis with a biopsy of the contralateral artery.

In an elderly patient complaining of stiffness and proximal myalgia the diagnosis of polymyalgia rheumatica should be considered. An elevated ESR would make this diagnosis quite likely. If any of the symptoms of temporal arteritis present, then a biopsy would be indicated. In an otherwise asymptomatic patient with polymyalgia rheumatica the likelihood of an associated temporal arteritis is probably under 20%. Since the patient will probably be treated with low doses of corticosteroids, a temporal artery biopsy in this setting is not routine.

Management. Corticosteroids are the drug of choice for temporal arteritis and should be instituted as soon as the diagnosis is made, either clinically or by biopsy. Since visual loss can be sudden and permanent, steroids should be started pending the results of a biopsy if the clinical suspicion is strong. In particular, jaw claudication in an elderly patient with an elevated ESR should be treated immediately, while arrangements are made for biopsy confirmation. Treatment with steroids probably does not alter the biopsy findings as long as biopsy is done within a week of starting treatment.[9] Biopsies can be done within 48 hr in most institutions.

The usual steroid dosage is 40 mg of prednisone once daily. In general, this dose will prevent vascular complications and rapidly make the patient asymptomatic. If there have been visual symptoms, then up to 60 mg can be used. If there has been recent visual loss, then parenteral steroids every 6 hr can be tried initially to see if any improvement can be obtained. If the initial dosage does not result in rapid symptomatic improvement, a higher dose can be utilized.

The patient should be continued on the lowest effective dose of prednisone for about a month. Close clinical follow-up and laboratory monitoring consisting of blood counts and ESR are important. If the patient is relatively asymptomatic and the laboratory parameters have normalized, then a slow and steady taper of the steroids can be attempted. The dose can generally can be reduced by 5 mg every week to ten days until the 20 mg level is reached. At that point, decrements are made in 2.5 mg intervals. At a 10 mg dosage, decrements of 1 mg may be necessary.

Patients who have responded should continue to be followed both clinically and with periodic determinations of the ESR. Relapses occasionally occur, particularly if the steroid taper has been too rapid. If relapse occurs, treatment should be reinstituted in a higher dosage. Very rarely, patients suffer a vascular complication while on therapy. Although treatment can be tapered and stopped in some patients within six months, many patients will require at least a year of treatment.

Complications of Therapy. The elderly seem more prone to complications of corticosteroid treatment. These include thinning of the skin, bruising, worsening of cataracts and osteoporosis with vertebral collapse. In one five-year follow-up study, patients treated with steroids had a six-fold increase in fractures and a four-fold increase in cataracts when compared to age-matched controls.[8] Treatment with calcium, 1000 mg per day, and vitamin D, 50,000 units three times a week, has been used for patients with rheumatoid arthritis to prevent steroid-induced osteopenia. Whether this regimen would be effective in the elderly is unknown. The high rate of steroid complications makes a positive biopsy reassuring in the face of the need for continued treatment.

A difficult clinical problem can arise when an elderly patient develops significant complications of steroid therapy or the treatment seriously interferes with the control of diabetes. If the patient is asymptomatic, then a rapid taper can be attempted. The ESR may not be the best guide in these circumstances, and the patient should be carefully assessed clinically. If there is clear need for continuing treatment, then methotrexate,[25] azathioprine,[26] and cyclosporine[27] have all been described as being effective as steroid-sparing agents. The numbers of patients studied with steroid-sparing immunosuppressive regimens are small.

The Case in Context. This patient had many features characteristic of temporal arteritis. Her jaw claudication and visual disturbance were symptoms very suggestive of temporal arteritis. Her complaints of fatigue, malaise and weight loss were very nonspecific. In all likelihood, arteritis was present in the weeks or months preceding the onset of jaw claudication. Diagnosis at that early stage would have been difficult, but an ESR might have been helpful.

Interestingly, she had no complaint of headache or any symptoms suggestive of polymyalgia rheumatica. Her temporal arteries were normal to physical examination. In the setting of jaw claudication and an elevated ESR, it would have been most appropriate to begin steroid therapy while arranging consultation and temporal artery biopsy. Her biopsy did not show characteristic giant cells, but otherwise was quite consistent with temporal arteritis.

The patient's symptoms responded nicely to the steroid therapy. The HCT and ESR normalized rapidly. Her weight increased. However, she developed emotional lability, probably due to the high dose of prednisone. At this point, the steroid should be rapidly tapered to a dose that could be better tolerated. If the psychiatric symptoms persisted, then consultation with a geriatric psychiatrist might be appropriate.

References

1. Calamia K, Hunder G: Clinical manifestations of giant cell (temporal) arteritis. Clin Rheum Dis. 1980;6:389-403.
2. Fauchald P, Rygvald B, Systease, B: Temporal arteritis and polymyalgia rheumatica. Ann Intern Med. 1982;77:845-852.
3. Bengtsson B-A, Malmvall BE: The epidemiology of giant cell arteritis including temporal arteritis and polymyalgia rheumatica. Arthritus Rheum. 1981;24:895-904.
4. Huston K, Hunder G, et al: Temporal arteritis. A 25-year epidemiologic, clinical and pathologic study. Ann Intern Med. 1978;88:162-167.
5. Goodman B: Temporal arteritis. Am J Med. 1979;67:839-852.
6. Bengtsson B-A: Clinical manifestations of giant cell arteritis. Acta Med Scand Suppl. 1982;658:18-28.
7. Biller J, Asconape J, et al: Temporal arteritis associated with normal sedimentation rate. JAMA. 1982; 247:486-487.

8. Robb-Nicholson C, Chang RW, et al: Diagnostic value of the history and examination in giant cell arteritis: A clinical pathological study of 81 temporal artery biopsies. J Rheumatol. 1988;15:1793-1796.

9. Fernandez-Herlihy L: Temporal arteritis: Clinical aids to diagnosis. J Rheumatol. 1988; 15:1797-1801.

10. Klein R, Hunder G, et al: Larger artery involvement in giant cell (temporal) arteritis. Ann Intern Med. 1975;83:806-812.

11. Editorial: Mr. Rumbold's headache. Lancet. 1982;2:858-859.

12. Calamia K, Hunder G: Giant cell arteritis (temporal arteritis) presenting as fever of undetermined origin. Arthritis Rheum. 1981;24:1414-1418.

13. Healey L, Wilske K: Presentation of occult giant cell arteritis. Arthritis Rheum. 1980; 23:641-643.

14. Bengtsson B-A: Eye complications in giant cell arteritis. Acta Med Scand Suppl. 1982; 658:38-43.

15. Editorial: Temporal artery biopsy. Lancet. 1983;1:396-397.

16. Allsop C, Gallagher P: Temporal artery biopsy in giant-cell arteritis. Am J Surg Pathol. 1981;5:317-323.

17. Klein R, Campbell RT, et al: Skip lesions in temporal arteritis. Mayo Clin Proc. 1979; 51:504-510.

18. Klein R, Hunder G, et al: Larger artery involvement in giant cell (temporal) arteritis. Ann Intern Med. 1975;83:806-812.

19. Kantor S: Temporal arteritis, in Griner P, Panzer R, Black E (eds): Diagnostic Strategies for Common Medical Problems. American College of Physicians 1991, in press.

20. Bedell S, Bush B: Erythrocyte sedimentation rate from folklore to facts. Am J Med. 1985;78:1001-1009.

21. Hall S, Hunder G: Is temporal artery biopsy prudent? Mayo Clin Proc. 1984;59:793-796.

22. Hall S, Lie JT, et al: The therapeutic impact of temporal artery biopsy. Lancet. 1983; 2:1217-1220.

23. Albert DM, Hedges TR III: The significance of negative temporal artery biopsies. Trans Am Ophthalmol Soc. 1982;80:143-154.

24. Ponge T, Barrier JH, et al: The efficacy of selective unilateral temporal artery biopsy versus bilateral biopsies for diagnosis of giant cell arteritis. J Rheumatol. 1988;15:997-1000.

25. Krall P, Mazanec D, Wilke W: Methotrexate for corticosteroid resistant polymyalgia rheumatica and giant cell arteritis. Cleveland Clin J Med. 1989;56:253-257.

26. Silva M, Hazleman B: Azathioprine in giant cell arteritis polymyalgia rheumatica: A double blind study. Ann Rheum Dis. 1986;45:136-138.

27. Wendling D, Hory B, Blanc D: Cyclosporine: A new adjuvant therapy for giant cell arteritis? (letter). Arthritis Rheum. 1985;28:1078-1079.

28. Cid M, Campo E, Ercilla G, et al: Immunohistochemical analysis of lymphoid and macrophage cell subsets and their immunologic activation markers in temporal arteritis. Influence of corticosteroid treatment. Arthritis Rheum. 1989;32:884-893.

Case 15

Evaluation After Acute Myocardial Infarction

James M. Ryan, MD, FACC

Case History

A 57-year-old local business executive had been in excellent health his entire life until the day of admission. On that day, he had worked his usual day at the office, and exercised for 90 minutes at his local health club as he had done three times weekly for the previous five years. Later that evening, he and his wife dined out, and both retired for the night at their usual time. At 3:00 am, he awoke with an uncomfortable heavy burning feeling in his chest. He was unable to sleep, and thinking he had a severe case of indigestion, took several doses of antacids throughout the rest of the night with no significant relief. Unable to sleep, he eventually showered, dressed and left for work at 7:00 am. Later that morning, he spoke with his wife by telephone and told her never to make reservations at the same restaurant again, and explained his miserable night in detail. His wife, a secretary at a physician's office, became quite concerned about his symptoms and demanded that he see his physician immediately.

Despite feeling much better, he made an appointment and saw his doctor later that afternoon. In the physician's office, an ECG showed evidence for an evolving inferior myocardial infarction, and he was immediately transferred by squad to the Ohio State University Hospital emergency room where a second ECG confirmed the likelihood of an acute myocardial infarction. By the time of his arrival, the patient was pain-free with stable vital signs. The ECG showed deep inferior Q waves in leads II, III, and AVF, with residual ST elevation in these leads of 1.5 mm. Precordial T wave inversions were also noted in V1 through V4. Due to the late presentation (at least 12 hours after onset of symptoms), a lack of ongoing chest pain, and an ECG consistent with a completed event, a decision was made not to treat with a thrombolytic agent or to proceed with urgent cardiac catheterization, and the patient was admitted to the coronary care unit.

Further historical points of interest included a family history of atherosclerotic coronary artery disease. The patient's father died from a myocardial infarction at age 65, and his older brother underwent coronary artery bypass grafting at age 61. The patient was a nonsmoker, and had no history of diabetes or hypertension. One total cholesterol level checked four years earlier was "normal" at 270. The patient's past medical history and review of symptoms were otherwise unremarkable.

Physical Examination. On physical examination, his pulse was 80 and regular and his blood pressure was 130/60. The head and neck exam was normal. His lungs were clear. Cardiovascular exam revealed a normal jugular venous pulse and normal carotid upstrokes. The precordium was normal to palpation. S1 and S2 were both normal, and a soft S4 gallop was noted. A grade II/VI holosystolic murmur was found at the apex. His abdominal, musculoskeletal and neurologic exams were normal. All baseline laboratory work was normal, and the chest radiograph showed no abnormalities. However, CPK enzymes rose to a peak of 2,100 with 16% MB fraction before returning to normal 72 hours after admission.

While in the CCU, he was treated with bed rest, supplemental oxygen, intravenous nitroglycerin, and beta blockade. His immediate post-myocardial infarction course was uncomplicated and he was transferred to the stepdown unit for progressive cardiac rehabilitation three days after admission.

On day seven, the patient underwent a submaximal exercise study. He was allowed to complete state II of the Bruce protocol and achieved a heart rate of 110, 60% of his age-predicted maximum. The patient did note mild "chest heaviness", in stage II, and his ECG demonstrated 2.0 mm of horizontal ST segment depression in leads V1 through V5. No ventricular ectopy was noted. Thallium-201 was injected at peak exercise, and thallium images demonstrated partial redistribution of defects in the inferior and posterior walls, with complete redistribution in the septum and anterior walls. Impressive lung uptake of thallium was also noted.

As a result of the exercise thallium study, a cardiac catheterization was performed the following day. Left ventriculography demonstrated reduced left ventricular function with hypokinesia of the inferior wall and mild mitral regurgitation. The ejection fraction calculated at 40%. Coronary arteriography revealed total occlusion of the proximal right coronary artery, with collaterals from the left coronary system. The left anterior descending artery had a 99% proximal stenosis, and significant branch vessel disease was noted in the circumflex vessel.

Thus, this middle-aged businessman had suffered an acute inferior infarction and had three-vessel coronary disease with reduced left ventricular function. The exercise study demonstrated ongoing ischemia at a relatively low exercise level. He was felt to be at high risk for a second cardiac event, and his physicians recommended coronary bypass surgery despite his recent myocardial infarction. A three-vessel coronary bypass was successful, and his recovery was uneventful. He has subsequently returned to work and remains active and asymptomatic two years following surgery.

Discussion

Despite a continued fall in the death rate from coronary artery disease in the 1970s and 1980s, coronary disease is likely to remain the leading cause of death in the 1990s. As we enter this new decade, the projected number of individuals who will suffer a myocardial infarction is 1.5 million per year, with 500,000 yearly deaths from coronary disease expected.[1] Historically, following a first myocardial infarction, the risk of death in the first 24 hours is 25-40%. Of those patients reaching the hospital, 10-15% die before discharge. Following hospital discharge, the death rate falls to an annual rate of 10% for the first six months and then stabilizes at 3-5% per year.[2,3] Thus, although the rate of death from a first myocardial infarction is highest prior to hospital discharge, a large number of patients will die in the following five years, especially in the first few months after discharge. It should be emphasized that the above figures represent only the risk of death after a first myocardial infarction and do not include patients with prior myocardial infarctions. If the figures for hospitalization due to reinfarction, congestive heart failure, or arrhythmia are combined with statistics for cardiac death, the total mortality and morbidity is staggering.

Selection of Patients for Catheterization. Fortunately, not all patients with a recent myocardial infarction are at significant risk for a second cardiac event. Risk appears to be a function of the degree of left ventricular dysfunction, the amount of residual ischemic myocardium, and the potential for ventricular arrhythmia. Not surprisingly, some "high-risk" patients can be identified by clinical parameters alone. Clinical markers such as congestive heart failure, postinfarction angina, and complex ventricular arrhythmia have been demonstrated to be predictive of poor outcome. However, the ability to separate other "high-risk" patients from "low-risk" patients cannot be done on clinical grounds alone. Since it has been well established that coronary bypass surgery can prolong life[4,5,6] and since advances in percutaneous transluminal technology continue to occur, it becomes increasingly important to identify those patients who might benefit most from revascularization. At the same time, it is equally important to identify the lower-risk population who can be spared the risk and expense of invasive procedures. Moreover, while cardiac catheterization accurately identifies left ventricular function and coronary anatomy, it as yet cannot provide adequate information regarding ischemic or arrhythmic potential. Furthermore, it is simply not reasonable or possible to send all postinfarction patients for catheterization prior to hospital discharge.

There is little question that those individuals suffering from congestive heart failure, hypotension, or recurrent angina after infarction are at highest risk and should undergo early catheterization prior to hospital discharge for the purpose of defining therapeutic options. However, since 75% of all hospitalized patients with an acute myocardial infarction have an uncomplicated course, it would be beneficial to direct only the "high risk" patients to early catheterization. It is within this framework that exercise evaluation with and without nuclear imaging has become a useful method in identifying critical prognostic factors prior to hospital discharge in the postinfarction patient.

Risk Stratification Using Exercise Testing. Despite early concerns, numerous studies have demonstrated that submaximal exercise electrocardiography can be performed safely within five to seven days of acute infarction.[7-15] These same studies clearly demonstrated that significant prognostic information could be identified with such submaximal testing. In the above studies, each of the following factors was found to carry significant prognostic value: Poor exercise capacity (i.e. a work load of < 5.0 mets), exercise induced angina, exercise-induced ST segment changes, abnormal blood pressure response to exercise, and exercise-induced complex ventricular arrhythmia. Although each of these parameters may yield statistically significant prognostic data, large numbers of patients with "normal" submaximal exercise studies still suffer early cardiac events post myocardial infarction. Fortunately, the improved ability of exercise nuclear imaging techniques to detect ischemia and identify multivessel disease can lead to improved risk stratification.

Thallium Exercise Testing. In 1983, Gibson published an important prospective study comparing the prognostic utility of exercise thallium criteria to exercise electrocardiography and cardiac catheterization in patients who had had uncomplicated transmural myocardial infarction and who were followed at least 15 months[16]. He noted that while the development of angina and/or ST segment depression on a predischarge submaximal exercise study did identify a population of patients at increased risk for future cardiac events (49-73%), 26% of cardiac events occurred in patients who developed neither angina nor ST segment changes (Fig. 1). Thus, while submaximal, nonnuclear, exercise electrocardiography can be helpful in identifying increased risk, it is not sensitive enough to identify all patients at increased risk or to identify those who are at lower risk.

On the other hand, when he used thallium scintigraphic criteria to identify underlying multivessel disease (multiple thallium defects), exercise-induced ischemia (thallium redistribution), and/or evidence for left ventricular dysfunction (thallium lung update), high-risk populations with event rates from 59 to 86% could be identified. Of equal importance was the finding that individuals with one vascular defect, no ischemia, and no evidence of left ventricular dysfunction—the low-risk population—had an event rate of only 6%. Thus, thallium scintigraphy not only identified the high-risk group, it accurately separated out the low-risk group as well (Fig. 2).

Risk Stratification Using Angiography. In comparison, when coronary anatomy alone was used to risk-stratify, patients with two- and three-vessel disease did have a significant risk for cardiac events (47 and 42%), but the group initially considered to be at lower risk (those with single vessel disease) also had a 22% event rate. Thus, coronary arteriography, like exercise electrocardiography, failed to adequately separate the low-risk population from those at high risk (Fig. 3). Surpris-

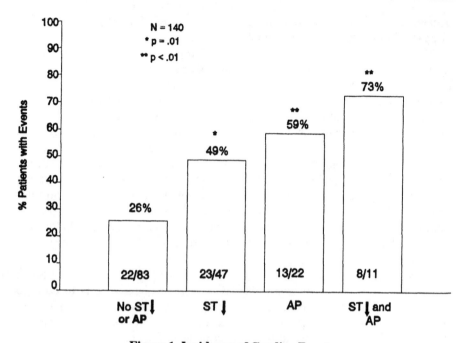

Figure 1. Incidence of Cardiac Events
Based on the presence or absence of exercise-induced ST segment depression (ST ↓) or angina pectoris (AP). Reprinted with permission of Circulation and the authors.[16]

ingly, left ventricular ejection fraction (by resting radionuclide angiography) had little correlation with future cardiac events.

To summarize, Gibson's work demonstrated that all three diagnostic studies could identify a population at increased risk for future cardiac events, but thallium scintigraphy was far superior in also identifying the low-risk population (Fig. 4). In conclusion, submaximal exercise thallium scintigraphy is an excellent method to risk- stratify patients transmural infarction, and can be used to intelligently direct high-risk patients to early cardiac catheterization, and low-risk patients to hospital discharge.

Exercise Radionuclide Ventriculography. Corbett,[17,18] Wasserman,[19] and Nicod[20] have performed similar risk stratification work post myocardial infarction using exercise radionuclide ventriculography. These studies have indicated that individuals with low ejection fractions (EF < 40%), flat or falling ejection fractions with submaximal exercise, or abnormal left ventricular volume changes with exercise are at higher risk for future cardiac events. As in Gibson's work, the ability to

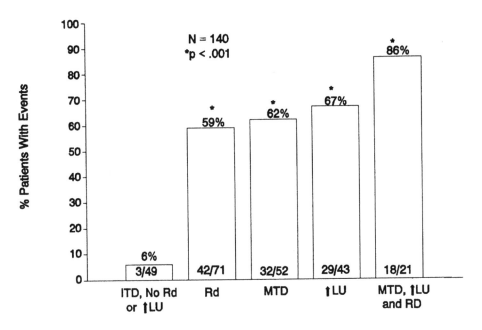

Figure 2. Incidence of Cardiac Events

Based on Tl scintigraphic findings. 1TD, thallium defect in one vasuclar region; Rd, redistribution; MTD, thallium defects involving multiple vascular regions. ↑LU, increased lung uptake of Tl. See text for further explanation. Reprinted with permission of Circulation and the authors.[16]

separate the low- and high-risk patient populations appears far superior with exercise radionuclide ventriculography than with exercise electrocardiography alone. Little comparative work exists between exercise thallium scintigraphy and exercise radionuclide ventriculography for risk stratification post myocardial infarction, but clearly, both are superior to exercise electrocardiography alone.

It should be pointed out that all of the above data were accumulated in the prethrombolytic era for the treatment of acute myocardial infarction. It was not until 1980 that Dewood's[21] landmark publication describing thrombotic occlusion as the etiology of acute infarction forever changed our concept of the pathophysiology of this process. Since that time, scores of studies have been devoted to the treatment of acute coronary thrombosis with numerous thrombolytic agents. Despite the demonstrated efficacy of these agents, early reocclusion has been a persistent problem in up to 20% of patients, especially when high-grade residual

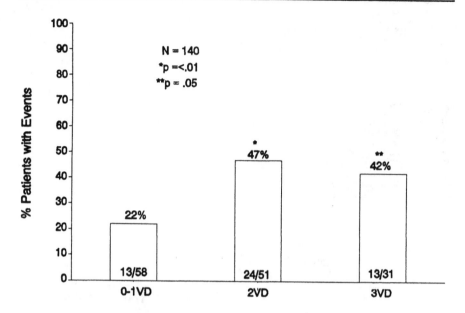

Figure 3. Incidence of Cardiac Events
Based on the extent of angiographic coronary artery disease. VD, vessel disease.
Reprinted with permission of Circulation and the authors.[16]

coronary stenosis remained.[22] As a result of this relatively high reocclusion rate, numerous trials have been conducted employing early recatheterization and angioplasty when indicated to reduce this risk. More recently, the large, randomized TIMI phase II trial demonstrated that after thrombolytic treatment of acute infarction, noninvasive exercise testing followed by appropriately directed cardiac catheterization and revascularization, was of equal efficacy to early catheterization in all patients.[23]

Non-Q Wave Infarction and Future Risk. It should also be noted that all of the above studies concern transmural or Q wave infarctions, as opposed to subendocardial or non-Q wave infarctions. While a large collection of data exists describing the noninvasive evaluation of non-Q wave infarctions with combined exercise and nuclear techniques, it is the author's opinion that such infarctions most often represent subtotal coronary thrombosis, and that the high risk for future total occlusion and subsequent completed transmural infarction deserves urgent cardiac catheterization.

Summary. Using all of the above information it is possible to arrive at a flow chart for the evaluation of a patient post myocardial infarction (Fig. 5). Nontrans-

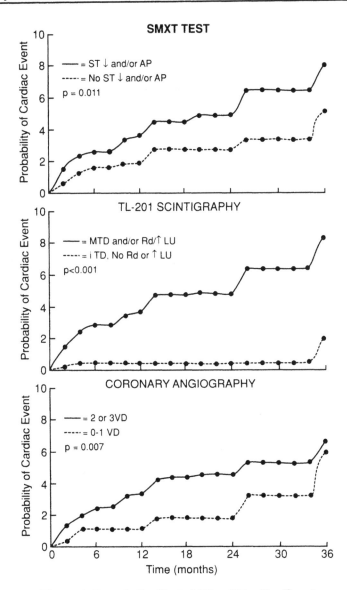

Figure 4. Cumulative Probability of Cardiac Events

As a function of time for different subgroups formed by the exercise test response (top), scintigraphic findings (middle), or angiographic findings (bottom) before hospital discharge. the solid and dashed lines represent the high-risk and low-risk cumulative probability, respectively. Reprinted with permission of Circulation and the authors.[16]

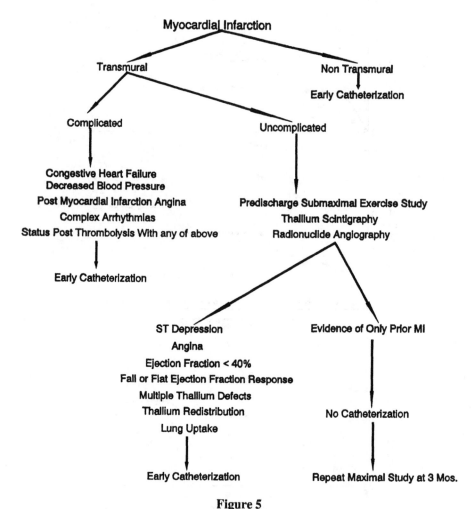

Figure 5

Prognostic approach to the post myocardial infarction patient prior to hospital discharge.

Table 1

High-Risk Criteria for Catheterization

High Risk Exercise ECG Variables Post Infarction
   1. Angina
   2. ST Segment Changes
   3. Low Exercise Tolerance (< 5.0 METS)
   4. Abnormal Blood Pressure Response
   5. Complex Ventricular Arrhythmia

High Risk Exercise Thallium Scintigraphic Variables Post Infarction
   1. Multiple Thallium Defects
   2. Redistribution
   3. Lung Uptake

High Risk Exercise RNA Variables Post Infarction
   1. Ejection Fraction < 40%
   2. Flat or Fall in Ejection Fraction
   3. Increased Systolic and/or Diastolic Volumes

mural and complicated transmural infarctions demand early catheterization. Uncomplicated infarctions require an in-hospital submaximal exercise evaluation, preferably with nuclear cardiac imaging prior to hospital discharge. Those individuals demonstrating any of the high-risk criteria discussed above should go on to catheterization prior to discharge (Table 1). Those with evidence of only their recent infarction, the low-risk population, need not go on to early catheterization and can be safely discharged to return in two to four months for a maximal exercise study.

The patient presented finally sought medical attention 12 hours after the probable onset of acute coronary occlusion. Due to his late and stable presentation, neither thrombolytic therapy nor urgent catheterization was required. His postinfarction hospital course was uncomplicated, and he underwent submaximal exercise thallium scintigraphy prior to discharge. This examination demonstrated numerous high risk criteria, angina at low work load, marked ST segment depression, multiple thallium defects with redistribution and impressive lung uptake. Early catheterization was recommended and subsequent coronary arteriography demonstrated severe three-vessel coronary disease amenable to revascularization with coronary bypass grafting. Due to his perceived increased risk of a future cardiac event, he underwent bypass surgery prior to hospital discharge. His surgical outcome was uneventful and he is presently in excellent health two years following his hospitalization.

References

1. American Heart Association: 1987 Heart Facts. Dallas, Texas, 1986.
2. Luria MH, Knoke JD, Margolis RM, et al: Acute myocardial infarction: Prognosis after recovery. Ann Intern Med. 1976;85:561.
3. Weinblatt E, Shapiro S, Frank CW, et al. Prognosis of men after first myocardial infarction: Mortality and first recurrence in relation to selected parameters. Am J Public Health. 1968;58:1329.
4. Rogers WJ, Russell RO, Foster ED, et al. Coronary artery surgery study (CASS): A randomized trial of coronary bypass surgery. J Am Coll Cardiol. 1984;3:128.
5. Detre KM, Peduzzi P, Takara T, et al: Eleven-year survival in the Veterans Administration's randomized trial of coronary bypass surgery for stable angina. N Engl J Med. 1984;311:1339.
6. Julian DG, Lorimer AR, Oakley CM, et al: Long term results of prospective randomized study of coronary bypass surgery in stable angina pectoris. Lancet. 1982;:1180.
7. Starling MR, Crawford MH, O'Rourke RA, et al: Exercise testing early after myocardial infarction: Predictive value for subsequent unstable angina and death. Am J Cardiol 1980;46:914.
8. Weld FM, King-Lee C, Rolnitzky LM. Risk stratification with low level exercise testing two weeks after acute myocardial infarction. Circulation. 1981;64:314.
9. Fuller CM, Raizner AC, Verani MS: Early post myocardial infarction treadmill testing. Ann Intern Med. 1981;94:739.
10. Debusk RF, Haskell W: Symptom-limited vs. heart-rate-limited exercise testing soon after myocardial infarction. Circulation.1980;61:743.
11. Davidson DM, Debusk RF: Prognostic value of a single exercise test three weeks after uncomplicated myocardial infarction. Circulation.1980;61:242.
12. Koppes GM, Kruger W, Jones FG, et al: Response of exercise early after uncomplicated acute myocardial infarction, long term follow up. Am J Cardiol. 1980;46:769.
13. Theroux P, Waters DD, Mizgala HF: Prognostic value of exercise testing soon after myocardial infarction. N Engl J Med. 1979;301:345.
14 .Sami M, Kraemer N, Debusk R: The prognostic significance of exercise testing after myocardial infarction. Circulation. 1979;60:1246.
15. Smith JW, Dennis CA, Marcus FI: Exercise testing three weeks after myocardial infarction. Chest. 1979;75:16.
16. Gibson RS, Watson DD, Beller GA, et al: Prediction of cardiac events after uncomplicated myocardial infarction: A prospective study comparing predischarge exercise thallium-201 scintigraphy and coronary angiography. Circulation. 1983;68:321-336.
17. Corbett JR, Dehmer GJ, Lewis SE, et al: The prognostic value of submaximal exercise testing with radionuclide ventriculography before hospital discharge in patients with recent myocardial infarction. Circulation. 1981;64:544.
18. Corbett JR, Nicod P, Lewis SE, et al: Prognostic value of submaximal exercise radionuclide ventriculography after myocardial infarction. Am J Cardiol. 1983;52:91A.

19. Wasserman AG, Katz RJ, Cleary P, et al: Noninvasive detection of multivessel disease after myocardial infarction by exercise radionuclide ventriculography. Am J Cardiol. 1982; 50:1247.

20. Nicod P, Corbett JR, Firth BG, et al: Prognostic value of resting and submaximal exercise radionuclide ventriculography after myocardial infarction in high risk patients with single and multivessel disease. Am J Cardiol. 1983;52:91A.

21. Dewood MA, Spres J, Nostske R, et al: Prevalence of total coronary artery occlusion during the early hours of transmural myocardial infarction. N Engl J Med. 1980;303:902.

22. Harrison DG, Ferguson DW, Collins SM, et al: Rethrombosis after reperfusion with streptokinase: Importance of geometry of residual lesions. Circulation. 1984;69:999.

23. The TIMI Study Group: Comparison of invasive and conservative strategies after treatment with intravenous tissue plasminogen activator in acute myocardial infarction. N Engl J Med. 1989;320:627.

Case 16

Unusual Skin Lesions in a Patient with Diarrhea

Scott Miller, MD and Fred Thomas, MD

According to Thomas Jefferson, "The disorders of the human body and the exanthems indicating them are as various as the elements of which it is composed." Nowhere in medicine is this more true than in diseases of the gastrointestinal tract. Diseases of the skin and gastrointestinal tract do not necessarily occur together by mere coincidence. Rather, they may be manifestations of the same entity, or may occur as a consequence of one another. It is an irony of our medical era that, in spite of the fact that the skin is the most observable, readily accessible, easily invadable "window" to the body, physicians frequently fail to see the clues it provides to gastrointestinal diseases. Indeed, the following case illustrates how nearsighted we are in this respect, for rather than providing a reflection of the patient's underlying disease, her skin lesions only served as a draperylike barrier to those initially caring for her.

Case History

A 28-year-old white female from southeastern Ohio presented to the Ohio State University Hospitals (OSUH) emergency room for the evaluation of very large ulcers on her face, extremities, and abdomen. She was in her usual state of what she perceived as excellent health until six weeks prior to admission when she developed an "intestinal flu-like" illness characterized by abdominal cramping, frequent loose watery bowel movements (3-4 times daily), two episodes of frank hematochezia, low-grade fever (100-101°F), and ill-defined arthralgia in her knees, ankles, and wrists. She saw her local physician who treated her for a suspected urinary tract infection on two separate occasions. However, no significant relief was noted by the patient. An IVP 4 weeks before admission was normal. Eight days prior to admission she developed daily fevers to 101°F, orally. She was empirically begun on ampicillin by her physician. Five days prior to admission she developed a painful "pimple" on her left cheek. Over the ensuing four days, this lesion rapidly enlarged and ulcerated. Similar eruptions subsequently occurred over her scalp, abdomen, and lower extremities. These lesions ranged in size from a nickel to a quarter. She was eventually admitted to her local hospital and started on Penicillin G intravenously with no significant improvement in either her fever or the skin lesions. She was then transferred to OSUH for further evaluation. On admission, she denied nausea, vomiting, headaches, or abdominal pain, and no longer complained of joint pain. Her initial diarrheal symptoms were not elicited by her physician. She had no unusual exposure to infectious diseases except that, approximately eight weeks earlier, she had participated in the Ohio State Fair sheep exhibit. Additionally, she had a pet dog and rabbit at home.

Past medical history included surgery for repair of a perforated viscus after a motor vehicle accident three years prior to admission. She was on no additional medications and denied any allergies. Her family history was not remarkable. Specifically, none of her family members had been ill with similar symptoms and none had had any significant gastrointestinal disease. Her social history was remarkable for her occupation as a sheep farmer. She denied alcohol or illicit drug use. Review of systems was otherwise not remarkable.

Physical Examination. On physical exam, she was a pleasant, thin female in no acute distress. Her blood pressure was 110/76 mm Hg, respiratory rate 24/minute, and pulse 120/minute. Her HEENT exam showed a 0.5-cm flat ulcerated lesion in her right buccal mucosa. Her integument exam demonstrated necrotic, exudative ulcers with surrounding violaceous induration and edema on her face, abdomen, scalp, and lower extremities. These ulcerations ranged in size from 0.5 to 1.5 cm with the largest ones appearing over her left cheek and right mandible (Fig. 1). She also had several other smaller pustules on an erythematous base scattered elsewhere. Her lungs were clear to auscultation and percussion. The heart rhythm was regular with a normal S_1 and S_2 and no murmurs were present. There was no lymphadenopathy present. Examination of the abdomen revealed mild tenderness to palpation in the left upper quadrant. Her bowel sounds were normal. Rectal exam was normal, but the stool was hemoccult positive. Her extremities were normal with the exception of the ulcerative lesions. The neurologic exam was normal.

Laboratory Data. WBC 13,600/mm^3, (28% bands, 38% neutrophils with toxic granulation), hemoglobin 9.6 gm/dl, hematocrit 27.3%, platelet count 523,000/mm^3, sodium 139 mEq/dl, potassium 3.6 mEq/dl, chloride 105 mEq/dl, CO_2 23 mEq/dl, BUN 6 mg/dl, creatinine 0.6 mg/dl, glucose 104 mg/dl, AST 40 U/liter, ALT 44 U/liter, LDH 138 U/liter, total bilirubin 1.3 mg/dl, alkaline phosphatase 168 U/liter, erythrocyte sedimentation rate (Westergren) 54, C reactive protein 2.1 mg/dl, rheumatoid factor negative, ANA 1:20. Urinalysis revealed 1+ blood, sp. gr. 1.008, pH 6.0; urinary microscopy demonstrated 12 WBC/hpf, 3 RBC/hpf, and no bacteria. A Gram stain of the exudate from the skin ulcers showed large numbers of neutrophils and the absence of bacteria. Blood cultures were

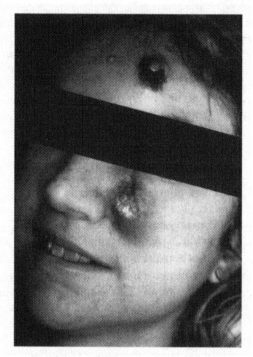

Figure 1
Note two pyoderma gangrenosum lesion on forehead and malar area respectively.

negative. The chest radiograph was normal. Upper GI series with small-bowel follow-through was normal.

Hospital Course. The patient was admitted to the Infectious Disease service with a presumptive diagnosis of multiple bacterial skin ulcers, possibly due to anthrax, and empirically placed on intravenous nafcillin. Dermatological consultants suggested that her skin ulcers might be due to one of the following: pyoderma gangrenosum (PG), Sweet's syndrome, staphylococcal, streptococcal, or atypical mycobacterial infection, Behcet's syndrome, or halogenoderma. A punch biopsy of the ulcer margin was performed. Histologically, this showed diffuse suppurative dermatitis with dense follicular suppuration consistent with PG. Special stains for bacteria, fungi, viruses, and mycobacteria were negative. Once the diagnosis of PG was established, gastroenterology was consulted in an effort to determine whether the patient had inflammatory bowel disease. Prior to this time, her primary physicians had overlooked her history of diarrhea and were more mindful of her impressive skin lesions. In retrospect it was discovered that in addition to her recent acute intestinal symptoms the patient had had episodes of diarrhea, hematochezia, and crampy abdominal pain for the past ten years. Moreover, she had had a 20-lb weight loss over the past two years. A flexible sigmoidoscopic examination was performed which revealed discrete but intermittent areas of mucosal erythema and ulceration in the rectosigmoid and left colon. Nevertheless, the rectum appeared relatively "spared" compared to the remainder of her sigmoid colon. At 50 cm (splenic flexure), there were more prominent multiple mucosal ulcerations, as well as mucosal edema, granulation tissue, and hemorrhage. Multiple biopsies were obtained. These revealed mixed inflammation, including plasma cells, extending into muscularis mucosa. No granulomas were present. All stool cultures, including those for Yersinia, ova and parasites, were negative. At this point, the diagnosis of Crohn's disease with PG seemed certain and the patient was begun on high-dose prednisone, 120 mg daily. She demonstrated remarkable improvement in the skin lesions, diarrhea and abdominal pain. She was discharged after five days on prednisone, 40 mg/day. Unfortunately, one month after discharge she required re-admission to OSUH. At that time, the PG lesion on her left cheek had extended to her periorbital area. Additionally, she had developed disabling sacroileitis. The patient was again placed on high-dose intravenous steroids (hydrocortisone 120 mg daily) with the addition of 6 mercaptopurine (6-MP), 75 mg daily. She has since responded well to this therapy with improvement in the PG lesions and sacroileitis

Discussion

Differential Diagnosis. This patient is particularly interesting since her primary complaint was not a gastrointestinal one, but rather a relatively uncommon dermatologic complication of inflammatory bowel disease (IBD), pyoderma gangrenosum. It cannot be overemphasized that when a patient presents with dermatologic findings similar to hers, a thorough search for gastrointestinal disease should be undertaken, even if the patient has no gastrointestinal symptoms! There are a variety of disorders that can closely resemble PG, both histopathologically and grossly. These entities generally fall under the category of neutrophilic vascular reactions. Sweet's syndrome (acute febrile neutrophilic dermatosis) is a disorder of unknown etiology characterized by inflammatory cutaneous plaques, fever, arthralgia, neutrophilia, and histologic evidence of neutrophilic dermal infiltration in the absence of infection.[1] Moreover, it is often associated with one of several myeloproliferative disorders.[2] Behcet's disease is a multisystem disease of unknown etiology, characterized by oral aphthous ulcers, genital aphthae, synovitis, ocular inflammation, and pustular vasculitis.[3] While our patient failed to meet the diagnostic criteria for either of these diseases, the histopathology of her skin disorder was nevertheless consistent with a diagnosis of either Sweet's syndrome or Bechet's disease.

Obviously, the appearance of PG itself leads most clinicians to suspect an infectious etiology such as may occur with infections due to staphylococci, streptococci, mucormycosis, sporotrichosis, cat-scratch disease, tularemia, plague, and mycobacteria. In patients with a strong exposure to animals and animal products, a zoonosis such as anthrax should be considered.[4] In fact, this was an initial and indeed primary consideration of the physicians caring for our patient. However, the time course for the development of the skin lesions in relation to her exposure was inconsistent with anthrax (i.e., the usual incubation period is 3-10 days for anthrax skin lesions). In our patient, the exposure to a potential anthrax infection occurred some eight weeks prior to the development of her skin lesions. Additionally, gastrointestinal manifestations of anthrax are extremely rare in the United States, but when they do occur there is almost always abdominal pain, vomiting, and bloody diarrhea. As was noted earlier, special stains of the ulcer debris, as well as the punch biopsy, were negative for infecting organisms. A final possible etiology for the type of dermatosis in our patient would be a halogenoderma, a disorder seen in patients previously exposed to iodinated dyes.[5] As already noted in this patient's history, she had an IVP four weeks prior to admission. Although the histopathology of the skin lesion was consistent with this diagnosis, it did not explain the patient's gastrointestinal complaints.

Obviously, the most likely diagnosis for this patient's skin disorder is PG, an ulcerating disease of unknown etiology characterized by pronounced tissue necrosis and a neutrophilic vascular reaction.[6] These lesions may expand in an explosive manner and on occasion lead to significant morbidity. When healed, they often leave significant residual deforming scars, particularly those that occur on the face.[1] The diagnosis of PG is principally made by exclusion of other lesions with a similar appearance, e.g., infectious ulcers (fungal, bacterial, mycobacterial), collagen vascular disease, malignant tumors of the skin, folliculitis syndromes (vasculitis associated with SLE, rheumatoid arthritis, Wegener's granulomatosis, and neutrophilic vascular dermatoses). Typically, the pyoderma lesion begins as a raised purplish "boil", which is quite tender, but initially contains very few leukocytes. Over ensuing days or weeks, the lesion enlarges and cavitates until the typical PG lesion is fully developed. Histologically, the lesion resembles a sterile abscess, in which venous and capillary thrombosis, arteritis, hemorrhage, fibrinoid necrosis and massive cell infiltration are present. In the majority of instances, the appearance of PG in patients with IBD indicates the presence of moderate to severe disease activity. While colectomy has occasionally been recommended for patients with ulcerative colitis (UC) who have severe multiple lesions unresponsive to drug therapy, it must be emphasized that colon resection does not always prevent recurrent pyoderma. This case is unusual in that the dermatologic manifestations of Crohn's disease overshadowed the patients intestinal complaints and in fact led her physician to overlook them.

In addition to PG, which occurs in approximately 0.5%, there are a variety of skin and mucous membrane lesions that more commonly occur in IBD (Table 1). Erythema nodosum is probably the most common cutaneous complication of IBD and may occur with either Crohn's disease or ulcerative colitis. However, it seems to occur more frequently in the latter (2-4 %). These raised, tender, erythematous

Table 1

Extraintestinal Manifestations of Inflammatory Bowel Disease

Cutaneous
Erythema nodosum
Pyoderma gangrenosum
Contact dermatitis
Miscellaneous
    Cutaneous granulomas (Crohn's disease only),
    Erythema multiform, lichen planus, vascular thrombosis

Mucous Membranes
Oral aphthous ulcers

Ocular
Conjunctivitis
Iritis, uveitis
Episcleritis
Keratitis

Musculoskeletal
Peripheral arthritis
Spondyloarthropathy

Hepatobiliary
Steatosis
Pericholangitis
Sclerosing cholangitis
Chronic active hepatitis
Gallstones
Cholangiocarcinoma

Renal
Nephrolithiasis (urate,
  oxalate)
Obstructive uropathy
Amyloidosis

Hematologic
Hypercoagulopathy
Arterial and venous thromboses
Vasculitis

Miscellaneous
Amyloid
Growth retardation

swellings usually occur along the extensor surfaces of the arms and legs and measure 2 to 5 cm in diameter.[7] Erythema nodosum tends to occur when the bowel disease is active, particularly when arthritis accompanies the condition. The major differentiating feature of erythema nodosum from PG is the lack of ulceration in the former. Treatment consists of appropriate management of the IBD.

Granulomas (metastatic cutaneous Crohn's disease) may involve the skin, mouth, lips, anus, as well as ileostomy and colostomy ostia.[8] Oral aphthous ulcers occur in approximately 8-10% of patients with ulcerative colitis, and 6-8% of patients with Crohn's disease.[9,10] Since these lesions may antedate the development of the bowel disease, any patient with recurring and otherwise unexplained aphthous ulcerations should have appropriate gastrointestinal tract studies done (barium enema, small bowel x-rays, flexible sigmoidoscopy, or colonoscopy) to rule out UC or Crohn's disease. Other dermatological manifestations can also be seen in inflammatory bowel disease but their incidence is very low. These include vascular thrombosis, erythema multiform and lichen planus. Additionally, rashes at colostomy or ileostomy sites are occasionally seen and are thought to be due to allergic contact dermatitis and/or "digestion" of the skin tissue by gut enzymes.

As noted in the case presentation, our patient had a 10-year history of intermittent diarrhea and two episodes of hematochezia. It is significant and indeed a mild indictment of today's superspecialized state of medicine that this history had been completely overlooked by her primary physicians who had "zeroed in" on a diagnosis of anthrax. In this regard, all of us would do well to remember the admonishment of Sir William Osler, "Rare diagnoses are usually the refuge of the diagnostically destitute." Only after dermatological consultation suggested that she had PG did the patient have the appropriate diagnostic gastrointestinal studies done. Although upper gastrointestinal and small bowel x-rays were normal, a flexible sigmoidoscopic exam demonstrated "skip" areas of friability and ulceration with more severe areas of mucosal damage seen just distal to the splenic flexure. It is axiomatic that once a diagnosis of IBD is established, two questions must be answered as completely as possible: (1) What is the disease—UC or Crohn's disease? (2) What is the anatomical extent of the disease? The answers to these questions provide more than a diagnostic academic exercise, for they not only dictate what the patient's long-term prognosis and quality of life will be, but they also provide some scientific rationale for medical therapy. Differentiation of UC and Crohn's disease can be quite difficult (Table 2). Indeed, in 25-30% of the patients with IBD the specific disease is indeterminable.[11] Usually sigmoidoscopic or colonoscopic exams and barium studies will document the distribution of the disease and the nature of the lesions. The endoscopic appearance of these two diseases is usually, but not always, quite different. In Crohn's disease, the mucosa appears thickened, with deep round, linear, or serpiginous ulcerations which appear between areas of normal appearing mucosa. In UC the mucosa is diffusely involved in a uniform, continuous pattern characterized by denuded, friable mucosa often with pinpoint excrescences. Although it is helpful to find crypt abscesses in UC and granulomas in Crohn's disease on mucosal biopsy, it is not unusual to see only an inflammatory infiltrate in both conditions. Although granulomata are found in less than 25% of rectal biopsy specimens in patients with Crohn's disease, all patients being evaluated for IBD should have rectal biopsies

Table 2

	Crohn's Disease	Ulcerative Colitis
Differentiation of Crohn's Disease and UC		
Anorectal	80%	20%
Complex fistulae	Common	Never
Massive bleeding	Uncommon	3%
Internal fistulae	Common	Rare
Toxic megacolon	Rare	2-5%
Strictures	Very common	< 10%
Free perforation	Rare	More common
Endoscopic:		
Rectal sparing	Common	Very rare
Friability	Uncommon	Very common
Ulceration	Solitary	Diffuse
Skip areas	Characteristic	Never
Pseudopolyps	Uncommon	Very common
Histology:		
Granuloma	Common	Absent
Fissure ulcers	Common	Rare

obtained at the time of sigmoidoscopy or colonoscopy even if the mucosa appears to be normal.[12]

In our patient, it seems reasonably certain that she had Crohn's disease based on the following: (1) predominant diarrhea history rather than a dysenteric one; (2) rectal sparing on sigmoidoscopic examination; and (3) clearly defined skip areas of colonic involvement. While her small bowel x-rays were thought to be normal, we should emphasize that normal radiological studies do not preclude small bowel involvement and further tests to more completely determine the presence of small intestinal involvement need to be performed. All patients with Crohn's disease should have upper gastrointestinal endoscopy looking for antral or duodenal involvement. Furthermore, it should be pointed out that functional testing for ileal involvement is clearly a more sensitive marker of ileal disease than are x-rays. Such functional testing should include a ^{14}C-cholyglycine breath test and a Schilling's test. Abnormalities of either of these indicate ileal disease and usually mandate treatment with corticosteroids. While our patient was treated with high daily doses of prednisone, this was done for her PG, and not from complete knowledge about the anatomical extent of her Crohn's disease.

As illustrated by this patient, IBD often presents with symptoms and signs which to the nondiscerning eye appear to be independent diseases rather than manifestations of underlying bowel disease. The most significant and frequent of these are ocular, joint, vascular, hepatobiliary and renal manifestations.

Ocular Manifestations. The most common ocular manifestations seen in patients with either Crohn's disease or UC are conjunctivitis, episcleritis, and uveitis (iritis). The incidence of ocular involvement is approximately 11% for UC and 3% for Crohn's disease.[13,14] Clinically, all three ocular conditions typically present with a "red eye"; however, pain and photophobia are usually seen with uveitis only.[15] Additionally, only uveitis is associated with an abnormal pupillary response to light. The precise role of IBD in triggering the ocular problem is only speculative, but seems most likely related to immune complex formation, particularly with anterior nongranulomatous uveitis.[15] Treatment of conjunctivitis and episcleritis is best accomplished with local hydrocortisone solutions, but the diagnosis of uveitis should prompt emergency ophthalmologic consultation.

Arthritis. IBD is frequently complicated by arthritic manifestations, which fall under the general category of the seronegative (rheumatoid factor negative) spondyloarthropathies. Of interest is the frequent occurrence of HLA-B27 positivity in 50-60% of patients with arthritis associated with IBD.[15] IBD-associated arthritis is generally described as either spondylitis and/or peripheral arthropathy.

A recent review of the literature demonstrated a 15-25% incidence of radiographic sacroileitis in patients with IBD.[15] While clinically apparent ankylosing spondylitis has a much lower incidence of 2%-6%, sacroileitis was a predominant complaint on the subsequent hospital admission by our patient.[16] The clinical course of the spondylitis is independent of the extent, location, duration, or severity of the IBD. In addition, it may become manifest prior to, or after the development of IBD.[15] The peripheral arthropathy complicating IBD has been reported in up to 22% of the patients.[17] In contrast to the spondylitis associated with IBD, the peripheral arthropathy is more frequently seen during exacerbations of the bowel disease, and is more common in those with a chronic course as opposed to its lower frequency in those with acute fulminant colitis. Additionally, the peripheral arthropathy seems to occur more often in those with left sided or universal colitis than in those with disease limited to the rectosigmoid area.[15]

Vascular Manifestations. Although thromboembolic disease has long been recognized as an important extraintestinal manifestation of IBD, its exact incidence is not known. Best estimates of the occurrence of this complication were reported in a recent review by Talbot et al in which they found an incidence of vascular complications of 1.3%.[18] The most commonly encountered problems were deep vein thrombophlebitis and pulmonary emboli followed by arterial thrombosis (only in postoperative cases), and cardiovascular accidents which were associated with both venous and arterial thromboembolic disease. Although elevated levels of factor VIII and thrombocytosis have been frequently reported, the precise underlying etiology of the thromboembolic complications remains an enigma. Recent evidence does, however, suggest an incompletely understood abnormality in fibrinolysis.[19]

Hepatobiliary Manifestations. The most common hepatobiliary complications of IBD include steatosis of the liver, pericholangitis, primary sclerosing cholangitis (PSC), and cholelithiasis. Less common are secondary biliary cirrhosis, postnecrotic cirrhosis, chronic active hepatitis, and cholangiocarcinoma. Rarely, one may see granulomatous hepatitis or secondary amyloidosis.

Approximately 5-10% of patients with IBD have clinically significant liver disease but up to 50% may have minor abnormalities in hepatic function.[15] The most common abnormality is steatosis of the liver which is reported to occur in 20-45% of patients with IBD.[20] Contributing factors to the development of this entity include corticosteroid therapy and malnutrition. The major importance of IBD-associated fatty liver is that it must be distinguished from the other more serious complications which often have similar clinical and biochemical presentations.

Pericholangitis is characterized by portal edema and varying degrees of bile duct proliferation and inflammation. It has a reported incidence of up to 30%.[15] It is best to think of this entity as part of the spectrum of PSC. Simply put, pericholangitis is nothing more than sclerosing cholangitis confined to small intrahepatic bile ducts with no involvement of the extrahepatic biliary tree. However, some patients with pericholangitis may progress to typical PSC, secondary biliary cirrhosis, and even cholangiocarcinoma.[20] The exact etiology of pericholangitis and PSC remains obscure. Diagnosis requires visualization of both the intra- and extrahepatic bile ducts by means of liver biopsy and either ERCP or percutaneous transhepatic cholangiography. Additionally, serologic tests for antimitochondrial antibodies, anti-smooth muscle antibodies, and antinuclear antibodies are useful to exclude other secondary causes of liver disease. There is no established effective treatment for either of these two conditions at the present time, but recent evidence suggests that ursodeoxycholic acid may be beneficial for PSC.

Cholelithiasis occurs in 30-35% of patients with Crohn's disease and is almost exclusively confined to those patients with ileal disease or ileal resection. Malabsorption of bile acids and the associated excessive fecal bile acid loss, especially in those patients with large segment ileal disease or resection of 100 cm, result in a diminished bile acid pool, and bile that is supersaturated with cholesterol as a result of disruption of the normal enterohepatic circulation of bile acids.

Renal Disease. Renal function may be impaired by a variety of mechanisms in patients with IBD. First, contiguous extension of the inflammatory process to involve the ureter (almost always the right side) has been reported to cause an obstructive uropathy in patients with Crohn's disease.[21] Second, nephrolithiasis is common in patients with IBD and has a reported incidence of 2-10%. Overall, nephrolithiasis occurs more frequently in Crohn's disease than in ulcerative colitis. The most common type of stone is the uric acid stone. Such stones form as a consequence of the hypercatabolic state of patients with active IBD, often in association with dehydration from diarrhea or excessive ileostomy fluid losses. Calcium oxalate stones are also common in patients with small intestinal Crohn's disease, particularly in those who have had an ileal resection. Normally intraluminal oxalate is bound to calcium which limits intestinal oxalate absorption. However, in those patients with steatorrhea, there is increased binding of calcium to unabsorbed fatty acids (steatorrhea), which decreases calcium oxalate formation. Thus, "free" oxalate is readily absorbed from the colon and results in hyperoxaluria. Treatment for this condition includes a diet high in calcium (to bind to oxalate), low oxalate diet, substitution of long-chain dietary fat with medium-chain triglyceride, and maintenance of a high urine volume. Finally, kidney function can be impaired by the development of secondary amyloidosis in patients with Crohn's disease. This diagnosis is established by renal biopsy.

Treatment. Although our particular patient had a clear cut need for corticosteroid treatment, primarily due to the severity of the skin lesions, this is not always the case. We shall now discuss an overview of the general therapeutic approach to the patient with IBD (Table 3).[22]

Sulfasalazine was originally developed in the 1940s but remains the mainstay of therapy for Crohn's colitis. It consists of sulfapyridine linked to 5-aminosalicylic acid (5-ASA) by an azo bond. Although the mechanism of action is incompletely understood, it is known that the sulfapyridine moiety serves merely as a vehicle for delivery of the active portion, 5-ASA, to the colon at a concentration higher than can be achieved with 5-ASA alone. Both molecules, however, seem to have a synergistic action. Sulfasalazine profoundly affects arachidonic acid metabolism at several different sites including inhibition of thromboxane B_2 formation, increased synthesis of PGF_2 and PGE_2 and inhibition of synthesis of other active postaglandins. In addition to these effects on the cyclooxygenase pathway, sulfasalazine also inhibits the lipoxygenase pathway leading to decreased synthesis of leukotrienes, and 5-HETE.[23,24] Sulfasalazine is currently recommended as initial therapy in patients with ulcerative colitis with mild to moderate symptoms or in patients with distal colitis who fail to respond to topical therapy with steroid enemas or ASA enemas.[25] The usual therapeutic dose is 2-4 gm/day. In patients with UC, therapy should be continued indefinitely, usually at a lower dose, for maintenance of remission. Except for maintenance therapy the same general recommendation for use of sulfasalazine is used for Crohn's colitis. Unlike the situation in UC, sulfasalazine has not been demonstrated to maintain remissions in Crohn's colitis. Moreover, sulfasalazine has no therapeutic efficacy in patients who have only small bowel disease. Topical salicylate enemas (4-ASA and 5-ASA) are useful as primary therapy in patients with proctitis, proctosigmoiditis and left-sided UC or limited Crohn's colitis (less than 60 cm of activity). Both drugs are relatively safe, well

Table 3

Medical Treatment

IBD

	UC Distal	Universal	Remission Maintenance
Sulfasalazine	+	+	+
5-ASA	+	−	−
Steroid enema	+	−	−
Oral aminosalicylate	+	+	+
Oral corticosteroid	+	+	+

Crohn's Disease

	Colon	Small Bowel	Colon and Small Bowel	Remission Maintenance
Sulfasalazine	+	−	+	−
5-ASA enema	+ (distal only)	−	−	−
Steroid enema	+ (distal only)	−	−	−
Oral aminosalicylate	+	?	+	−
Oral corticosteroid	+	+	+	−
Metronidazole	+ (perineal fistulae)	+	+	−
6-MP	+	+	+	+
Cyclosporin	+	+	+	−

tolerated, and effective. It should be remembered that patients with left-sided colitis who have active disease despite talking sulfasalazine must be continued on sulfasalazine when adding enemas to the regimen. Clinical response to aminosalicylic enemas varies from rapid to gradual depending on the particular patient.[26]

Corticosteroids have had a dramatic impact on the prognosis of patients with IBD. The development of steroid retention enemas has enabled patients to benefit from the local anti-inflammatory and/or immunosuppressive actions of steroids with minimal systemic effects. Steroid enemas are used primarily in the treatment of mild to moderate disease involving the distal colon. During severe bouts of IBD, oral or systemic forms of corticosteroids must be used in relatively high doses. However, once the acute or fulminant manifestations of the disease come under control, then a gradual dose reduction and discontinuation must be attempted as there is no evidence that continuous steroid therapy prolongs remission in either UC or Crohn's disease. Failure to respond to high dose steroids occurs in up to 25% of patients with fulminant IBD and should prompt immediate surgical consideration.[27]

Finally, there exist on the horizon a few new oral aminosalicylic preparations that have shown promise in the treatment of IBD. Olsalazine is a compound of two molecules of 5-ASA coupled by a diazo bond. Mesalamine is an encapsulated form of 5-ASA. Both preparations avoid rapid absorption in the small intestine by virtue of their unique delivery systems and deliver adequate doses of the active component, 5-ASA, to the colon while avoiding the frequent side effects seen with the sulfapyridine moiety of sulfasalazine.[28]

Metronidazole was initially introduced as an antibacterial agent in 1960. However, in recent years it has gained relatively widespread use in the treatment of IBD, especially Crohn's disease. The mechanism of its effect in IBD has not been satisfactorily elucidated but in addition to its antibacterial properties, it has moderate immunosuppressive activity. Metronidazole appears to have significant benefit for certain patients with IBD, particularly those with Crohn's colitis with perianal Crohn's disease, or in those with fistulae. However, it should be emphasized that there is a disturbing tendency of the perianal disease to relapse when the drug is stopped.[29]

Two antineoplastic drugs, 6-MP and azathioprine, have gained increasing popularity among gastroenterologists for the treatment of refractory IBD. Recent studies on 6-MP have demonstrated its safety and effectiveness providing close observation of the patient's blood count and clinical status is established.[30,31] Current recommendations for the use of 6-MP in the treatment of Crohn's disease include: (1) patients with chronic active disease who have failed to respond to sulfasalazine, steroids, or metronidazole; (2) in cases of steroid toxicity or steroid therapy lasting greater than 6 months in doses of 15 mg/day or more; (3) the presence of fistulae which do not respond to other medical approaches; (4) prior to extensive surgery; (5) maintenance remission. To date 6-MP has not been routinely used in UC since colectomy is curative.

Cyclosporin has been used over the past decade to depress cellular immunity in patients undergoing organ transplantation. The exact mechanism of action is not fully understood, but is felt to involve reversible inhibition of helper T-lymphocytes and possibly lymphokine production. In a recent prospective study, cyclosporin administration to patients with active Crohn's disease resulted in improvement in 59% of patients versus 32% with placebo.[32] Although its onset of action is rapid, further studies are needed to demonstrate long-term efficacy.

References

1. Jorizzo JC, Soloman AR, Zanelli MD, et al: Neutrophilic vascular reactions. JAAD. 1988;19:983-1005.

2. Su WPD, Liu HNH: Diagnostic criteria for Sweet's syndrome. Int J Dermatol. 1987; 26:178-180.

3. Jozzio JC: Bechet's disease: An update based on the 1985 international conference in London. Arch Dermatol. 1986;122:556-558.

4. Brachman PS: Anthrax, in Evans A, Feldman H (eds): Bacterial Infections of Humans: Epidemiology and Control. New York, Plenum Medical Book Co, 1982, pp 63-74.

5. Boudoulas O, Siegle RJ, Grimwood RE: Ioderma occurring after orally administered iopanoic acid. Arch Dermatol. 1987;123:387-388.

6. Hideman JG: Pyoderma gangrenosum. Clin Dermatol. 1983;1:102-113.

7. Greenstein AJ, Janowitz HO, Sachar DB: The extra-intestinal complications of Crohn's disease and ulcerative colitis: A study of 700 patients. Medicine. 1976;55:401.

8. McCallum DI, Kinmono PDC: Dermatologic manifestations of Crohn's disease. Br J Dermatol. 1968;80:1.

9. Edwards FC, Truelove SC: The course and prognosis of ulcerative colitis. Gut. 1964;5:1.

10. Croft CB, Wilkinson AR: Ulceration of the mouth, pharynx, and larynx in Crohn's disease of the intestine. Br J Surg. 1972;59:249.

11. Schacter H, Kirsner J: Definitions of inflammatory bowel disease of unknown etiology. Gastroenterology. 1975;68:591.

12. Donaldson RM Jr: Crohn's disease, in Sleisenger MH, Fordtran JS (eds): Gastrointestinal Disease, Philadelphia, 4 ed. WB Saunders Co, 1989.

13. Wright R, Lunsden J, Luntz MH, et al: Abnormalities of the sacroiliac joints and uveitis. Q J Med. 1965;34:229-236.

14. Rankin GB, Watts HD, Melynk CS, et al: The National Cooperative Crohn's Disease Study: Extraintestinal manifestations and perianal complications. Gastroenterology. 1979; 77:914-920.

15. Danzi JT: Extraintestinal manifestations of idiopathic inflammatory bowel disease. Arch Intern Med. 1988;148:297-302.

16. Moll JM: Inflammatory bowel disease. in Pancyi GS (ed): Clinics in Rheumatic Disease. Philadelphia, WB Saunders Co, 1985, pp 87-105.

17. Neuman V, Wright V: Arthritis associated with inflammatory bowel disease. in Losowsky MS (ed): Clinics in Rheumatic Disease. Philadelphia, WB Saunders Co, 1983, pp 767-795.

18. Talbot RW, Helppell J, Dozios RR, et al: Vascular complications of inflammatory bowel disease. Mayo Clin Proc 1986;61:140-145

19. Conlan MG, Haise WD, Burnett DA: Prothrombotic abnormalities in inflammatory bowel disease. Dig Dis Sci. 1989;7:1089-1093.

20. Wee A, Ludwig J: Pericholangitis in chronic ulcerative colitis: Primary sclerosing cholangitis of the small bile ducts. Ann Intern Med. 1985;102:581-587.

21. Kyle J: Urinary complications of Crohn's disease. World J Surg. 1980;4:153-160.

22. Summers RW, Switz DM, Sessions JT, et al: National Cooperative Crohn's Disease Study: Results of drug treatment. Gastroenterology. 1979;77:847-869.

23. Hawkey CJ, Boughter-Smith NK, Whittle BJR: Modulation of human colonic arachidonic acid metabolism by sulfasalazine. Dig Dis Sci. 1985;30:1161-65.

24. Dreyling KW, Hoppe V, Peskar BH, et al: Leukotrienes in Crohn's disease: Effect of sulfasalazine and 5-aminosalicylic acid. Adv Prostaglandin Thromboxane Leukotriene Res. 1987;17:339-343.

25. Das K: Sulfasalazine therapy in inflammatory bowel disease. Gastroenterol Clin North Am. March 1989.

26. Ginsberg AL: Topical salicylate therapy (4-ASA and 5-ASA enemas). Gastroenterol Clin North Am. March 1989.

27. Jewell DP: Corticosteroids for the management of ulcerative colitis and Crohn's disease. Gastroenterol Clin North Am. March 1989.

28. Robinson M: New Oral Salicylates in the therapy of chronic idiopathic inflammatory bowel disease. Gastroenterol Clin North Am. March 1989.

29. Brandt LJ, Bernstein LH, Boley SJ, et al: Metronidazole therapy for perianal Crohn's disease: A follow-up study. Gastroenterology. 1982;23:383-387.

30. Present DH: 6-Mercaptopurine and other immunosuppressive agents in the treatment of Crohn's disease and ulcerative colitis. Gastroenterol Clin of North Am. March 1989.

31. Present DH, Meltzer SJ, Krumholz MP, et al: 6-Mercaptopurine in the management of inflammatory bowel disease: Short- and long-term toxicity. Ann Intern Med. 1989; 111:641-649.

32. Brynshov J, Freund L, Rosmussensiv, et al: A placebo controlled, double-blind, randomized trial of cyclosporin therapy in active chronic Crohn's disease. N Engl J Med. 1989; 321:845-850.

Case 17

Acute Pancreatitis: Diagnosis and Complications

David B. Thomas, MD and John J. Fromkes, MD

Case History

This was the first admission to Ohio State University Hospitals for this previously healthy 38-year-old white male. Four days prior to admission he began manifesting epigastric pain with radiation to the back. The discomfort began in the morning shortly after eating, and persisted throughout the day. He presented to his local hospital where he was admitted with an amylase of 250 U/dl and a triglyceride level of 2,500 mg/dl.

Shortly after admission, he began experiencing nausea and vomiting and a nasogastric tube was placed. Intravenous hydration was also begun and analgesics administered as needed. The presumed diagnosis was acute cholecystitis. An ultrasound exam was performed and demonstrated the gallbladder to be normal in appearance without evidence of gallstones or inflammation. The pancreas could not be visualized. A hepatobiliary iminodiacetic acid (HIDA) scan demonstrated patency of the cystic duct and good visualization of the gallbladder. An acute abdominal series was unremarkable. A repeat amylase was 114 U/dl.

Forty-eight hours after hospitalization, nasogastric suction was discontinued and the patient was placed on clear liquids. His abdominal pain worsened, and the patient was then transferred to University Hospital for further evaluation and therapy.

His past medical history was unremarkable for diabetes, peptic ulcer disease, hypertension, or heart disease. He was on no medications and denied any drug allergies. His family history was significant only for atherosclerotic heart disease. He denied tobacco or drug use, but drank approximately one to two beers a day.

Physical Examination. The patient was noted to be in mild painful distress but cooperative, alert, and oriented. Vital signs were notable for a temperature of 100.2, pulse of 88, blood pressure of 147/87, and respirations of 16. Examination of the head, eyes, ears, nose, and throat was unremarkable. The lungs were clear to auscultation and percussion. The heart exam was normal. The abdomen was mildly distended and demonstrated normoactive bowel sounds. There was mild epigastric tenderness to palpation but no rebound. There was no hepatosplenomegaly or masses. Cullen's and Gray-Turner signs were absent. Rectal exam revealed normal sphincter tone and the stool was hemoccult negative. Neurological exam was physiologic.

Laboratory Data. The hemoglobin was 13.6 g/dl and the hematocrit was 40.1 %: the white blood cell count was 14,100/mm^3. The amylase was 96 U/liter, lipase 172 U/liter, and the amylase-creatinine clearance ratio was abnormal at 8%. A timed urinary amylase was elevated at 604 U/liter. Alkaline phosphatase (ALP) was 155 U/liter, serum aspartate aminotransferase (AST) 130 IU/l, alanine aminotransferase (ALT) 35 IU/l. Total bilirubin was 1.4 mg/dl with a direct fraction of 0.4 mg/dl. Triglycerides and cholesterol were 1200 and 274 mg/dl, respectively. The protime was 11.5 seconds (control 11 seconds). Serum protein electrophoresis revealed evidence of hypoalbuminemia. Blood urea nitrogen (BUN), creatinine, glucose, and serum electrolytes revealed the following: sodium 127 mmol/liter, potassium 3.9 mmol/liter, chloride 101 mmol/liter, carbon dioxide 25 mmol/liter, calcium 9.6 mmol/liter, BUN 13 mg/dl, creatinine 0.8 mg/dl, glucose 105 mg/dl. An acute abdominal series demonstrated linear atelectasis in the left lung and a moderate small bowel ileus in the region of the duodenal loop. No free air could be visualized.

An abdominal ultrasound was performed and demonstrated a normal-appearing gallbladder. The pancreas was poorly visualized secondary to the small bowel gas. Abdominal computerized tomography (CT) revealed the liver and biliary tree to be normal. However, the pancreatic head and uncinate process were enlarged and there was infiltration of the peripancreatic fat. There was also evidence of a low-density collection extending from the anterior prerenal space to the iliac crest. Because a pancreatic phlegmon was demonstrated the patient was continued NPO and low-fat total parenteral nutrition initiated. The patient's pain resolved over the following two weeks and a clear liquid diet begun. His diet was then advanced to high carbohydrate, low protein, and low fat and this was tolerated without difficulty. A lipoprotein electrophoresis was then performed and demonstrated a Type V hyperlipoproteinemia. Furthermore, it was felt that both serum amylase and lipase activity were reduced because of the hypertriglyceridemia. The patient was started on a Type V diet and lopid begun. The patient continued to do well; however, a follow-up abdominal CT noted a 2-cm pancreatic pseudocyst. Repeat exam at six weeks showed complete resolution of the pseudocyst. Because of the abnormal liver function studies, outpatient endoscopic retrograde cholangiopancreatography (ERCP) was performed and demonstrated a normal biliary tree and pancreatic duct.

Discussion

This case highlights several important aspects of acute pancreatitis that will be discussed in a general review of this illness. When acute pancreatitis is being considered, several questions should be asked. What is the etiology? What is the differential diagnosis? Are complications arising? What is the prognosis? The proper management of a patient with pancreatitis relies on addressing each of these questions.

Pathogenesis. Acute pancreatitis is a process of autodigestion caused by premature activation of zymogens to active proteolytic enzymes within the pancreas. The pathophysiology of chronic pancreatitis is quite different, and beyond the scope of this discussion.

What initiates acute pancreatitis is unknown. Several hypotheses have been made but unfortunately, experimental studies have been conflicting. Currently held theories include: (1) obstruction to secretion (2) reflux of duodenal contents (3) bile reflux, and (4) intracellular protease activation.[1-12] Current evidence would suggest that trypsin activates other proenzymes (plasminogen, prothrombin, kininogen, and elastase) in the pancreas. It also activates phospholipase A_2 which appears to be integral in the inflammatory mediation of pancreatitis. Phospholipase A_2 causes severe parenchymal and adipose tissue necrosis in the presence of low concentration of bile acids. The cytotoxic nature of phospholipase A_2 is caused by its ability to hydrolyze cell membrane phospholipids, among which products include arachidonic acid and lysolecithin. The former may cause clotting (via PGI_2 and thromboxane) and the latter causes coagulation and fat necrosis. In addition, lipase activation may cause fat necrosis.[13,14]

Diagnosis. When acute pancreatitis is in the differential, three important considerations should be made: (1) ruling out other causes of epigastric pain and hyperamylasemia; (2) never totally exclude acute pancreatitis in patients with normal amylase activity; (3) always consider acute pancreatitis in the patient with shock or coma of unknown cause.

Diseases as diverse as perforated ulcer, acute cholecystitis, mesenteric infarction, and ascending cholangitis may all need to be considered for their medical and surgical management are very different.

A perforated peptic ulcer may have striking similarities to acute pancreatitis, including hyperamylasemia. However, the perforated viscus patient has more abrupt pain and signs of peritoneal irritation on physical examination. Radiologic examination is diagnostic of a perforated peptic ulcer. Acute pancreatitis may also be confused with acute cholecystitis. A TC-HIDA scan may help in differentiating between the two. Choledocholithiasis must also be considered especially with a steadily rising serum bilirubin, ALP, and ALT. CT and ultrasound may be unable to detect stones in the biliary tree. In a patient with jaundice and a clinically worsening condition, ERCP with endoscopic sphincterotomy is the procedure of choice. If any stones fail to pass, then endoscopically introduced baskets are used to remove these stones.[15,16] Ascending cholangitis in a patient with acute pancreatitis may appear similar to a stone impaction but will usually be associated with high fever (101-104°F) and signs of gram-negative sepsis. Thus, although acute pancreatitis remains a clinical diagnosis, laboratory studies as well as radiographic imaging provide useful diagnostic as well as prognostic information. In addition, such data have a direct bearing on patient management.

Laboratory Data. The serum amylase rises approximately 2 to 12 hours after the onset of symptoms and remains elevated typically for three to five days. Although still considered the "gold standard" the use of the serum amylase as the sole diagnostic criterion and prognosticator for acute pancreatitis has several shortcomings. First, the level may remain elevated for prolonged periods with no evidence of clinical illness. Furthermore, the magnitude of elevation does not correlate with the severity of disease or prognosis. In fact, 10% of lethal pancreatitis patients had normal amylase levels.[17]

In addition, patients with marked hypertriglyceridemia (serum values greater than 2000) and acute pancreatitis frequently have normal serum amylase and lipase activity.[18] This relates to an inhibitor of enzyme activity in the serum. Finally, there are other reasons for elevated amylase activity which should always be considered in the differential diagnosis (Table 1).

Table 1

Conditions Other Than Acute Pancreatitis Associated with Hyperamylasemia
Pancreatic pseudocyst
Carcinoma of pancreas
Perforation of stomach, duodenum, jejunum
Mesenteric infarction
Opiate administration
After ERCP
Common bile duct obstruction
Acute cholecystitis
Salivary adenitis
Postoperative state
Renal insufficiency
Metabolic including diabetic acidosis
Acute and chronic hepatocellular disease
Anorexia nervosa, bulimia
Ovarian Neoplasm
Salpingitis, ruptured ectopic pregnancy
Macroamylasemia

Another laboratory marker utilized in acute pancreatitis is the timed urinary amylase. The measurement of urinary amylase, however, provides little additional information except in the setting of hypertriglyceridemia. Elevation of serum triglycerides in acute pancreatitis will characteristically show normal serum amylase and lipase activity (as in this patient). Finally, patients with elevated serum amylase concentrations secondary to the rare condition of macroamylasemia will have low concentrations of urinary amylase because of their inability to clear these macromolecular aggregates of amylase.

The serum lipase activity is elevated in approximately 87% of patients with acute pancreatitis. It remains normal in those patients with amylase elevations caused by extrapancreatic disease and is therefore considered more specific. It, however, is not a more sensitive test.[19,20] Finally, serum immunoreactive trypsinogen/trypsin concentrations have been measured in patients with acute pancreatitis but its sensitivity and specificity are about the same as amylase.

The remaining laboratory tests performed during acute pancreatitis are useful more in terms of prognostication rather than in disease diagnosis. These laboratory tests are utilized in Ranson's criteria of prognostic signs (Table 2). Five measured at the time of admission reflect the intensity of the inflammatory process. Six measured at 48 hours reflect end organ failure, shock, and third space loss. Individual signs are present in only 15-30% of patients; thus, assessment requires

Table 2

Ranson's Criteria

At admission

(1) Age 55 years
(2) White blood cell count $> 16,000$ cells/mm^3
(3) Blood glucose > 200 mg/dl
(4) Serum LDH > 350 IU/liter
(5) AST (SGOT) > 250 Sigma

During initial 48 hours

(6) Hematocrit drop > 10
(7) BUN rise > 5 mg/dl
(8) Arterial $< PO_2$ 60 mm Hg
(9) Base deficit > 4 mEq/liter
(10) Serum calcium < 8.0 mg/dl
(11) Estimated fluid sequestration < 6 liters

---

measurement of all 11 signs. When less than three signs are present, all patients survive. While mortality increases with four or more signs, the majority of fatalities occur when six or more signs are positive. It must be noted that these signs are only useful in predicting increased mortality if utilized at the time of admission and at 48 hours. It is also important to note that the purpose of Ranson's criteria is to identify those at risk for such complications as pancreatic necrosis, infection, and overall high mortality at an early enough stage that intervention may affect the outcome.

Finally, a preliminary study has suggested that marked elevation in the C-reactive protein on the first day of hospitalization predicts progression to severe necrotizing pancreatitis with an accuracy of 95%.[21] It remains to be seen whether this will replace Ranson's criteria.

Radiologic Studies. Initial evaluation should include standard chest x-ray as well as upright and supine abdominal films.

More definitive imaging techniques include abdominal ultrasound (US) and CT imaging. Clearly, abdominal CT is the imaging procedure of choice for acute pancreatitis. However, the two tests are more complementary than exclusive. US imaging is indicated in diagnosing cholelithiasis as a contributory cause for pancreatitis. CT is superior in identifying changes consistent with acute pancreatitis as well as pancreatic abscess. It should also be noted that US and CT show a morphologically normal pancreas in approximately 10% and 28% respectively, of patients with acute, uncomplicated pancreatitis.[22]

Finally, diagnostic CT during the first 48 hours appears to have some utility in predicting an adverse outcome. With mild pancreatitis, CT is frequently normal during the initial 48 hours. Thus, an indication during the first 48 hours would be in assessing those patients with normal amylase and epigastric pain or in those with greater than three of Ranson's signs. A grading system proposed by Balthazar classifies five grades of acute pancreatitis: Grade A — normal; Grade B — focal or diffuse pancreatic edema with no parapancreatic disease; Grade C — intrinsic pancreatic abnormality with inflammatory changes restricted to peripancreatic fat; Grade D — simple phlegmon; Grade E — two or more fluid collections. Patients with Grade D or E pancreatitis within the first 48 hours have an unfavorable prognosis with a high likelihood of eventual infection. In studies performed recently, patients with D or E pancreatitis and a high Ranson's score were noted to have an infection rate between 25 and 67% with a mortality of 33-58%. On the other hand, in those patients with severe pancreatitis (D or E) on CT and a low Ranson score, infection still occasionally occurs but almost all patients survive.[23-26] In addition, diagnostic CT guided needle aspiration is also now recommended in patients with clinical toxicity and Grade D or E changes.

The term phlegmon has also grown out of favor. In its place the terms interstitial pancreatitis and necrotizing pancreatitis have emerged. The difference is based on assessment of the vascular supply. Should a pancreatic enlargement be present on

Table 3

Conditions Associated with Acute Pancreatitis

Cholelithiasis
Ethanol abuse
Idiopathic
Abdominal operations
Hyperlipidemia
Injection into pancreatic duct
Trauma
Hypercalcemia
Pregnancy
Peptic ulcer
Outflow obstruction
Pancreas divisum
Organ transplantation
End-stage renal failure
Hereditary (Familial pancreatitis)
Drugs
Scorpion bile
Miscellaneous: viral infection,
   mycoplasma, hypoperfusion,
   intraductal parasites

CT, IV contrast should be utilized to assess whether the vascular supply is intact (interstitial pancreatitis), or whether the vascular supply has been interrupted (necrotizing pancreatitis)[27-30]

Associated Conditions. Table 3 lists the etiologies of acute pancreatitis. A discussion of each of these conditions is beyond the scope of this chapter; however, several important points should be made. Alcohol abuse and gallstones account for 85% of all cases of acute pancreatitis in the USA. Although ethanol is the leading cause of chronic pancreatitis, gallstones rarely lead to chronic disease. In addition, choledocholithiasis may be confused with acute pancreatitis especially if it is associated with hyperamylasemia. One must strongly suspect gallstone disease if the: (1) alkaline phosphatase is greater than twice the upper limit of normal, (2) ALT level is greater than 2.2 times the upper limit of normal, and (3) serum bilirubin level is greater than 2.5 mg/dl.

If cholecystitis is coincident with pancreatitis and requires emergent surgery, laparotomy should not be delayed. In those patients with gallstones and alcohol-related pancreatitis, however, removal of the gallstones will not prevent further attacks.[31]

The pancreatitis associated with hyperparathyroidism and other hypercalcemic states is acute and severe in one third, and chronic in the remainder. Because relative hypocalcemia may develop during acute pancreatitis, hypercalcemia cannot be ruled out until several weeks after the acute process has resolved.

General Treatment. Once the diagnosis of acute pancreatitis is certain, therapy is initiated. The obvious goal is cessation of pancreatic autodigestion and symptom resolution. Currently, the mainstay of therapy is supportive and involves intensive critical care management if the disease is severe. Controlled clinical trials have shown no significant benefit from using H-2 blockers, anticholinergics, glucagon, calcitonin, somatostatin, prostaglandin synthetase inhibitors, or proteolytic enzyme inhibitors. Thus, standard therapy includes nothing by mouth, nasogastric suction (if there is nausea and vomiting), and narcotics for pain relief. A most important consideration is adequate volume replacement. As a general rule, all patients with greater than three of Ranson's criteria and all patients with hypotension or oliguria should be admitted to the ICU. The main causes of early death with acute pancreatitis are cardiovascular collapse, adult respiratory distress syndrome (ARDS), acute intraabdominal hemorrhage, renal failure, and complicating acute cholangitis. Complications occurring after the first week of pancreatitis include sepsis, pneumonitis, and pancreatic abscess.

In those patients with a necrotic pancreas and hypotension, several uncontrolled clinical studies have been performed in order to determine if removal of pancreatic tissue would improve mortality. These include peritoneal lavage, peritoneal dialysis, sump drainage, and partial to total pancreatectomy.[32-36] The majority of evidence argues against their use in decreasing mortality.[37,38] As a rule, surgical intervention should be reserved for those patients in whom pancreatic abscess and/or contiguous infection is documented or suspected.

The complication of ARDS generally occurs in those patients with hyperlipidemia, marked hypocalcemia and in those patients who require large amounts of colloid. Early recognition and prompt treatment of this complication generally results in a favorable response. Renal insufficiency, on the other hand, is associated with a 50% mortality rate. Acute tubular necrosis is usually the etiology of the renal insufficiency and is associated with hypovolemia and shock. A very similar type of acute renal failure may develop in the absence of hypotension but the prognosis is good.[39] Here, the pathogenesis is selective renal vasoconstriction.

Management of Local Complications. Pseudocysts complicate the course of acute pancreatitis in 10-20% of cases.[21] Overall, there is an approximately 10% mortality for patients with acute pseudocysts primarily due to hemorrhage, sepsis, and rupture. Their formation is a result of pancreatic ductal disruption. Complications have been reported in 30 to 55% of patients with pseudocysts.[40] The decision as to management depends on both size and duration. Secondly, the course of a pseudocyst secondary to acute pancreatitis is much different than one related to chronic pancreatitis. The former have a much higher degree of resolution. As a rule, pseudocysts which persist greater than six weeks and/or are greater than 6 cm in diameter and not decreasing in size require surgical drainage. Few pseudocysts resolve after six weeks and complications increased significantly beyond this period.[41] The initial approach to a pseudocyst is that of percutaneous aspiration or the surgical formation of a cystoenteric anastomosis for drainage.

The etiology of bleeding in acute pancreatitis results from several mechanisms: (1) contiguous pancreatic head inflammation resulting in antral and duodenal erosions; (2) intrapancreatic and/or peripancreatic hemorrhage; (3) intracystic hemorrhage leading to the formation of pseudoaneurysm; (4) bleeding from a pseudocyst into the pancreatic duct leading to gastrointestinal hemorrhage (hemosuccus pancreaticus); (5) variceal bleeding from portal hypertension secondary to portal and/or splenic vein obstruction, and (6) fistulization of an abscess or pseudocyst into the stomach, duodenum, or colon.

With regard to pancreatic infection, accurate and quick identification can lead to decreased morbidity and mortality. The organisms involved are enteric and usually polymicrobial. Thus, good antimicrobial coverage should include coverage for E. coli, Enterococcus, Proteus, Klebsiella, Pseudomonas, Staphylococcus, Streptococcus faecalis, and Bacteroides. The timely diagnosis of infection in acute pancreatitis remains a clinical challenge. Many of the physical exam abnormalities and laboratory studies found in acute pancreatitis are similar in the setting of pancreatic abscess. It is recommended that a patient with a temperature greater than 101, leukocytosis, and a toxic appearance undergo needle aspiration with Gram stain and culture. In those with infection and pancreatic necrosis, surgical debridement should be undertaken. On the other hand, pancreatic pseudocysts which are infected may be treated with external surgical drainage or pigtail catheter drainage and followed.[42,43] If unsuccessful, surgical debridement may be necessary.

Prevention of Recurrence. Once a patient has recovered from his first attack of acute pancreatitis, he has a 25 to 60% chance of recurrent pancreatitis in the next one to two years. This emphasizes the importance of identifying correctable conditions which predispose the patient to acute pancreatitis. Furthermore, it is important for therapeutic reasons to distinguish between acute and chronic pancreatitis. This differentiation can be made by radiographic pancreatic calcifications, diabetes, fat malabsorption, and secretory pancreatic testing. US and CT may also make this distinction. However, ERCP is the most useful in making the diagnosis of chronic pancreatitis.

The incidence of "idiopathic" cases has been reduced in number with the advent of ERCP and sphincter of Oddi manometry. In those cases that were described as idiopathic, diagnostic ERCP detected surgically remediable abnormalities in 35 to 40% of patients.[44,45] The abnormalities found include US negative choledocholithiasis and cholelithiasis, obstruction of the pancreatic duct by calculi, strictures, small pseudocysts, annular pancreas, carcinoma, tumors of the papilla of Vater, choledochocole, and pancreatic divisum. Short of carcinomatosis, many of these findings may be amenable to endoscopic correction.

In addition to lesions demonstrated by ERCP, many patients who have been described as having idiopathic pancreatitis may have sphincter of Oddi dysfunction either due to fibrosis or inflammation as well as functional sphincter abnormalities (dyskinesia). Several studies have been suggested in establishing the diagnosis of sphincter dysfunction but unfortunately, they have had poor sensitivity and specificity. Currently, the procedure of choice is sphincter of Oddi manometry. Unfortunately, this test is technically demanding and is offered only in a few centers. When it has been properly performed, abnormal sphincter function has been identified in approximately 20% of patients with idiopathic pancreatitis and normal ERCP.[46-48] Surgical sphincteroplasty combined with septectomy or endoscopic sphincterotomy of the pancreatic sphincter has eliminated further attacks of pancreatitis in a good number of patients with sphincter of Oddi dysfunction.[49]

References

1. McDermott WV Jr, Bartlett MK, Culver PJ: Acute pancreatitis after prolonged fast and subsequent surfeit N Engl J Med 1956;254:379.
2. Venu RP, Geenen JE, Hogan WJ, et al: Role of endoscopic retrograde cholangiopancreatography in the diagnosis and treatment of cholecochocele. Gastroenterology. 1984;87:1144.
3. Nakamura K, Sarles M, and Payan H: Three-dimensional reconstruction of the pancreatic ducts in chronic pancreatitis. Gastroenterology. 1972;62:942.
4. Lotveit T, Aune S, Johnsrud NK, et al: The clinical significance of juxta-papillary duodenal diverticula. Scand J Gastroenterol. 10(1975;suppl. 34)22.
5. Farmer RC, Maslin SC, and Reber HA: Acute pancreatitis - Role of duct permeability Surg Forum. 1983;34:224.
6. Creutzfeldt W, Schmidt H: Aetiology and pathogenesis of pancreatitis Scand J Gastroenterol. 1970;5(suppl 6):47.
7. Geenen JE, Hogan WJ, Dodds WJ, et al: Intraluminal pressure recording from the human sphincter of Oddi. Gastroenterology. 1980;78:317.
8. Opie EL: The etiology of acute hemorrhagic pancreatitis. Bull Johns Hopkins Hosp 1901;12:182.
9. Acosta JM, Rossi R, Ledesma CL: The usefulness of stool screening for diagnosing cholelithiasis in acute pancreatitis. A description of the technique Am J Dig Dis. 1977;22:168.
10. DiMagno EP, Shorter RG, and Taylor WF: Relationships between pancreaticobiliary ductal anatomy and pancreatic ductal parenchymal histology. Cancer. 1982;49:361.
11. Anderson MC, Mehn WH, Methad HL: An evaluation of the common channel as a factor in pancreatic or biliary disease. Ann Surg. 1960;151:379.
12. Steer ML, Meldolesi J, Figarella C: Pancreatitis: The role of lysosomes Dig Dis Sci. 1984;29:934.
13. Geokas MC, Rinderknecht H, Swanson V, et al: The role of elastase in acute hemorrhagic pancreatitis in man. Lab. Invest 1968;19:235.

14. Lasson A: Acute pancreatitis in man A clinical and biochemical study of pathophysiology and treatment. Scand J Gastroenterol. 1984;19(suppl 99):1.

15. Peterson LM, Brooks JR, Lethal pancreatitis: A diagnostic dilemma. Am J Surg 1979; 127:491.

16. Dickson AP, O'Neill J, Imrie CW: Hyperlipidaemia alcohol abuse and acute pancreatitis. Br J Surg 1984;71:685.

17. Eckfeldt JH, Kolars JC, Elson MK, et al: Serum tests for pancreatitis in patients with abdominal pain. Arch Pathol Lab Med. 1985;109:316.

18. Steinberg WM, Goldstein SS, Davis ND, et al: Diagnostic assays in acute pancreatitis. A study of sensitivity and specificity. Ann Intern Med. 1985;102:576.

19. Buchler M, Malfertheiner P, Uhl W, et al: A new staging system in patients with acute pancreatitis. (abstract). Gastroenterology. 1986;90:1361.

20. VanDyke JA, Stanley RJ, Berland LL: Diagnosis and treatment. Pancreatic imaging. Ann Intern Med. 1985;102:212.

21. Balthazar EJ, Ranson JHC, Naidich DP, et al: Acute pancreatitis: Prognostic value of CT. Radiology. 1985;156:767-772.

22. Sostre CF, Flournoy JG, Bova JG, et al: Pancreatic phlegmon clinical features and course. Dig Dis Sci 1985;30:918-927.

23. Nordestgaard AG, Wilson SE, Williams RA: Early computerized tomography as a predictor of outcome in acute pancreatitis. Am J Surg. 1986;152:127-132.

24. Vernacchia FS, Jeffrey RB, Federle MP, et al: Pancreatic abscess: Predictive value of early abdominal CT. Radiology. 1987;162:435-438.

25. Jeffrey RB, Grendell JH, Federle MP, et al: Improved survival with early CT diagnosis of pancreatic abscess. Gastrointest Radiol. 1987;12:26-30.

26. Gerzof SG, Banks PA, Robbins AH, et al: Early diagnosis of pancreatic infection by computed tomography-guided aspiration. Gastroenterology. 1987;93:1315-1320.

27. Bittner R, Block S, Buchler M, et al: Pancreatic abscess and infected pancreatic necrosis; different local septic complications in acute pancreatitis. Dig Dis Sci. 1987;32:1082.

28. Banks PA, Gersoz SG, Robbins AH, et al: Diagnosis of pancreatic infection by CT-guided aspiration: An update. Pancreas 3. 1988;5:590.

29. Howard MJ: Gallstone pancreatitis, in Howard JM, Jordan GL Jr, Reber HA (eds): Surgical Diseases of the Pancreas Philadelphia Lea & Febiger 1987 p. 269.

30. Goodman AJ, Neoptolemos JP, Carr-Locke DL, et al: Detection of gallstones after acute pancreatitis. Gut. 1985;26:125.

31. Safrany L, Cotton PB: A preliminary report: urgent duodenoscopic sphincterotomy for acute gallstone pancreatitis. Surgery. 1981;89:424.

32. Mayer AD, McMahoy MJ, Corfield AP, et al: Controlled clinical trial of peritoneal lavage for the treatment of severe acute pancreatitis. N Engl J Med. 1985;312:399.

33. Stone HH, Fabian TC: Peritoneal dialysis in the treatment of acute alcoholic pancreatitis Surg Gynecol Obstet. 1980;150:878.

34. Waterman NG, Walsky R, Kasdan ML, et al: The treatment of acute hemorrhagic pancreatitis by sump drainage Surg Gynecol Obstet. 1968;126:963.

35. Nordback IH and Auvinen OA: Long-term results after pancreas resection for acute necrotizing pancreatitis Br J Surg. 1985;72:687.

36. Beger HG, Bittner R, Block S, et al: Bacterial contamination of pancreatic necrosis A prospective clinical study. Gastroenterology. 1986;91:433.

37. Pellegrini CA: The treatment of acute pancreatitis: A continuing challenge (editorial). N Engl J Med. 1985;312:436.

38. Reber HA: Surgical intervention in necrotizing pancreatitis (editorial). Gastroenterology. 1986;91:479.

39. Goldstein DA, Llach R, Massry SG: Acute renal failure in patients with acute pancreatitis. Arch Intern Med. 1976;136:1363.
40. Dickson AP, Imrie CW: The incidence and prognosis of body wall ecchymosis in acute pancreatitis. Surg Gynecol Obstet. 1984;159:343.
41. Clavien PA, Hauser H, Meyer P, et al: Value of contrast-enhanced computerized tomography in the early diagnosis and prognosis of acute pancreatitis. A prospective study of 202 patients. Am J Surg. 1988;155:457.
42. Pubols MH, Bartelt DC, Greene LJ: Trypsin inhibitor from human pancreas and pancreatic juice. J Biol Chem. 1974;249:2235.
43. Warshaw AL, Lesser PB, Rie M, et al: The pathogenesis of pulmonary edema in acute pancreatitis. Ann Surg. 1975;182:505.
44. Cotton PB, Beales JSM: Endoscopic pancreatography in management of relapsing acute pancreatitis Br Med J. 1974;1:608.
45. Feller ER: Endoscopic retrograde cholangiopancreatography in the diagnosis of unexplained pancreatitis. Arch Intern Med. 1984;144:1797.
46. Geenen JE, Hogan WJ, Dodds WJ, et al: Intraluminal pressure recording from the human sphincter of Oddi. Gastroenterology. 1980;78:317.
47. Toouli J, Roberts-Thomson IC, Dent J, et al: Sphincter of Oddi motility disorders in patients with idiopathic recurrent pancreatitis. Br J Surg. 1985;72:859.
48. Venu RP, Geenen JE, Hogan WJ, et al: Idiopathic recurrent pancreatitis (IRP): Diagnostic role of ERCP and sphincter of Oddi manometry. Gastrointest Endosc. 1985;31:141.
49. Moody FG, Berenson MM, McCloskey D: Transampullary septectomy for postcholecystectomy pain. Ann Surg. 1977;186:415.

Case 18

Evaluation of Erectile Dysfunction

Cynthia G. Kreger, MD and Jeffrey P. York, MD

Case History

A 68-year-old male was seen in the ambulatory setting at the Ohio State University Hospitals, for general medical evaluation after his primary care provider had retired. He had long-standing Type II diabetes mellitus managed with insulin and an oral agent. He also had moderate systolic hypertension treated with a diuretic and beta blocker. Although he denied any known cardiovascular disease, evaluation of his resting EKG revealed evidence of an inferior myocardial infarction.

Upon detailed questioning, this patient admitted to a several year history of erectile dysfunction. He recalled mentioning it to his physician and being told this was due to the medications he was on and also that "this happens at your age." No subsequent evaluation of this problem was undertaken.

The patient stated that he noted the gradual onset of erectile dysfunction over approximately an eight-year period, shortly after the diagnosis of diabetes was made. This progressed incrementally from a marked decrease in frequency of erections, to an inability to achieve an erection with rigidity sufficient for intercourse. Early morning erections remained present. The patient then had total cessation of erectile functioning after starting a beta blocker for hypertension, although he did not mention this to his physician because of discomfort and what he perceived to be an inevitable fact of aging.

The patient reported no change in configuration of his penis such as bowing or curvature with erections, and no ejaculatory dysfunction. His past medical history was negative for trauma, pelvic surgery, ethanol or tobacco use. He was circumcised in 1982 (because of recurrent cutaneous infections), which he felt coincided with worsening of his erectile dysfunction. He otherwise denied angina, claudication, paresthesias, problems with gait or balance, or symptoms of bladder dysfunction. He also denied coexistent depression, or associated life stressors.

He stated that his libido had not changed and that both he and his wife wanted to resume sexual intimacy. His partner appeared supportive and there were no extramarital partners involved.

Physical Exam. On physical exam the patient was afebrile, with BP and pulse in the recumbent position of 164/88 and 76, respectively, with no significant change upon standing. Chest exam revealed no gynecomastia and was otherwise unremarkable. His cardiovascular system was normal except for diminished posterior tibialis pulses bilaterally. Genital exam revealed no inguinal hernias, a circumcised phallus without fibrosis or plaques, bilaterally descended testes (approx 20 gm) without masses and of firm consistency. Rectal exam revealed normal sphincter tone and a benign prostate. Perineal pin prick sensation was intact. Screening neurologic exam revealed diminished vibratory sense in the lower extremities; however, knee jerk, ankle jerk, and proprioception were intact.

Laboratory Data. Laboratory evaluation revealed normal prolactin, thyroid, renal, and hepatic studies. In addition, CBC and serum chemistries were within normal limits. A fasting blood sugar was 137 mg/dl while HG A1C was 10.6. Initial testosterone determination was borderline low with a value of 2.7 ng/ml (normal 3 to 10). However, a repeated testosterone level was 3.1 ng/ml.

After history, physical examination, and laboratory determination, the patient was referred for further urologic evaluation.

Additional Diagnostic Studies. Based on history and physical examination, it was felt this patient had a form of organic impotence, as opposed to psychogenic, and thus evaluation for possible vasculogenic causes was begun. Measurement of the dorsal penile brachial index (PBI), a noninvasive screening test for penile arterial insufficiency, revealed an index of 0.95. Such a value made arteriogenic erectile dysfunction less likely, but, did not rule this out entirely. Thus, a more physiologic evaluation of the penile arterial system, using intracorporal injection of a vasoactive agent (papaverine hydrochloride), was offered to the patient; however, he declined this evaluation

The patient then underwent evaluation for venous incompetence, as a cause of erectile dysfunction, with dynamic infusion cavernosometry. This study revealed an abnormally rapid fall of intracorporal pressure after saline-induced erection, consistent with a severe venous leak. Cavernosography (radiologic imaging of the penile venous system) revealed drainage via the right corporal vein with abnormal run off from the circumflex and deep dorsal vein. Cavernosal arteries were noted to be normal during this study. In light of the abnormal results of the above test, and without evidence for an underlying neurologic disorder, formal testing of the afferent penile neuro-pathway was not undertaken.

Based on history, physical examination, laboratory evaluation, PBI, and cavernosography-cavernosometry, the etiology of this patient's erectile dysfunction was believed to be at least in part venous incompetence. Therapeutic alternatives offered to this patient included: venous ligation, insertion of a penile prosthesis, use of a vacuum-assisted device, or trial of intracorporal vasodilator injections. The patient is still considering his options.

Discussion

Impotence, or erectile dysfunction, is defined as the inability to obtain and sustain an erection satisfactory for intercourse during 50% of sexual encounters. Historically, impotence has been viewed either as a "natural" consequence of aging, and as a problem that should just be accepted by the patient, or alternatively as a problem with a psychogenic etiology, characteristically poorly responsive to psychotherapy. Consequently, the primary care physician as well as the sub-specialist had limited options to offer the patient with erectile dysfunction who desired potency.

In the last decade there has been dramatic progress in the understanding of normal erectile physiology and the mechanisms potentially responsible for erectile dysfunction. As a consequence, our diagnostic tests and therapeutic options for the treatment of impotence have become significantly more sophisticated. Current-ly, there is much a physician can do to help the impotent patient desiring potency; but the first hurdle is identification of the problem.

Prevalence

Impotence is a common problem, affecting up to 10 million American men.[1,2] The Kinsey data of 1943 suggest that prevalence increases with increasing age such that 10% of 55-year-old men are impotent as compared to 20-25% of those 60-70 years old, and 55-75% of those 75-80 years old.[3] In a more recent study, 34% of men surveyed in a medical outpatient clinic were impotent; the average age in this study was 59.4 years.[4] Certain patient populations appear to be particularly vul-nerable to this problem. It has been estimated that 50-75% of diabetic men will suffer erectile dysfunction at some point in their lives.[5,6]

Given the large number of Americans suffering from diabetes mellitus, and the estimate that 21% of the US population will be over age 65 in the year 2000,[7] impotence will be an increasingly important issue for many of our patients. With greater understanding of the pathophysiology of erectile dysfunction and greater diagnostic and therapeutic options, it becomes the responsibility of the primary care physician to discuss issues pertaining to sexual function with patients in order to identify this problem and thus initiate the workup and appropriate referral for those patients desiring sexual potency.

What are the critical steps in approaching this problem? In order to best evaluate the salient features of the history, physical exam, and workup of impotence with reference to the above case, a familiarity with erectile physiology and the differential diagnosis of impotence is needed.

Erectile Anatomy and Physiology

Penile erection is a complex phenomenon dependent upon the synergistic interplay of an intact vascular, hormonal, peripheral and central nervous system. There are both reflexogenic erections, elicited by local stimulation of the genitalia, and psychogenic erections mediated by central stimuli. The afferent and efferent pathways for reflexogenic erections are mediated by the pudendal nerve and the sacral parasympathetics (which carry fibers to the penile nerve), respectively.[8] The central pathways for psychogenic erections are not as well delineated but appear to be primarily sympathetic. While much is still to be understood about the neurophysiologic initiation and maintenance of erection, significant advances in understanding the hemodynamic components of the erectile response have been made in the last ten years.

The blood supply to the penis is derived from the internal pudendal artery (arising from the internal iliac artery), which becomes the penile artery and then branches into the dorsal, spongiosal, cavernosal, and bulbar arteries. The dorsal and spongiosal arteries are responsible for engorgement of the glans penis and corpus spongiosum, while the cavernosal arteries supply the main erectile bodies, i.e. the corpora cavernosa. Within the corpora cavernosa, the deep penile arteries end in multiple helicine arterioles which empty into the sinusoidal spaces (vascular spaces with a smooth muscle lining). In the flaccid state, the terminal arterioles as well as the sinusoidal spaces are contracted.[9]

Venous drainage of the corpora cavernosa is primarily by numerous small venules originating in the sinusoidal spaces. These venules form a subtunical venous plexus which drains via emissary veins running obliquely through the tunica albuginea (the thick fibrous sheath which encases the cavernosal tissue). Distally, the emissary veins coalesce into circumflex veins which drain into the dorsal vein. Proximally the cavernosal bodies drain directly into the cavernosal vein and the internal iliac system.[9,10]

Penile tumescence and rigidity are thought to be the result of neurologically mediated sinusoidal smooth muscle relaxation with subsequent dilation and increased compliance of the sinusoidal spaces. Such changes are most likely accompanied by a decrease in cavernosal vascular resistance and a marked increase in blood flow via the internal pudendal artery and branches. Expansion of the blood-filled sinusoidal system against the noncompliant tunicae albuginea causes passive compression of the venous outflow with entrapment of blood and maintenance of erection. The neurologic stimuli leading to all of the above-mentioned actions are still controversial. There is combined cholinergic and adrenergic interplay but also a nonadrenergic, noncholinergic neurotransmitter which acts directly on the smooth muscle cells to secrete an "endothelial derived relaxation factor", causing relaxation and dilation of the sinusoidal spaces. The exact role of psychic stimuli as well as hormonal input in this schema needs further delineation.[9-12]

After ejaculation or cessation of stimuli, there is sympathetically mediated contraction of smooth muscles around the sinusoids and arterioles, hence diminishing arterial flow. In addition, blood is probably actively expelled from the sinusoidal spaces and, as venous channels reopen, flaccidity returns.[9,10,12]

Differential Diagnosis

Given the complex physiology of the erectile response, any process that interferes with the penile vascular system, innervation, or hormonal and psychic input may produce impotence (Table 1). Currently, the vast majority of cases of impotence, despite coexisting psychogenic factors, have an organic basis. In contrast to our thinking of just 15 years ago, impotence with solely a psychogenic basis is probably uncommon. Vascular disease and diabetes mellitus account for the majority of impotence. More specific estimates for other etiologies are influenced by the clinic population studied and by the realization that a majority of cases are probably multifactorial in origin.[4,7]

Diabetes Mellitus. Diabetes mellitus may be the single most common disease entity associated with erectile dysfunction.[13] As in the patient under discussion, diabetic patients characteristically complain of gradual onset of loss of erectile capability with preservation of libido. The loss of erections is not always a late

Table 1

Differential Diagnosis of Impotence	
Diabetes Mellitus	**Endocrine (other than diabetes)**
	Hypogonadism
Vasculogenic	Primary
Arterial insufficiency	Secondary
Venous incompetence	Hyperprolactinemia
Iatrogenic disruption of	Pituitary adenoma
vascular supply	Medication-induced
	Hypothyroidism
	Hyperthyroidism
Neurogenic	**Anatomic**
Cerebral vascular accidents	Phimosis
Multiple sclerosis	Penile fibrosis
Parkinson's disease	Peyronie's disease
Spinal cord injuries	
Medications	**Psychogenic**

manifestation of the disease, but may in fact be the presenting complaint in a previously undiagnosed diabetic patient.[5,6]

The loss of erections in the diabetic is probably due to a combination of the neurogenic and vasculogenic abnormalities associated with this disease. There is evidence to indicate that diabetes may cause collagen deposition on the sinusoidal smooth muscle. This leads to a noncompliant sinusoidal system precluding neurotransmitter-induced relaxation, and thus an inability to increase vascular inflow.[5,6,11,14] These alterations in smooth muscle functioning have been demonstrated in ultrastructural anatomic studies[15] and are implied by the relative resistance of diabetic impotent patients to respond to intracavernosal injection of vasodilating agents.

Endocrinologic. Endocrine clinics, with predominantly referral based populations, have reported a 6 to 45% incidence of impotence due to endocrine causes. In the general population, however, these cases probably account for less than 2% of the impotent patients.[4,16] Despite this small number, evaluation of the hypothalamic-pituitary-gonadal axis is fairly uncomplicated and inexpensive. Importantly, abnormalities of this axis are usually easily treated.

Endocrinologic causes of impotence include primary and secondary hypogonadism, hyperprolactinemia, and thyroidal disorders. Although spontaneous nocturnal erections may be affected by testosterone levels, it is libido and desire for sexual activity that is most exquisitely depressed in patients with hypogonadism.[16]

Hyperprolactinemia is usually caused by medications known to increase the prolactin level (e.g., estrogens, phenothiazine, etc.). Hyperprolactinemia due to primary pituitary abnormalities or adenomas is usually associated with a depressed testosterone level, libido, and erectile function. It is thought that the high levels of prolactin may alter the pulsatile LH secretion by the pituitary gland and secondarily affect the pituitary-gonadal axis. Lastly, erectile dysfunction has been associated with hypothyroidism as well as hyperthyroidism; however, the physiologic basis for this is unclear.[16]

Vasculogenic. Primary arterial ageing factors such as macro- and micro-atherosclerotic vascular disease probably account for the majority of organic causes of erectile dysfunction. The patient may complain of total lack of erections, but more commonly will complain of decreased hardness, frequency, and early loss of erections. Risk factors include hypertension, tobacco usage, hyperlipidemia, and diabetes mellitus.[17] Other causes of arteriogenic erectile dysfunction include pelvic or abdominal surgery, penile or pelvic trauma, or external beam irradiation to the pelvis; all of which may interfere with penile blood flow.[18]

Patients with isolated venous incompetence, or excessive venous outflow, will often describe partial erections or erections that are quickly lost and inadequate for vaginal intercourse. Venous leakage appears to correlate with increasing age, Peyronie's disease, and may be a major factor in primary erectile dysfunction of young men. The patient in the case under discussion related a history most compatible with vasculogenic impotence.

Neurogenic. Any disease state which interferes with the central or peripheral innervation of the penis may cause erectile dysfunction. Although some patients suffering from a complete or incomplete traumatic spinal cord injury may exhibit erectile function, less than 25% are able to have satisfactory vaginal intercourse.[19] The majority of these patients have reflexogenic erections induced by sexual or noxious stimulation of the genitalia. In this setting, the corporal cavernosal bodies engorge without involvement of the spongiosum or glans penis and thus tumescence is extremely short-lived. Nontraumatic spinal injury, such as spinal stenosis, disc disease, and infectious etiologies, can also cause erectile dysfunction. In addition, demyelinizing or supratentorial disease such as cerebral vascular accidents, multiple sclerosis, or Parkinson's disease have been implicated in erectile dysfunction. Nondiabetic neuropathy (particularly due to alcohol abuse) may cause posterior column abnormalities and exacerbate preexisting concomitant disease states.[19] The patient in the current case did not have a history which suggested an underlying neurologic disorder existed.

Drugs. A combination of vascular, neurologic, hormonal, and psychic influences are needed to obtain normal penile erection. Understanding this, it is easy to see that erectile function may be adversely affected by pharmacologic agents which influence any one of these components. Evidence to support pharmacologic causes of impotence, however, is meager and mostly subjective, based upon questionnaires or case reports. Very few double-blind studies have been performed with objective criteria for erectile dysfunction as a side effect. In addition, the

Table 2

Drugs Associated With Impotence	
Antihypertensives	**Others**
Sympatholytics	Cimetidine
Aldomet	Ranitidine
Clonidine	Clofibrate
Reserpine	Digoxin
Guanethidine	Anticholinergics
Alpha blockers	Ethanol
Beta blockers	Cocaine
	Marijuana
Major tranquilizers	Nicotine
Antidepressants	
Anxiolytics	**Chemotherapeutic agents**

mechanism by which most drugs cause erectile dysfunction is unknown. Nevertheless, many medications have been associated with impotence (Table 2).

The antihypertensive medications are the group most commonly implicated in erectile dysfunction. The sympatholytics (primarily alpha methyldopa, clonidine, reserpine, and guanethidine) are frequently accused of interfering with sexual functioning. The alpha blockers are relatively infrequently cited and the beta adrenergic agents primarily influence libido and not erectile capacity. The calcium channel blockers, angiotensin-converting enzyme inhibitors, and the diuretics probably do not affect erectile functioning.[20,21]

Other categories of drugs reported to cause disturbances in libido, erectile capacity, and ejaculation include the major tranquilizers, antidepressants, anxiolytics, and chemotherapeutic agents. A whole host of other medications have been implicated in impotence (cimetidine, ranitidine, clofibrate, digoxin, anticholinergic medications, baclofen). As previously stated, the majority of these implications have been case reports and poorly documented in terms of cause and effect. It is prudent, however, when initiating a new medication to determine the status of the patient's erectile capacity prior to starting the medication.[20,21] Medication-induced impotence is less likely an etiologic factor in the current case.

Alcohol also has a tendency to decrease both libido and sexual capability. The central sedative properties of alcohol probably play a role in this, as well as the polyneuropathy and alteration in estrogen metabolism seen with chronic abuse.[22] Chronic use of marijuana has been associated with decreased libido and erectile dysfunction. It is thought that this is due to estrogen like activities of the pesticides used on this drug and not due to the marijuana itself. Cocaine is often used for its aphrodisiac effect, and prolonged erection to the point of priapism has been reported with its use. Chronic cocaine usage, however, has been associated with loss of both libido and erectile capacity. This may be due to a decrease in the reuptake of catecholamines or a vasoconstrictor effect.[23]

Cigarette smoking has long been viewed as detrimental to erectile dysfunction, but only recently has the effect of nicotine been shown to cause local penile vasoconstriction. It is also felt that nicotine may inhibit the nonadrenergic, noncholinergic neurotransmitter found within the corporal cavernosal body, diminishing the ability for relaxation of the sinusoidal smooth muscles.[24]

Psychogenic. Psychologic factors clearly influence erectile capacity and cannot be overlooked even in the presence of an obvious organic cause. Anxiety, depression, and stressful life situation are most commonly found in these cases. Preoccupation during a stressful life event may decrease sexual arousal which otherwise would lead to a normal erection. Anxiety in small amounts may actually improve sexual function; however, as the anxiety increases, both arousal and sexual functioning decrease.[25] It is important to attempt to distinguish between anxiety that causes erectile dysfunction and anxiety that is due to erectile dysfunction. Such factors did not appear to be playing a role in the above-mentioned case.

Patients will often describe the phenomenon of performance anxiety. This is a fairly natural state, in which an inability to perform at one point in time leads to concern over future performance capability, and hence may be self-defeating. This oftentimes happens during a midlife crisis or in a younger man. Usually, with sufficient understanding and support by the sexual partner, this problem resolves spontaneously. Without support from the partner, neither psychotherapy nor reassurance from the primary care physician or urologist will alleviate this problem.[26]

Unfortunately, psychiatric evaluation to determine a nonorganic cause for erectile dysfunction is extremely difficult and oftentimes is not successful in delineating a cause-and-effect relationship.

Evaluation of the Impotent Patient

As mentioned above, penile erection is a neurovascular phenomenon dependent upon sufficient arterial inflow to achieve erection, venous impedance to outflow to maintain it, and appropriate neurologic mediation of these events. In the last ten years much has been written on the various diagnostic modalities to evaluate these components. However, there is no systematic approach to evaluation of the impotent patient documented in the literature. In addition, the sensitivity and specificity of various diagnostic tests have not been clearly determined. Thus, what follows are common strategies for evaluating a patient with erectile dysfunction.

History and Physical Exam. Patient evaluation starts with a fairly detailed sexual, medical, and psychosocial history, as well as physical exam and screening laboratory tests. A thorough history and physical exam, while rarely establishing a specific etiology, will help direct the subsequent work up.

Unlike a complaint of chest pain, a concern over sexual dysfunction is often not volunteered spontaneously by the patient. Instead, this history must be explicitly sought in high risk populations (e.g. diabetics, geriatric patients). The first goal in taking the history is to be sure the problem is indeed impotence as opposed to another form of sexual dysfunction such as diminished libido, ejaculatory failure, or premature ejaculation. Once the problem is established as impotence, as in the case under discussion, it is important to delineate the onset, duration, and exact character of the problem, distinguishing pathologic processes from the normal changes of aging.[18,27] Such normal changes of ageing include: requiring more stimulation to achieve an erection, shorter-lived erections, longer latency time, and a general decrease in frequency of coital activity.[28]

While organic and psychogenic impotence may overlap, the history may at times be helpful in sorting this out. A patient who has psychogenic impotence is more likely to describe the problem as having an abrupt onset, often associated with a life stressor. In addition, this patient usually describes total loss of erectile function which upon further questioning may be partner specific. Usually there is preservation of nocturnal tumescence and rigidity, although reported loss of libido.[18,26,27]

In contrast, erectile dysfunction which is gradual in onset, progresses incrementally from a decrease in frequency of erections to an inability to obtain an erection sufficiently rigid for intercourse (yet with full preservation of libido), tends to be organic. There may be preservation of partial, although weak, nocturnal erections.[18,27] Such a history is similar to the history obtained from the patient under discussion.

In addition to course and onset, the clinician needs to ascertain if it is a problem of attaining or maintaining an erection, what the quality of the erection is, and if the orgasmic response is intact. This may help somewhat in differentiating various organic etiologies. Specifically, if the patient describes weak erections or early loss of rigidity without ejaculation, this is suggestive of venous incompetence. In contrast, if patients describe little or no erectile response, without loss of libido, this may represent arterial insufficiency. In this situation, morning erections may be weak or absent, and the ejaculatory mechanism is usually intact. Risk factors for penile vascular insufficiency should be sought. These include cigarette smoking, hypertension, hyperlipidemia, diabetes mellitus, history of coronary artery disease or peripheral vascular disease.

An underlying neurologic cause may be suggested by a history of known neurologic disease, changes in bowel and bladder function, decreased penile sensation, or symptoms of a peripheral neuropathy (none of which were elicited from the patient under discussion).

Given the association of many medications with impotence, a detailed medication history should also be sought. Although the patient under discussion related further worsening of erectile functioning after starting an antihypertensive medication, it was most likely coincidental, as his erectile capacity had been steadily declining for some time.

It is also important to ascertain the presence of social or economic stressors, as well as any past history suggestive of mental illness. Lastly, the patient's relationship with his sexual partner needs to be explored in some detail. The attitude of the sexual partner may well influence diagnostic as well as therapeutic options.

Physical Exam. The physical exam may provide clues to the cause of the erectile dysfunction. Specifically, the exam should focus on evaluation of the neurologic, endocrine, and vascular systems as well as the genitalia. The autonomic and peripheral nervous system (including sensory testing of the penis and perineum) should be evaluated for evidence of possible neurogenic impotence. In addition, the patient should be examined for gynecomastia (possible evidence of hyperprolactinemia) and the presence of small soft testes (possible evidence of hypogonadism), as well as overall development of secondary sex characteristics. Evidence of widespread vascular disease should be sought. Occasionally, an anatomic cause of erectile dysfunction will be found when careful genital exam reveals phimosis, fibrosis, or the plaques of Peyronie's disease. In the current case, the physical exam was helpful in ruling out signs of an endocrinopathy, widespread vascular disease, or anatomic cause of impotence.

Laboratory Evaluation. The laboratory evaluation may be used to screen for diabetes mellitus as well as other endocrinopathies. A normal urinalysis and fasting blood sugar should rule out diabetes mellitus in the majority of patients. Laboratory data can also be used to rule out hyperprolactinemia, hypogonadism, and disorders of thyroid function. In most cases, a serum testosterone, if normal, should be a sufficient screening test for hypogonadism. It should be remembered, however, that testosterone is secreted in diurnal and cyclic fashion.[16] Thus, a low level of testosterone should be either repeated, as was done in the current case, or a "pooled" specimen (three blood drawings over an hour) sent to smooth out the diurnal pattern. Most clinicians also obtain a complete blood count, liver panel, and renal panel.

NPT (Nocturnal Penile Tumescence) Testing. In normal males, nocturnal erections lasting 25-35 minutes occur periodically during REM sleep.[28] In 1970, Karacan suggested that formal evaluation of tumescence during REM sleep may be used as a tool in the evaluation of impotence.[29] Since that time, NPT testing has been utilized to differentiate psychogenic from organic erectile dysfunction. Historically, it has been believed that men with psychogenic impotence display normal patterns of REM-associated erections whereas patients with organic impotence lack this.[29,30] Importantly, however, this procedure fails to distinguish among various etiologies of erectile dysfunction.

NPT testing has traditionally taken place in a formal sleep lab over two to three nights. Penile strain gauges, EEG, and EOG (electrooculogram) patches are placed in order to monitor changes in penile circumference, as well as the pattern of sleep since disturbances in the latter may affect erectile activity. Because Wein and co-workers[31] described functionally inadequate rigidity in some patients with adequate tumescence, it is routine practice during NPT testing to physically evaluate the quality of erection with either a strain gauge or manual compression of the penis.[30]

Because of the inconvenience and expense of nonambulatory testing, a number of home devices have been designed to take the place of NPT testing, although they do not document sleep patterns. These include the stamp test,[32] the Snap-Gauge band,[33] and the Rigiscan[30] device. All evaluate tumescence but only the Snap-Gauge band and the Rigiscan formally provide data regarding rigidity of erection.

NPT monitoring may still be the best means of differentiating organic from functional erectile dysfunction. However, there are reports that depression may interfere with nocturnal erections and that treatment of the underlying depression may restore erectile capacity. In addition, in selected other organic conditions a patient may have seemingly normal nocturnal tumescence and yet be unable to perform adequately sexually.[30] NPT was not performed in the current case.

Vasculogenic Evaluation. Leriche first directed attention to the association of arterial insufficiency with impotence in 1923.[18] Much later, Karacan[34] in his hallmark studies of NPT reported that more than 50% of the cases of impotence he evaluated had an organic etiology, the majority of which were due to arterial lesions. Recent advances in the understanding of the physiology of erection highlight the importance of the venous as well as the arterial tree, in obtaining and maintaining an erection adequate for vaginal intercourse. Thus, it is necessary to evaluate the integrity of these two systems often employing both noninvasive and invasive diagnostics, as was done in the case under discussion.

PBI. In 1971, Gaskell evaluated blood flow through the glans penis using a spectroscopic measurement of oxyhemoglobin absorption.[35] Since that time, mercury strain gauge plethysmography, Doppler measurements of dorsal artery pressure, pulse wave analysis, thermography, and radionuclide blood flow studies have been utilized to determine the adequacy of penile arterial blood flow.[36] All of these techniques are suboptimal in that penile blood flow is measured in the flaccid state and does not reliably reflect the functional capacity of the arterial tree during erection.

The most common screening test to evaluate arteriogenic impotence, the PBI, is performed by placing a 2-cm pneumatic cuff around the base of the penis. The systolic pressure distal to the cuff is measured and compared to the brachial systolic blood pressure. Britt[37] determined that normal subjects had a penile systolic blood pressure, in the flaccid state, greater than or equal to the brachial pressure. A ratio less than 0.6 is considered abnormal and correlates with arterial insufficiency.[36-38]

One can also screen for pelvic steal phenomenon by measuring PBI before and after lower extremity exercise. A normal study shows minimal depression of PBI following exercise. A severe depression indicates aorto-iliac occlusive disease with shunting of blood from the hypogastric to the external iliac system resulting in erectile loss.[36,38]

There are several drawbacks to PBI as a measure of arterial insufficiency. Pressure readings may be altered by inappropriate cuff size. In addition, PBI measures flow in the dorsal arteries which contribute little to filling of the main erectile bodies, the corpora cavernosa. Moreover, flow is measured in the flaccid state and may not correlate with events during erection. Despite these shortcomings, a doppler penile brachial index is a good noninvasive screening test, as an abnormal result may define penile arterial insufficiency with a positive predictive value of 91%.[39] A negative test, however, does not exclude vascular insufficiency as angiographic studies and PBI measurements do not always correlate.[36] In the case under discussion, the PBI was 0.95. While arterial insufficiency is less likely to be playing a major role in this patient's impotence, a more physiologic evaluation of the integrity of the arterial system may be attempted as described below.

Vasodilator Studies. Virag[40] first demonstrated that a combination of papaverine hydrochloride, phentolamine, and phenoxybenzamine could cause an erection when injected into the cavernosal spaces. These medications act via an antinicotinic effect at the ganglionic receptor or by direct dilation of the sinusoidal smooth muscles, leading to engorgement of the cavernosal bodies and thus pharmacologic erection. Response to these drugs requires an intact arterial system and veno-occlusive mechanism, as well as the capability of the sinusoidal smooth muscles to relax. Thus, many clinicians feel that evaluating the response to intracavernosal injection of a vasodilating drug is the single best screening test to rule out arteriogenic impotence.[36,40,41] The patient under discussion declined this diagnostic study.

Papaverine is the most common medication used for intracavernosal injection with the normal response being penile lengthening, tumescence, and rigidity within five to ten minutes, lasting approximately one to four hours.[39,42,43] Both penile plethysmography and pulse Doppler analysis demonstrate a significant increase in penile arterial inflow and arterial diameter in normal subjects after injection. Arteriographic studies have confirmed this finding.[36,42]

Intracavernosal test injections of papaverine can thus be used to measure directly the vascular component of erection. It is generally accepted that attainment of a rigid erection after a standard dose of papaverine eliminates significant vasculogenic abnormalities as the cause of erectile dysfunction. However, the response to vasodilating agents does not differentiate between neurogenic and psychogenic impotence as in both cases pharmacologically induced erections may be normal.[39,42,43]

A very weak or delayed erection, or no erectile response, may be consistent with arteriogenic impotence. It should be noted, however, that extreme anxiety may dampen the response to intracavernosal injection while sexual stimulation enhances it. For this reason, a lack of response to papaverine injection by no means guarantees a vasculogenic etiology.[39]

Intracavernosal papaverine injection is not without risk. If a significant venous leakage exists, the bolus of papaverine may become systemic very quickly and there have been reported cases of severe hypotension, facial flushing, and loss of consciousness.[41] The major side effect in the use of this diagnostic tool is the small incidence of priapism (prolonged erection greater than five to six hours in duration). In these cases it is necessary to pharmacologically reverse the erection with a direct intracavernosal injection of a sympathomimetic agent such as phenylephrine after removing a corresponding amount of blood from the cavernosal body. There have been no reported cases of an inability to pharmacologically reverse the papaverine-induced erection.

In summary, many feel that injection of low-dose papaverine is a very useful diagnostic test to rule out significant vasculogenic erectile abnormalities. Importantly, if the pharmacologic erection is not fully rigid and/or is quickly lost, further evaluation for possible venous incompetence is warranted.

Arteriography. Pelvic arteriography is utilized to define the penile arterial inflow in those patients in whom a discrete lesion is anticipated and who may be candidates for a penile arterialization procedure. The instillation of intracavernosal vasoactive agents during the study allows for optimal visualization of the arterial tree in the dilated state.

Arteriography, however, is an invasive procedure requiring femoral arterial catheterization with the use of contrast medium. In addition, it is necessary to visualize both internal pudendal, inferior epigastric, cavernosal, and dorsal arteries. For these reasons, very few "normal" men have been studied in this manner and thus normal anatomy and variances have not been adequately described. Because of associated risk and the difficulty of revascularization procedures, careful selection of patients undergoing arteriography is required.[36,39]

Evaluation for Venous Incompetence. Lue[44] in 1983 provided evidence that venous outflow decreases during normal erections. Since then, several investigators have provided evidence that an intact veno-occlusive mechanism is necessary for the production and maintenance of normal erections. Cavernosometry can measure the functional capability of the veno-occlusive mechanism while cavernosography can provide anatomical information regarding individual drainage systems.[45,46]

Normal saline is infused into the cavernosal body and the rate needed to obtain and maintain an artificial erection is measured. Pretreatment with intracavernosal papaverine provides a more physiologic test and reduces the rate of flow and volume of saline needed. If no vascular abnormality is present, a corporal pressure approaching the mean brachial pressure will be obtained within 10 to 15 minutes and cavernosography will show nonvisualization of the venous system. When intracavernosal pressure becomes suprasystolic, infusion slows to maintain that set pressure. Once the infusion is stopped, intracorporal pressure slowly returns to normal.[36,45-47]

In contrast, in venous incompetence quite high flow rates and substantial volumes may be needed and then only a weak erection observed. Venous incompetence may also be manifest by a markedly rapid pressure drop once the infusion is stopped, as was the case with the patient under discussion. If venous leakage occurs, dilute contrast medium is instilled and plain films of the pelvis taken. In this manner, penile venous tributaries can be seen and suitability for surgical correction ascertained.[36,45-47]

Dynamic infusion cavernosometry is an invasive test. Indications for performance of the test include (1) primary erectile dysfunction, (2) no response to intracavernosal vasoactive drugs, and (3) poor response to vasoactive drugs with intact penile Doppler studies (i.e. adequate arterial dilatation with administration of vasoactive drugs intracorporally).[46] Risks are minor, but potentially can be devastating. This is a relatively new diagnostic test and findings are still being analyzed. This test should be used only on patients deemed suitable candidates for venous surgery.

Neurogenic Evaluation. A neurogenic etiology for erectile dysfunction is said to exist if there is an alteration in either central or peripheral neurologic stimulation of the penis leading to failure of the normal hemodynamic response. Less than 20% of cases of impotence are neurogenic in origin and are primarily seen in patients with underlying neurologic disease.[48] However, the complaint of impotence may reflect an undiagnosed neurologic condition which may be subsequently discovered with careful evaluation.

Unlike the evaluation of arteriogenic and psychogenic impotence, neurogenic evaluation has not progressed substantially. The efferent autonomic cavernosal nerves cannot be directly tested, although impairment may be suggested by a complaint of bowel or bladder dysfunction. The afferent somatic pathway of the dorsal nerve may be tested by penile biothesiometry; a subjective but reproducible test of vibratory proprioception at the head of the penis. Perception of vibration was found to be an age dependent phenomenon perhaps reflecting degeneration of Pacinian corpuscles or age-related dermal changes.[48]

If there is evidence of sensory loss, a more objective assessment may be obtained by evaluating the conduction velocity of the dorsal nerve or the latency of the bulbocavernosus reflex. It has been implied that patients with a prolonged dorsal nerve root response may be able to obtain normal erections but have difficulty in maintaining their erections without constant glandular stimulation.[48]

Therapeutic Options

As our diagnostic capabilities have increased, so have the therapeutic options for restoring penile tumescence and rigidity. The traditional treatment of impotence in the last 15 years has been the penile prosthesis. Although this is still the mainstay of therapy, several new options exist including oral pharmacotherapy, intracavernosal injection of vasoactive compounds, penile revascularization procedures, and hand-held mechanical devices to augment erection. The therapy chosen needs to be tailored to the patient and may involve a multidisciplinary approach, employing the primary care physician, urologist, endocrinologist, and psychologist when appropriate.

Elimination of Adverse Medications. A careful history must always be taken with consideration of changing or stopping medications that may be interfering with erectile function. Surprisingly, this can sometimes alleviate the need for invasive diagnostic or therapeutic interventions.

Hormonal Treatment. Hormonal therapy is advisable only in that subset of patients with a clearly documented endocrine deficiency. Testosterone therapy may prove beneficial in the impotence of hypogonadal origin. The most effective dose appears to be 200-300 mg given intramuscularly every two to three weeks. Side effects include fluid retention, possible worsening of hypertension, and polycythemia due to the androgen stimulated erythropoietin production. Since testosterone is peripherally converted to estradiol, there may be resultant gynecomastia. Importantly, testosterone may stimulate prostate growth which may be a significant problem for men with BPH, or undetected adenocarcinoma of the prostate. As a result, the use of testosterone in impotent men with low normal or borderline testosterone levels remains controversial.[16] It is for these reasons that testosterone injection was not a therapeutic alternative offered to the patient under discussion.

In patients with hyperprolactinemia, assuming no pituitary tumor is found, bromocriptine may be used and may improve erectile function, but exogenous androgens are often also needed. Lastly, treatment of underlying hypo- or hyper-thyroidism may be of some benefit.[16]

Oral Vasoactive Drugs. Yohimbine, an indole amine alkaloid found in the bark of the yohimbine tree, has long been thought to be an aphrodisiac. Morales et al[49] in 1987 reported that 42.6% of patients believed to have organic impotence reported a positive response to oral yohimbine after a ten-week course of therapy. As an alpha adrenergic blocking agent, with selectivity for alpha-2 receptors, the physiologic basis for improved erectile capacity with this agent remains obscure. Because of its safety, oral route of administration, and reported effectiveness in some men, one could argue that a trial of yohimbine is warranted. However, further studies are needed to clarify the efficacy, and possible physiologic mechanism of this agent.[49,50]

Intracavernosal Vasoactive Drugs. Zorgniotti[51] found that many patients evaluated for vasculogenic impotence with papaverine testing had posttest improvement in erectile capacity for weeks to months. Thus began the use of intracavernosal vasoactive agents, primarily papaverine alone or with phentolamine, for therapeutic purposes. This has proved to be one of the most important advances in the treatment of impotence to date. Initially, vasoactive drugs were injected by physicians on a periodic basis in the ambulatory setting. However, more recently, autoinjection by the patient at home has gained wide acceptability.

The instillation of vasoactive agents directly into the corpora cavernosum pharmacologically mimics natural erections lasting approximately 30 minutes. As a result, this has been a very satisfactory therapeutic alternative for many patients, particularly those suffering from neurogenic impotence. In addition, many patients with mild arterial insufficiency as well as psychogenic erectile dysfunction are able to use autoinjection of a vasoactive agent to restore potency. While not acceptable to all patients, for those comfortable with autoinjection, there appears to be a fairly good degree of patient-partner satisfaction. In contrast, this is a less successful therapeutic alternative for patients with severe penile arterial insufficiency or venous incompetence, especially in the diabetic. Patients who lack manual dexterity, have poor visual acuity, or suffer from bleeding diatheses are not appropriate candidates for this therapy.[50,52]

Careful titration of dosage has limited the incidence of priapism to 2-4%.[52] Concern still exists over penile fibrosis, potential hepatotoxicity with these agents, and unknown long term consequences. In some, there is also the development of tolerance and thus higher doses may be needed or a combination of drugs (particularly papaverine, phentolamine, and prostaglandin E1).[51,52] Because of potential side effects and lack of FDA approval, dosage and frequency of use (limited to 3 times per week) must be monitored carefully by clinicians trained in the use of this as a therapeutic modality.

Vascular Surgery. The foregoing discussion has emphasized the common finding of vascular insufficiency in a large number of impotent patients. Unfortunately, arterial bypass for penile arterial lesions has remained fairly disappointing. This is primarily because of the diffuse, small-vessel nature of this abnormality in a majority of patients. Arterial revascularization may be a viable option, however, in patients with discrete lesions.[18,50] This is usually seen in young men who have sustained severe pelvic or perineal injury.

Newer techniques in microvascular surgery have resulted in higher success rates for revascularization of diffuse distal penile atherosclerosis, as is common in older men. The long-term results of such procedures, however, are not yet available. Importantly, this is a microvascular procedure, requiring extensive preoperative evaluation and understanding on the part of the patient and thus is not undertaken lightly.[50] Improved imaging techniques for distal vasculature and thus improved patient selection, may make penile revascularization a more viable option for some patients.

Patients with excessive venous outflow, as demonstrated by dynamic infusion cavernosometry, may be candidates for venous surgical correction of their erectile dysfunction. This is a procedure best performed on patients demonstrating normal arterial inflow, normal neurogenic control and who have demonstrated an organic basis on NPT testing.[50,53]

This surgery may be done as an outpatient, but more commonly a one-night stay in the hospital is preferred. The goal of the procedure is to increase the venous pressure of the deep dorsal and superficial dorsal systems by ligating the deep dorsal and all circumflex veins. It is probably a heroic measure to attempt venous ligation if cavernosal vein drainage, or a cavernosal-spongiosal shunt exists. Success rates for restoring potency with this procedure have been reported between 28 and 73%, however, there are as yet no studies of long-term follow-up of patients undergoing venous ligation.[53,54]

Penile Prostheses. Surgical correction of impotence in the form of a penile prosthesis has a long history. Initial trials included rib cartilage rolled in skin tubes or inserted between Buck's fascia and the dorsal penile skin. Goodwin in 1952 inserted an acrylic splint under the skin of the penis as a prosthesis and Beheri in the late 1950s inserted two rods intracavernosally.[55]

Further refinements were made with the introduction of silicone in 1973 and, in the same year, the age of modern penile prostheses was ushered in with the development of the inflatable device. Since then, new and improved devices have been developed which make insertion easier and safer, as well as improving patient satisfaction.[50,55]

As diagnostic strategies and therapeutic options have increased, insertion of a penile prosthesis is often the last resort. For patients with arteriogenic or severe venogenic impotence, however, it may be the best option. In considering prosthesis insertion, the patient must clearly understand what the prosthesis does and does not do. It gives the penis enough axial rigidity for vaginal intercourse. It is not designed to improve libido, orgasm, alter ejaculation, lengthen the penis beyond its normal length, or longer than the normal erect penis. Most prostheses do not increase the girth of the penis, although most patients have intact spongiosal arterial inflow and may have circumferential enlargement with sexual arousal. The patient and his sexual partner need to be counseled as to the limitations of the prosthesis and the surgeon should be assured of their expectations.[50,56]

There are several types of prostheses (malleable, multicomponent, and self-contained inflatable); each with its own risk and benefit. Complications of prosthesis insertion, in general, include: infection, edema, pain, urethral injury or erosion, hematoma formation, and mechanical breakdown of the inflatable devices. Mechanical failure, a particular problem of the multicomponent prosthesis in the past, is now less than 5% with a five-year follow-up. Infections seem to be statistically more frequent only in spinal cord injury or immunosuppressed patients. Regardless of the type of prosthesis, couples express satisfaction in greater than 85% of cases. Most dissatisfaction arises from inadequate physician-patient counseling.[50,56]

Vacuum Erectile Devices. Despite the previous discussion on the use of intracavernosal pharmacotherapy and penile prosthesis, there are significant numbers of men who prefer a less invasive treatment for their erectile dysfunction. The vacuum-assisted devices may fill this void.

These devices, in general, consist of a plastic cylinder which is placed over the flaccid penis and attached to a hand-held suction pump. Vacuum is applied to the entrapped penis causing vascular engorgement and resultant penile erection. A constricting rubber band is then placed over the base of the penis entrapping blood in the erect organ. Nadig found that over 90% of men with organic impotence can achieve erections satisfactory for intercourse in this manner.[57]

Several disadvantages exist with these devices. The penis becomes cool to touch and fairly cyanotic due to lack of blood flow. Thus, this is safe for only approximately 30 minutes before release of the constrictor device must occur. Rigidity is only distal to the rubber band, allowing for a pivot point at the base of the penis. Ejaculation cannot occur through the constrictor device and may lead to increased epididymitis or orchitis. Lastly, this device cannot be utilized in patients with coagulation defects.[57]

Despite these shortcomings, the vacuum-assisted devices give satisfactory erectile capacity to men who may not be surgical candidates for penile prosthesis and either who cannot or are not willing to embark on an intracavernosal pharmacologic erection program.

Conclusion

Over the last decade there have been several advances in basic science research which have clarified the neurovascular mechanisms of normal erectile functioning. With these advances have come an enhanced understanding of the etiologic factors of impotence, and in particular, recognition that most cases are organic in origin. As a result, the armamentarium of diagnostic and therapeutic options for the impotent patient has greatly expanded.

Evaluation of the patient with erectile dysfunction needs to begin with a careful history, physical exam, and screening laboratory evaluation. It is important to assess the nature and extent of the problem as well as the patient's desires and expectations. More sophisticated diagnostic evaluation should be directed toward elucidating vascular, hormonal, or neurogenic causes of the patient's erectile incapacity. Once cause is ascertained, the patient may be offered a whole host of treatment options, including medical, mechanical, or surgical therapies.

While additional investigation is needed to evaluate further the sensitivity and specificity of various diagnostic tests, as well as to evaluate the long-term outcome of therapeutic alternatives, the impotent patient desiring potency has several options not previously available. The first hurdle is for the clinician to identify that a problem exists and initiate further evaluation.

References

1. Shabsigh R, Fishman IJ, Scott FB: Evaluation of erectile impotence. Urology. 1988;32:83-90.
2. Furlow WL: Prevalence of impotence in the United States. Med Aspects Hum Sex. 1985; 19:13-16.
3. Kinsey AC, Pomerroy WB, Martin CE: Sexual behavior in the human male. Philadelphia. WB Saunders Co, 1948.
4. Slag MF, Morley JE, Elson MK, et al: Impotence in medical clinic outpatients. JAMA. 1983;249:1736-1740.
5. Kaiser FE, Korenman SG. Impotence in diabetic men. Am J Med. 1988;85:147-152.
6. Saenz de Tejada I, Goldstein I: Diabetic penile neuropathy. Urol Clin North Am. 1988; 15:17-22.
7. Morely JB: Impotence. Am J Med. 1986;80:897-905.
8. Malloy TR, Markowicz KB. Pharmacologic treatment of impotence. Urol Clin North Am. 1987;14:297-305.
9. Aboseif SR, Lue TF. Hemodynamics of penile erection. Urol Clin North Am. 1988;15:1-7.
10. Fournier GR, Juenemann KP, Lue TF, et al: Mechanisms of venous occlusion during canine penile erection: An anatomic demonstration. J Urol. 1987;137:163-167.

11. Saenz de Tejada I, Goldstein I, Azadzoi K, et al: Impaired neurogenic and endothelium-mediated relaxation of penile smooth muscle from diabetic men with impotence. NEJM. 1989;320:1025-1030.
12. Saenz de Tejada I, Goldstein I, Krane RJ. Local control of penile erection. Urol Clin North Am. 1988;15:9-15.
13. Montague DK, James RE, de Wolfe VG, et al: Diagnostic evaluation, classification and treatment of men with sexual dysfunction. Urology. 1979;14:545-549.
14. Maatman TJ, Montague DK, Martin LM: Erectile dysfunction in men with diabetes mellitus. Urology. 1987;24:589-592.
15. Jevtich MJ, Khawand NY, Vidic B: Clinical significance of ultrastructural findings in the corpora cavernosa of normal and impotent men. J Urol. 1990;143:289-293.
16. McClure RD: Endocrine evaluation and therapy of erectile dysfunction. Urol Clin North Am. 1988;15:53-63.
17. Virag R, Bouilly P, Frydman D. Is impotence an arterial disorder? A study of arterial risk factors in 440 impotent men. Lancet. 1985;1:182-184.
18. Krane RJ: Sexual function and dysfunction, in Walsh PC, Gittes RF, Perlmutter AD, Stamey TA (eds): Campbell's Urology. Philadelphia, WB Saunders Co, 1986; vol. 1, pp 700-735.
19. Torrens MJ: Neurologic and neurosurgical disorders associated with impotence, in Krane RJ, Siroky MB, Goldstein I (eds): Male Sexual Dysfunction. Boston: Little, Brown, 1983, pp 55-61.
20. Seagraves RT, Madsen R, Carter CS, et al: Erectile dysfunction associated with pharmacologic agents, in Seagraves RT, Schoenberg HW (eds): Diagnosis and Treatment of Erectile Disturbances. New York, Plenum Medical, 1985, pp 23-63.
21. Wein AJ, Van Arsdalan KN: Drug induced male sexual dysfunction. Urol Clin North Am. 1988;15:23-30.
22. Abel EL: A reveiw of alcohol's effects on sex and reproduction in drug alcoholic dependency. Drug Alcohol Depend. 1980;5:321-327.
23. Rodriques-Blazquez HM, Cardona PE, Rivera-Herrera JL: Priapism associated with the use of topical cocaine. J Urol. 1990;143:358.
24. Forsberg L, Gustavii B, Hojerback T, et al: Impotency, smoking and beta blocking drugs. Fertil Steril. 1979;31:589-594.
25. Barlow DH: Causes of sexual dysfunction: The role of anxiety and cognitive interference. J Consult Clin Psychol. 1986;54:140-148.
26. Smith AD: Psychological factors in the multidisciplinary evaluation and treatment of erectile dysfunction. Urol Clin North Am. 1988;15:41-51.
27. Padma-Nathan H, Goldstein I, Krane RJ: Evaluation of the impotent patient. Semin Urol. 1986;4:225-232.
28. Ware JC: Impotence and aging. Clin Geriatr Med. 1989;5:301-314.
29. Karacan I: Clinical value of nocturnal erection in the prognosis and diagnosis of impotence. Med Aspects Human Sex. 1970;4:27-34.
30. Kessler WO: Nocturnal penile tumescence. Urol Clin North Am. 1988;15:81-86.
31. Wein AJ, Fishkin R, Carpiniello VL, et al: Expansion without significant rigidity during nocturnal penile tumescence testing: A potential source of misinterpretation. J Urol. 1981;126:343-344.
32. Barry JM, Blank B, Boileau M: Nocturnal penile tumescence testing with stamps. Urology. 1980;15:171-172.
33. Anders EK, Bradley W, Krane RJ: Nocturnal penile rigidity measured by the Snap Gauge band. J Urol. 1983;129:964-966.
34. Karacan I, Moore CA: Nocturnal penile tumescence: An objective diagnostic aide for erectile dysfunction, in Bennett AH (ed): Management of Male Impotency. Baltimore, Williams & Wilkins, 1982, pp 62-72.

35. Gaskell P: The importance of penile blood pressure in cases of impotency. Can Med Assoc 1971;105:1047-1050.
36. Mueller SC, Lue TF: Evaluation of vasculogenic impotence. Urol Clin North Am. 1988; 15:65-74.
37. Britt DB, Kemmerer WT, Robison JR: Penile blood flow determination by mercury strain gauge plethysmography. Invest Urol. 1971;8:673-677.
38. Zorgniotti AW. Practical diagnostic screening for impotence. Urology. 1984;23:98-102.
39. Melman A: The evaluation of erectile dysfunction. Urol Radiol. 1988;10:119-128.
40. Virag R: Intracavernous injection of papaverine for erectile failure. Lancet. 1982;2:938.
41. Abber JC, Lue TF, Orvis BR, et al: Diagnostic tests for impotence: A comparison of papaverine injection with the penile-brachial index and nocturnal penile tumescence monitoring. J Urol. 1986;135:923-925.
42. Lue TF, Mueller SC, Jow R: Functional evaluation of penile arteries with duplex ultrasound in vasodilator-induced erection. Urol Clin North Am. 1989;16:799-807.
43. Virag R, Frydman D, Legman M, et al: Intracavernous injection of papaverine as a diagnostic and therapeutic method in erectile failure. Angiology. 1984;35:79-87.
44. Lue TF, Takamura T, Schmidt RA, et al: Human dynamics of erections in the monkey. J Urol. 1983;130:1237-1241.
45. Lue TF, Hricak H, Schmidt RA, et al: Functional evaluation of penile veins by cavernosography in papaverine-induced erection. J Urol. 1986;135:479-482.
46. Steif CG, Wetterauer U. Quantitative and qualitative analysis of dynamic cavernosographies in erectile dysfunction due to venous leakage. Urology. 1989;34:252-257.
47. Goldstein I, Krane RJ, Greenfield AJ, et al: Vascular diseases of the penis: Impotence and priapism, in Pollack HM (ed): Clinical Urography. Philadelphia, WB Saunders Co, 1990, vol 3, pp 2231-2247.
48. Padma-Nathan H. Neurologic evaluation of erectile dysfunction. Urol Clin North Am. 1988;15:77-80.
49. Morales A, Condra M, Owen JA, et al: Is yohimbine effective in the treatment of organic impotence? Results of a controlled trial. J Urol. 1987;137:1168-1172.
50. Orvis BR, Lue TF: New therapy for impotence. Urol Clin North Am. 1987;14:569-581.
51. Zorgniotti AW, Lefleur RS: Auto-injection of the corpus cavernosum with a vasoactive drug combination for vasculogenic impotence. J Urol. 1985;133:39-41.
52. Sidi AA: Vasoactive intracavernous pharmacotherapy. Urol Clin North Am. 1988;15:95-101.
53. Lewis RW: Venous surgery for impotence. Urol Clin North Am. 1988;15:115-121.
54. Treiber U, Gilbert P. Venous surgery in erectile dysfunction: A critical report on 116 patients. Urology. 1989;34:22-27.
55. Bretan PN: History of the prosthetic treatment of impotence. Urol Clin North Am. 1989;16:1-6.
56. Montague DK: Penile prosthesis: An overview. Urol Clin North Am. 1989;16:7-11.
57. Witherington R: Suction device therapy in the management of erectile impotence. Urol Clin North Am. 1988;15:123-127.

Case 19

Weight Gain and Muscular Weakness in a Young Man

Bhaskar Rao, MD, FACP

Case History

A 28-year-old man consulted his physician because of rapid weight gain and considerable difficulty in climbing stairs for the past 9 months. His family had noticed that his face appeared puffy. He developed severe acne over his face and upper back and felt very lethargic.

He had been well previously. He had no cardiorespiratory symptoms and his appetite was normal. He neither smoked nor used alcohol. There was a diminution in his libido but no symptomatology suggestive of thyroid disease or diabetes mellitus. He did not use recreational drugs.

Physical Examination. Comparison with photographs taken 2 years prior to his clinic visit revealed a distinct rounding of his face and a marked weight gain. The blood pressure was 160/112. There were multiple acneiform eruptions over his face and back. He exhibited broad violaceous striae in his axillae, groin, and flanks. There was no peripheral edema. He had no hepatomegaly or other features of congestive heart failure.

Neurological examination was remarkable only for diminished power in the proximal groups of muscles in all four limbs and a diminution of the biceps and the knee reflexes. There was no sensory change.

Laboratory Data. The white cell count was 9,900/mm^3, serum sodium 142 mEq/liter, chloride 99 mEq/liter, bicarbonate 34 mEq/liter, creatinine 0.7 mg/dl, fasting blood glucose 169 mg/dl, and calcium 4.2 mEq/liter. The 8 AM plasma cortisol was 34.8 μg/dl. Urinalysis revealed a trace of glucose but no proteinuria or abnormal features on microscopic examination.

Discussion

The occurrence of hypertension in a young individual will raise the question of a remediable underlying cause. In this young man, apart from obesity, acne, and purple striae, there were no remarkable clinical features. In particular, he had no bruits over the abdomen or chest. There were no features of renal disease. With this presentation, hypercortisolism (Cushing's syndrome) is obviously the disease state to be considered. This condition is more common in women between the ages of 20 and 40. Although the so-called buffalo type of obesity is characteristic of Cushing's syndrome, generalized obesity may also be seen, especially in children. Table 1 lists the different clinical manifestations of Cushing's syndrome.[1,2] Although obesity, hypertension, and glucose intolerance are the most common features, they are not diagnostic since they occur commonly in middle-aged individuals either alone or in combination. However, additional features that strongly favor the diagnosis are: (1) hyperandrogenism in women, i.e., acne, menstrual dysfunction and hirsutism and (2) evidence of negative nitrogen balance, i.e., atrophy of the skin with striae, easy bruising, osteoporosis, and muscular wasting, especially in the proximal groups. Mental changes are seen in a significant number of patients.

The etiology of Cushing's syndrome is seen in Table 2. It is also worth emphasizing that the clinical features of Cushing's syndrome, in their classic form, may not be seen when the condition is due to an ectopic ACTH syndrome caused by a malignant tumor. The process is so rapid that the full-blown clinical picture does

Table 1

Clinical Features of Cushing's Syndrome

Feature	Incidence %
Obesity	85
Hypertension	75
Glucose intolerance/diabetes	75/20
Neuropsychiatric	85
Skin	
Facial plethora	80
Hirsutism	75
Superficial fungal infections	50
Striae	50
Acne	35
Bruising	30
Menstrual disorders	75
Impotence	65
Osteopenia	80
Weakness	50

Table 2

Etiology of Spontaneous Cushing's Syndrome

- **ACTH-dependent**
    - Pituitary adenoma (Cushing's disease) 72.4%
    - Ectopic ACTH 10.9%
    - Ectopic CRH from neoplasm (rare)
- **ACTH-independent**
    - Adrenal adenoma 7.4%
    - Adrenal carcinoma 5.8%
    - Primary adrenocortical nodular dysplasia 3.5%
- **Pseudo Cushing's syndrome (alcohol induced)**

---

not develop and the patient may only present with wasting and pigmentation. Table 3 lists the causes of the ectopic ACTH syndrome.

The striking laboratory abnormality in the patient described above was, of course, hypokalemia. This is seen in fewer than 5% of cases of Cushing's disease (due to a pituitary adenoma) but much more commonly with an ectopic ACTH syndrome or an adrenal carcinoma.[2]

The laboratory diagnosis usually consists of two steps: (1) confirmation of the diagnosis of Cushing's syndrome, i.e., hypercortisolism, (2) determination of the etiology of the syndrome.

Confirmation of Hypercortisolism. The screening test used to confirm the diagnosis of hypercortisolism is the overnight dexamethasone suppression test. The normal response to dexamethasone (1 mg given at 11 PM) is a plasma cortisol of

Table 3

Neoplasms Known to Produce Ectopic ACTH Syndrome

- Oat cell carcinoma of bronchus
- Carcinoid tumors:
    - Bronchial
    - Thymic
    - Pancreatic
- Pancreatic islet cell tumors
- Medullary carcinoma of the thyroid
- Pheochromocytoma
- Ovarian tumors

---

less than 5 μg/dl the next morning (8 AM). However, we observed the level to be 26.6 μg/dl in our patient. There are several factors which influence the results of the test and must be borne in mind to avoid drawing invalid conclusions.[3] First, obesity may cause an abnormal result with the overnight dexamethasone suppression test. High-estrogen states like pregnancy or estrogen therapy raise plasma cortisol levels due to an increase in corticosteroid binding globulin. Anticonvulsant drugs like phenytoin and phenobarbital induce the hepatic microsomal enzymes which accelerate dexamethasone metabolism, and may cause falsely abnormal results. Certain disease states may be associated with abnormal results even in the absence of Cushing's syndrome. These include: (1) endogenous depression, which appears to alter the hypothalamic pituitary adrenal axis, (2) alcoholism, usually with liver disease, which produces a clinical state, clinically and biochemically identical with Cushing's disease (the stigmata and the biochemical abnormalities reverse with abstinence), and (3) renal failure, which may result in an inadequate plasma cortisol suppression with oral dexamethasone. Defective oral absorption of dexamethasone in renal failure may explain the impaired suppression.

Periodic hormonogenesis (cyclic Cushing's syndrome)[4] can result in apparent normal suppression although the patient has features of Cushing's syndrome. Rarely, delayed clearance of dexamethasone with higher than usual plasma levels may also cause apparent suppression even in established disease.[5] Furthermore, normal cortisol suppressibility may exist early in the course of Cushing's disease. In all the above situations, a 24-hr urinary free cortisol must be done to confirm diagnosis. Urinary excretion of cortisol is expected to be normal in renal failure and obesity but abnormal in alcoholism and endogenous depression. The latter can usually be differentiated from Cushing's syndrome on clinical grounds. In depressed subjects, insulin-induced hypoglycemia will result in normal ACTH and cortisol responses. Thus, the urinary free cortisol measured in the 24-hr urine sample helps to confirm the diagnosis except in the presence of periodic hormonogenesis.

Determination of Etiology. The anatomical localization of the disease is the next step in the diagnosis, since endogenous Cushing's syndrome is usually due to a tumor. A helpful classification is based on the integrity of the pituitary-adrenal axis, i.e., whether the neoplasm is ACTH-dependent or ACTH-independent (Table 2).

In the ACTH-dependent disease, ACTH is secreted by the pituitary gland or an extrapituitary neoplasm that can synthesize hormones like ACTH and corticotropin releasing hormone (CRH). With pituitary tumors (Cushing's disease), the feedback relationship between the pituitary and adrenal glands is maintained, although it is abnormal. In contrast, in ectopic ACTH syndrome, pituitary ACTH release is suppressed by the excessive production of cortisol, which is stimulated in turn by an overproduction of ACTH from the ectopic source. In the ectopic CRH syndrome, the peptide produced by the tumor stimulates ACTH from the pituitary gland leading to hypercortisolism. In patients who have ACTH-independent types of Cushing's syndrome, the excessive cortisol from the adrenal tumors suppresses the pituitary ACTH secretion.

In the case described, the urinary free cortisol was over 800 μg/24 hr on more than one occasion. Hence, the diagnosis of Cushing's syndrome was hardly in doubt. The next step in diagnosis involves the delineation of the pathophysiologic mechanism, i.e., the biochemical study of the pituitary-adrenal axis to decide whether the lesion is ACTH-dependent or ACTH-independent. Radiological investigations are then used to determine the location of the lesion, as discussed below.

Biochemical Investigation. The principle behind biochemical tests is to demonstrate deranged feedback regulation of ACTH by cortisol. In the traditional dexamethasone suppression test, the drug is given in doses of 0.5 mg every 6 hr for 8 doses (low dose) followed by 2 mg every 6 hr for 8 doses (high dose). Lack of suppression of 24-hr urinary free cortisol or 8 AM plasma cortisol to less than 50% of baseline following low dose is found in all types of Cushing's syndrome, but the majority of patients with ACTH-dependent Cushing's syndrome due to a pituitary tumor suppress with high doses of dexamethasone. Fewer than 10% of patients with the ectopic ACTH syndrome and none with the ACTH-independent type respond in this manner.[6] There have been a number of refinements of the test and one that is getting to be popular consists of a single dose of 8 mg dexamethasone administered orally at 11 PM and serum cortisol measured the next morning at 8 AM.[7] The suppression of the plasma cortisol to less than 50% of the basal values is suggestive of pituitary etiology. A lack of suppression is indicative of an adrenal tumor or an ectopic ACTH syndrome. This appears to be as reliable as the classic test administered over a period of 48 hr.

Metyrapone acts by blocking the 11 – ß-hydroxylation in cortisol synthesis. Normal response to metyrapone consists of an increase in 11-deoxycortisol and ACTH and a fall in plasma cortisol. Only in the ACTH-dependent type will a normal response be seen. The metyrapone test consists of administering the drug in doses of 30 mg per kg body weight at midnight. The next morning at 8 AM, blood samples for ACTH, cortisol, and 11-deoxycortisol are obtained. Predictably, all the above tests have false- positives and false-negatives. Hence, several other tests have been introduced to aid diagnosis.

Plasma ACTH. Typically, the 8 AM plasma ACTH is low in patients with ACTH-independent Cushing's syndrome whereas it tends to be within or above the normal range in the majority of patients with Cushing's disease. In many patients with the ectopic ACTH syndrome, it is considerably elevated. Some cases of Cushing's disease, however, have low basal levels of ACTH. Likewise, patients with ectopic ACTH syndrome due to a benign tumor like a bronchial carcinoid, may have plasma ACTH levels which are only minimally elevated.[8] Hence, as a further refinement, the CRH test has been introduced.

CRH Test. This assesses the integrity of the hypothalamic-pituitary axis.[9] An intravenous injection of ovine CRH typically results in an increase of plasma ACTH in ACTH-dependent Cushing's syndrome. In contrast, patients with ACTH-independent syndrome exhibit no demonstrable increase over their low basal levels. However, the distinction between ectopic ACTH syndrome and ACTH-dependent tumors of the pituitary may be less well-defined with this test. Finally, to differentiate between pituitary tumors and the ectopic ACTH syndrome, inferior petrosal vein catheterization can be performed.

Inferior Petrosal Vein Catheterization. The inferior petrosal veins drain blood from the pituitary gland in a well-lateralized manner. They can be cannulated via the femoral veins and samples for ACTH are obtained from both sides and compared with the levels in the peripheral circulation. Normally, the petrosal vein/peripheral vein ACTH gradient is approximately 1.5. In the ectopic ACTH syndrome, the gradient is reversed and may even be 1 to 15. Thus, this test helps to locate the source of ACTH excess. Furthermore, the majority of pituitary adenomas are found in one or the other half of the pituitary gland and preoperative lateralization is of great help to the neurosurgeon. To achieve lateralization, the CRH test is performed after cannulating the petrosal vein. Injection of CRH will result in a greater increase in plasma ACTH on the side of the tumor. This procedure is especially helpful when the tumor is less than 10 mm (microadenoma).[10]

Imaging Procedures. CT scans and magnetic resonance imaging (MRI) are used for the diagnosis of Cushing's syndrome. CT scans of the head are positive in about 10% of pituitary microadenomas. MRI is more sensitive than CT, and tumors are demonstrated in 30% of cases. With contrast enhancement of MRI, another 15% of the tumors are seen. A further 15% may be detectable after the administration of gadolinium. Hence, even MRI can detect a pituitary tumor only in 60% of the cases and the remainder do not demonstrate a neoplasm regardless of the procedure employed.

Ectopic ACTH Syndrome. A tumor in the lung may be evident on conventional chest x-rays or in CT scans and, on occasion, may require repeated studies over a period of time before they are evident.

Adrenal Tumors. MRI of the abdomen is helpful not only in locating tumors of the adrenal gland but also in diagnosing adrenal carcinoma. As a rule, tumors greater than 6 cm are likely to be malignant while those which are less than 3 cm are benign. In masses of an intermediate size, T2 weighted imaging may cause brightening, if due to adrenal carcinoma.[11] CT scans are also very useful. It should be emphasized that radiological procedures, valuable as they are, must be used in conjunction with biochemical tests, since at least 1% of abdominal CT scans performed for other indications may reveal an adrenal mass without demonstrable hormonal derangement.[12]

Ectopic Tumors Producing CRH and Cushing's Syndrome. These include bronchial carcinoids, medullary thyroid cancer, and prostatic carcinoma. These patients may have features of ACTH-dependent disease in that they may respond to dexamethasone suppression or metyrapone although they exhibit very high levels of plasma ACTH. However, the clinical course is rapid in contrast to the more common pituitary microadenomas.[13]

Hospital Course. In the case described above, CT scans of the head, chest. and abdomen proved to be unremarkable. The patient did not respond to the high-dose dexamethasone suppression test. After 8 mg of dexamethasone at 11 PM, his plasma cortisol was 26.6 μg/dl in the morning, and his urinary cortisol did show an appreciable fall. He was diagnosed to have ACTH-dependent disease since his 8 AM plasma ACTH level was 43.8 (the upper limit of normal is 40 pg/ml).

Petrosal vein catheterization was recommended but the patient declined to have the procedure done. However, he was agreeable to a neurosurgical exploration.

In preparation for neurosurgery, the patient was given ketaconazole 600 mg/day in divided doses. His urinary cortisol was checked twice a week. It was necessary to increase his dose to 1200 mg/day since the urinary cortisol did not show a satisfactory fall. Three weeks later, the patient developed cough and chest discomfort with pulmonary infiltrates on x-ray. Bronchoscopy and bronchoalveolar lavage revealed nocardiosis, for which he was treated with trimethoprim/sulfamethoxyzole for 3 weeks. He then underwent a transsphenoidal partial hypophysectomy. The postoperative recovery was marked by diabetes insipidus which required arginine vasopressin for control. Evaluation after 4 weeks revealed that his diabetes insipidus persisted in a mild form, and the other clinical features of Cushing's syndrome had not abated. Ketaconazole was continued and metyrapone 1 g/day was added to the regimen. This helped to control his blood pressure and diabetes. As neurosurgery had not ameliorated his condition, he underwent a total bilateral adrenalectomy. He is currently on maintenance steroid replacement.

In our case, several treatment modalities had to be employed for the control of hypercortisolism. The three major forms of treatment for Cushing's syndrome include drug therapy, surgery, and irradiation. Whenever feasible, surgical removal of the offending tumor is the treatment of choice. Subjects who are unfit for surgery at diagnosis may be controlled with pharmacological therapy for a period of a few months before surgery is undertaken. If surgery is inadvisable or unsuccessful, we have the choice of treating the patient with radiotherapy in combination with a drug. Alternatively, bilateral adrenalectomy may be recommended as this is certain to cure the disease regardless of etiology. The different modalities of treatment and their success rates are discussed below.

Drug Therapy. There are several agents available to treat patients with hypercortisolism (Table 4). Cyproheptadine has been successful in 60% of cases in a series, in doses up to 24 mg a day.[14] It has been used in children and pregnant

Table 4

Pharmacotherapy in Cushing's Syndrome

Inhibition of ACTH secretion
    Cyproheptadine
    Bromocriptine
    Sodium Valproate
Inhibition of cortisol synthesis
    Ketaconazole
    Metyrapone
    Aminoglutethimide
    Mitotane
    Trilostane
Competitive inhibition at receptor site
    RU-486
    (investigational)

subjects. Bromocriptine has not been uniformly effective and like valproate is not the drug of choice.[15]

Ketaconazole, an imidazole derivative and antifungal agent, blocks cholesterol side chain cleavage and inhibits 11β-hydroxylation. The usual dose is 600-1200 mg a day in divided doses[16] and the effect is seen in 4 to 6 weeks. It is useful in Cushing's disease and adrenal tumors. GI upsets, hepatotoxicity, and iatrogenic adrenal insufficiency should be watched for and the dose adjusted with frequent urinary cortisol estimations.

Mitotane inhibits cortisol synthesis in the same manner as ketaconazole. In addition, it causes destruction of adrenal cortical tissue, largely the zona reticularis and fasciculata. It has been used successfully (80%) in combination with pituitary irradiation for Cushing's disease.[17] It is employed in doses of 2-4 gm daily; GI upsets, skin rashes, and hepatotoxicity may be encountered. However, this is the drug of choice in adrenal carcinoma.

Aminoglutethimide has been used effectively in adrenal cancer and in Cushing's disease.[18] It inhibits cholesterol side chain cleavage and blocks the conversion of cholesterol to pregnenolone in the adrenal cortex. The doses range from 0.5 to 1 gm/daily. Transient generalized rash, hypothyroidism, and GI upsets are some of the more important side effects.

Metyrapone, an 11β-hydroxylase inhibitor used for the diagnosis of Cushing's syndrome, has also been tried as adjunctive therapy for Cushing's disease in doses of 1-3 gm daily, especially in combination with aminoglutethimide. The resulting accumulation of the cortisol precursor 11-deoxycorticosterone may cause hypertension and hypokalemic alkalosis.

All the above drugs can be used for several weeks to months before surgery.

Surgery for Cushing's Disease. Transsphenoidal microsurgical removal of pituitary adenoma is the treatment of choice. Even when the tumor is not detectable by imaging techniques, transsphenoidal exploration may reveal the tumor in the majority and cure rates up to 80% have been reported.[19,20] Preoperative petrosal vein catheterization may help in lateralizing the tumor. If a well-defined tumor cannot be identified at surgery, total or subtotal hypophysectomy should be considered. However, this aspect must be discussed with the patient, preoperatively. In subjects wishing to have children, total hypophysectomy is obviously contraindicated. After selective adenomectomy, in successful cases, endocrine function returns to normal after an initial period of adrenal insufficiency. This form of surgery is also successful in children and adolescents. Diabetes insipidus, CSF rhinorrhea, and chronic sinusitis may complicate postoperative recovery.

Pituitary Irradiation. This is accomplished either with conventional megavoltage or heavy particle (proton beam) radiation. Conventional therapy is administered in doses of 180 rads daily over a 4 week period and the total dose must not exceed 4,500 rads. It is the treatment of choice in children and adolescents and successful in up to 80%. In adults, however, it is reserved for subjects with persistence or recurrence of disease after neurosurgery and used along with mitotane. It may also be employed prophylactically to prevent the development of a pituitary tumor (Nelson's syndrome) after bilateral adrenalectomy.

Radiation damage to the optic chiasm or the oculomotor nerves contained in the cavernous sinus can compromise vision. Though the normal pituitary tissue is radioresistant, it may suffer damage with heavy particle radiation.[21]

Bilateral Adrenalectomy. This is a major surgical procedure, albeit very effective in eradicating hypercortisolism. It is an option in subjects with persistent or recurrent disease following pituitary adenomectomy. Poor wound healing is characteristic of Cushing's disease and may complicate postoperative recovery. More importantly, permanent adrenal insufficiency is the inevitable consequence of surgery. In essence, one chronic disease is traded for another.

In the immediate postoperative phase, the management is that of an adrenal crisis. Steroid dosage is gradually tapered over several days until a maintenance dose of glucocorticoid (hydrocortisone, 30 mg a day) and a mineralocorticoid (Florinef, 0.1 mg a day) is reached. Intensive patient education regarding dosage adjustment during stress and the recognition of an impending crisis is essential.

A more dreaded complication of bilateral adrenalectomy is an ACTH-secreting pituitary adenoma (Nelson's syndrome). Clinical features include hyperpigmentation and visual compromise due to pressure on the optic chiasm and the oculomotor nerves in the cavernous sinus. The tumor is also prone to infarction, recognized by the onset of sudden, severe headache.

The diagnosis is confirmed by serial MRI of the pituitary gland and the demonstration of progressively increasing plasma ACTH despite "physiologic" replacement doses of steroids.

Prognosis. Untreated Cushing's disease may cause severe morbidity or mortality in up to 50% of cases. In subjects treated successfully, a reversal of the clinical features was seen in up to 75% of cases in different series. However, the disease may recur as early as 3 years after surgery. A second exploration is made difficult by scarring due to previous surgery. No single series has documented extensive experience with repeat surgery. Radiotherapy may be tried in this situation along with adrenal enzyme inhibitors.

Ectopic ACTH Syndrome. Surgical resection of primary neoplasm is the obvious therapy. The advisability and success of this procedure is dependent upon the histological type. A benign tumor or a slow-growing, malignant tumor offers the best chance. Postoperatively radiation therapy or chemotherapy may be needed. Where the primary tumor is not resectable, pharmacologic adrenal inhibition may ameliorate the symptoms. Bilateral surgical adrenalectomy is an option that is frequently impractical.

ACTH-Independent Cushing's Syndrome. Adrenocortical adenomas are surgically curable.[22] Adrenal insufficiency will ensue until recovery of the hypothalamic-pituitary- adrenal axis. Unfortunately, adrenocortical carcinomas are highly malignant, and their treatment has not been well standardized. Remission may be seen following surgery,[23] radiation therapy,[24] or mitotane therapy but the prognosis is poor.

References

1. Urbanic RC, George JM. Cushing's disease - 18 years experience. Medicine. 1981;60:14.
2. Aron DC, Findling JW, Tyrell JB. Cushing's disease. Endocrinol Metab Clin. 1987;3:15.
3. Schteingart DE: Cushing's syndrome. Endocrinol Metab. Clin North Am. 1989;3:311.
4. Atkinson AB, Chestnutt A, Crowthers E, et al. Cyclical Cushing's disease. Two distinct rhythms in a patient with basophil adenoma. J Clin Endocrinol Metab. 1985;60:328.
5. Kapcala LP, Hamilton SM, Meikle AW. Cushing's disease with "normal suppression" due to decreased dexamethasone clearance. Arch Intern Med. 1984;144:636.
6. Liddle GW. Tests of pituitary adrenal suppressibility in the diagnosis of Cushing's syndrome. J Clin Endocrinol Metab. 1960;12:1539.
7. Tyrell JB, Findling JW, Aron DC, et al: An overnight high dose dexamethasone suppression test for rapid differential diagnosis of Cushing's syndrome. Ann Intern Med. 1986;104:180.
8. Besser GM, Edwards CRW: Cushing's syndrome. J Clin Endocrinol Metab. 1972;1:451.
9. Chrousos GP, Schulte HM, Oldfield EH, et al. A corticotropin releasing factor stimulating test. An aid in the evaluation of patients with Cushing's syndrome. N Engl J Med. 1984;310:622.
10. Oldfield EH, Chrousos GP, Schulte MH, et al. Preoperative lateralization of ACTH-secreting pituitary adenomas by bilateral and simultaneous inferior petrosal venous sinus sampling. N Engl J Med. 1985;312:100.
11. Loriaux DL: in Cushing's syndrome. Oral presentation at the Annual Meeting of the Endocrine Society, 1989.

12. Siegelman SS, Fishman EK, Gatewood OMB, et al: CT of the adrenal gland. Contemp Issues Comput Tomogr. 1984;3:223.
13. Schteingart DE, Lloyd RV, Akil H, et al: Cushing's syndrome secondary to ectopic CRH-ACTH secretion. J Clin Endocrinol Metab. 1986;63:770.
14. Kreiger DT: Cyproheptadine for pituitary disorders. N Engl J Med. 1976;295:394.
15. DePinho MM, Antunes RC, Lima MB, et al. Cushing's disease. Clinical and laboratory response to Bromocriptine. J Endocrinol Invest. 1984;7:585.
16. Sonino N, Bascaro M, Merola G, et al: Prolonged treatment of Cushing's disease by ketoconazole. J Clin Endocrinol Metab. 1985;6:718.
17. Schteingart DE, Tsao HS, Taylor C, et al: Sustained remission of Cushing's disease with mitotane and pituitary irradiation. Ann Intern Med. 1980;92:613.
18. Schteingart DE, Conn JW. Effects of aminoglutethimide upon adrenal function and cortisol metabolism in Cushing's syndrome. J Clin Endocrinol Metab. 1967;27:1657.
19. Boggan JE, Tyrell JB, Wilson CB: Transsphenoidal microsurgical management of Cushing's disease. J Neurosurg. 1983;59:195.
20. Nakane T, Kuwayama A, Watanabe M, et al: Longterm results of transsphenoidal adenomectomy in patients with Cushing's disease. Neurosurgery. 1987;21:218.
21. Schteingart DE: The diagnosis and medical management of Cushing's syndrome, in: Thompson NW, Vinik AW (eds) Endocrine Surgery Update. New York. Grune & Stratton, 1983 p 187.
22. Scott HW, Abumrad NN, et al: Tumors of the adrenal cortex in Cushing's syndrome. Ann Surg. 1985;201:586.
23. Hajjar RA, Hickey RC, Samaan NA: Adrenal cortical carcinoma. A study of 22 patients. Cancer. 1975;35:549.
24. PerCarpio B, Knowlton AH. Radiation therapy of adrenal cortical carcinoma. Acta Radiol Oncol Radiat Phys Biol. 1976;15:288.

Case 20

The Antiphospholipid Syndrome

N. Paul Hudson, MD

Case History

A 31-year-old white male was first admitted to the Ohio State University Hospital after the sudden onset of expressive aphasia and right arm weakness. He had been healthy until several months prior when he developed scrotal edema followed by anasarca. While hospitalized elsewhere for evaluation he denied any symptoms of gastrointestinal, rheumatic, cardiopulmonary, or systemic illness as well as medications or allergies. Findings included anemia (Hct = 32%), thrombocytopenia (53,000/cm^3), renal insufficiency (creat = 2.2; creat clr = 58ml/min), nephrotic syndrome (32 gm protein/24 hr, cholesterol = 408, total protein = 3.5 gm), a normal IVP, and a cerebral CT that was reportedly negative. When focal neurologic deficits, appeared he was transferred.

His physical examination was notable for low-grade fever (100.8°F), mild alopecia, gingival bleeding, anasarca, a grade II/VI ejection murmur, an S4 gallop, abnormal cerebellar examination of the right hand, and expressive aphasia.

Laboratory evaluation detected 4+ proteinuria with oval fat bodies, 57,000 platelets, a hemoglobin of 9.6 gm, BUN = 24 mg/dl, creat = 2.3 mg/dl, a Westergren ESR of 132 mm/hr, a positive RPR with a negative FTA, mildly depressed C3, and an APTT of 55 sec. The chest x-ray showed bilateral pleural effusions, a blood smear was negative for schistocytes, a 24-hr urine demonstrated 26 gm of protein, and multiple ANA studies were negative. A lupus anticoagulant was detected and a strongly positive test for IgG antiphospholipid antibodies was reported.

A bone marrow aspirate showed normal megakaryocytes, and a screen for disseminated intravascular coagulopathy was negative. A renal echo was normal. Renal biopsy was considered but was not done because of a prolonged bleeding time (>15 min).

A neurological consultant diagnosed a left middle cerebral artery lesion and an MRI study documented a 3x5 cm lesion in the left posterior temporal region consistent with glioma, lymphoma, or infarction. A repeat examination demonstrated some resolution suggesting the latter. An initial echocardiogram showed mitral thickening or vegetation with mitral regurgitation and possibly a left ventricular mass, but a subsequent study showed only thickening of the aortic and mitral valves. Multiple blood cultures were negative, as were fungal and hepatitis serologies. An abdominal CT failed to demonstrate evidence of lymphoma, and a skin biopsy was negative for a lupus band.

The patient was treated for presumed ANA-negative lupus with prednisone doses of 1 mg/kg/day with fall of his renal protein loss to 17 gm/day. He was discharged after surgical correction of an inguinal hernia, resection of melanoma in situ from his chest, and diuresis of 30 lb.

The patient was readmitted four months later reporting a two-day history of sudden dyspnea, orthopnea, hemoptysis, fever, and chills. He denied chest pain, paroxysmal nocturnal dyspnea, palpitations, syncope, or wheezing. He also described the recent onset of frequent small-volume emesis unrelated to meals or any gastrointestinal symptoms. He denied skin rash, photosensitivity, mucous membrane ulcers, arthritis, arthralgias, serositis, or central nervous system disease. A chest x-ray showed marked cardiac enlargement with bilateral infiltrates and he was referred to OSU for evaluation.

On examination he was afebrile and chronically ill with a resting tachycardia, malar rash, alopecia, mottling of the skin over the flexor surface of the extremities, and an active precordium with a laterally displaced PMI, an S3, and a grade II/VI mitral regurgitant murmur.

Admission studies showed 4 + proteinuria, Hct = 30%, 93,000 platelets, ESR = 99 mm/hr, BUN = 46 mg/dl, creat = 2.1 mg/dl, APTT = 64 sec, pH = 7.45, pO_2 = 89, pCO_2 = 30, and cholesterol = 302 mg%. A chest x-ray showed massive cardiomegaly with pulmonary venous congestion, bilateral pleural effusions, and a right lower lobe infiltrate. The ECG showed nonspecific T-wave changes.

A repeat cardiac echo showed marked LV dysfunction and mitral regurgitation and possibly a left ventricular mural thrombus. Multiple cultures were again negative, including specimens obtained by bronchial alveolar lavage. A brain CT demonstrated changes in the left posterior parietal and the right frontoparietal regions consistent with subacute infarctions. The ANA and rheumatoid factors were again negative, and cryoglobulins were not found. The C3 was again mildly depressed.

The five-day hospital course was marked by rapid deterioration of renal function (creat = 2.1 to 4.3), progression of anemia (Hct = 30% to 20%), thrombocytopenia (93,000 to 23,000 platelets), and a persistently prolonged APTT (64 sec to 81 sec). The renal consultant felt that the data did not support a diagnosis of proliferative glomerulonephritis, but rather acute tubular necrosis superimposed on chronic glomerulonephritis. Infection was also considered, and immunosuppressive doses of prednisone and azathioprine were begun and then moderately reduced.

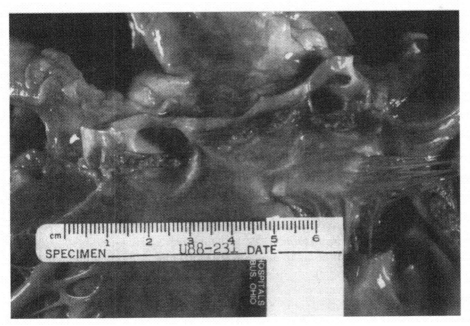

Figure 1
Libman-Sacks lesions.

On the fifth hospital day the patient became apneic without prior respiratory distress and could not be resuscitated. The postmortem examination demonstrated multiple vegetations along the line of closure of the aortic and mitral valves (Figure 1). These vegetations measured from 1 to 7 mm in greatest diameter and histologically were composed of bland fibrinous material with few inflammatory cells. These were consistent with vegetations of the Libman-Sacks type. Examination of the brain revealed gross evidence of infarction (Figure 2). Numerous microscopic bland thrombi and associated micro-infarcts were present in the heart (Figure 3), lungs, kidneys and brain (Figure 4). No evidence of vasculitis was seen. Microscopic findings diagnostic of membranous glomerulonephritis were present in the kidneys.

Discussion

This young man had a systemic illness that presented with nephrotic syndrome, thrombocytopenia, anemia, and a central nervous system lesion. The initial diag-

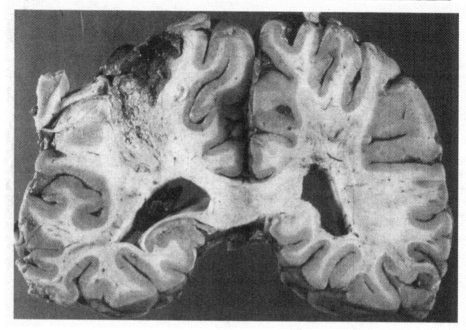

Figure 2
Cut section of the brain demonstrating ischemic lesions.

nostic considerations included subacute bacterial endocarditis, thrombotic thrombocytopenic purpura/hemolytic uremic syndrome, atrial myxoma, systemic infection, occult malignancy with marantic endocarditis, systemic vasculitis, and
systemic lupus erythematosus.

Subacute bacterial endocarditis (SBE), an often subtle but generally treatable
disease, should always be near the top of the differential of a systemic disorder.
Although this patient did not have persistent fevers or cutaneous findings of SBE,
multiple blood cultures and a search for valvular vegetations were undertaken.
With multiple negative cultures, this diagnosis was discarded as being both unlikely
and inadequate to explain this complex clinical disorder. Interestingly, both
echocardiograms were read as showing thickening of the mitral and aortic valves
rather than the extensive Libman-Sacks lesions found at postmortem examination.

A second uncommon disease, thrombotic thrombocytopenic purpura (TTP), or
hemolytic uremic syndrome (HUS) should be considered when a patient presents
with thrombocytopenia, renal, and central nervous system disease. Though fever
is typically present and the CNS lesion usually includes altered mental status rather
than a focal deficit, an evaluation of the peripheral smear for microangiopathic

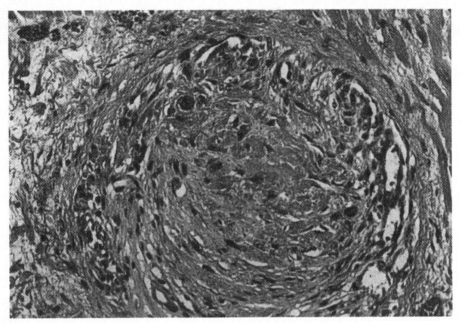

Figure 3
Organizing thrombus, myocardium.

hemolytic anemia (fragmented RBCs) was done and was negative. A related consideration was that of disseminated intravascular coagulopathy (DIC), but an assay for fibrinogen and fibrin split products ruled out this process.

A third important possibility is embolic disease from an intracardiac source, such as an atrial myxoma. Although neither echocardiogram suggested an atrial mass, the first study did suggest a possible intraventricular mass, but a follow-up study did not confirm this. Again, this possibility was discarded as unlikely and inadequate to explain this man's illness.

Systemic infections due to fungal organisms were also considered but were not supported by serologic studies. Hepatitis serologies were also negative and made the likelihood of post-hepatitis polyarteritis nodosa remote. Occult malignancy with marantic endocarditis was also considered, but computed tomography of the abdomen was negative for any evidence of lymphoma, and no other sources of malignancy were suggested by an exhaustive evaluation of other organ systems.

As one might safely predict, the possibility of vasculitis was considered in this puzzling case. Since there was no palpable purpura, the possibility of hypersensitivity vasculitis was essentially nil. Both forms of giant cell vasculitis (temporal arteritis and Takayasu's arteritis) were also eliminated due to the patient's age (too young for TA) and atypical presentation (absence of arterial disease). This left the

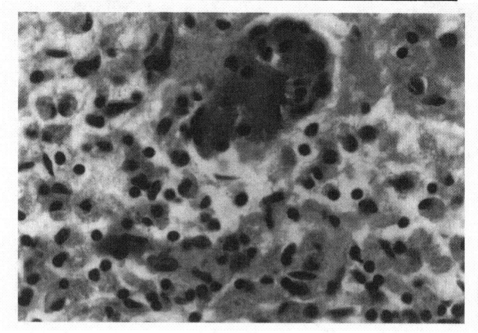

Figure 4
Recent thrombus, brain.

polyarteritis nodosa group, the necrotizing granulomatous diseases, and the vasculitides of the connective tissue diseases to consider.

Polyarteritis nodosa encompasses a spectrum of disease that ranges from classic periarteritis nodosa (involving renal and mesenteric vessels and sparing the pulmonary bed) to the Churg Strauss syndrome (characterized by pulmonary vasculitis with eosinophilia and a history of asthma). Indeed, overlaps of these two distinct disorders appear and can give the impression of a widespread vasculitic process. In this case, however, the absence of gastrointestinal symptoms and the pulmonary involvement without asthma or eosinophilia spoke eloquently against this diagnosis. A CT scan failed to suggest mesenteric artery disease, and an arteriogram was not done.

The necrotizing granulomatous diseases are Wegener's and lymphomatoid granulomatosis. Wegener's is a vasculitis of the pulmonary and renal beds that seldom extends beyond these areas, and usually causes progressive pulmonary and renal failure. Lymphomatoid granulomatosis also produces pulmonary and renal vasculitis, as well as cutaneous lesions. However, neither of these diseases is consistent with the prolonged history of renal disease nor the cardiac and neurologic problems encountered in this case.

Finally we come to the vasculitis associated with connective tissue diseases. When invoking this diagnosis, one is obligated to identify the connective tissue disease present. Systemic lupus erythematosus (SLE) was strongly suggested by the history of renal, pulmonary, hematologic, and central nervous system disease, but all involved in this case had problems with the persistently negative ANAs.

The literature on ANA-negative SLE suggests that most patients in this category have subacute cutaneous lupus erythematosus (SCLE) and are SS-A (Ro) and/or single-stranded DNA antibody-positive.[1] This subset of SLE is noted for its extensive photosensitive-distribution skin rash and paucity of internal organ involvement. These patients indeed produce anti-nuclear antibodies, but the antigens characteristic for this syndrome are not abundant in standard ANA test tissue substrate. Consequently, their ANA-negative status is an artifact of testing.

In this particular case, the diagnosis of ANA-negative SLE was made with some misgivings, since the clinical picture did not suggest SCLE. On the other hand, no other diagnosis seemed viable and it was clear that this man had a progressive multi-system disease. Thus, steroid treatment was begun.

In retrospect, he did not respond well to steroids except for some modest fall of his urinary protein loss. His terminal course was marked by cardiac failure, rapidly progressive renal failure, unexplained gastrointestinal symptoms, and sudden death. Although the postmortem examination explained his multisystem disease as the result of multiple emboli, a clear understanding of this case requires recognition of a newly described disorder: the antiphospholipid syndrome.

The Antiphospholipid Syndrome

The antiphospholipid syndrome has been defined over the past decade by case reports and descriptions of patients with recurrent thrombotic or thromboembolic disease.[2,3] Although most of the initial patients had SLE, some of these patients have had an ANA-negative lupus-like syndrome,[4-6] while some have had no evidence of any connective tissue disease.[2,7-9] Thus, the literature refers to a primary antiphospholipid syndrome, and to the antiphospholipid syndrome as an extension of the definition of SLE.

Laboratory Features. Antiphospholipid antibodies are IgG, IgA, or IgM immunoglobulins directed against phospholipid antigens.[10] Phospholipids in biologic systems are primarily cell membranes. While there could be many antibodies directed against cell membrane antigens, only three types have been defined. The most familiar are referred to as reagin: antibodies that produce positive VDRL and RPR tests, and are associated with syphilis, Lyme disease, and connective tissue disorders.

A second group of antiphospholipid antibodies is defined as an inhibitor of coagulation tests: the so-called lupus anticoagulant. Although originally described in a patient with a bleeding diathesis, this factor is neither unique to lupus, nor is it an anticoagulant. These antibodies are merely capable of inhibiting the completion of any in vitro coagulation study that depends on a phospholipid cofactor (like prothrombinase converting complex).

A third antiphospholipid antibody group is anticardiolipin. Although the substrate for this antigen-antibody reaction is specific, it appears that most antiphospholipid antibodies have some degree of affinity for this complex molecule and produce a positive result.[11] (Many laboratories use an anticardiolipin assay to detect antiphospholipid antibodies.)

Thus, there are three available tests to detect antiphospholipid antibodies: a VDRL or RPR serology, a lupus anticoagulant assay, and an anticardiolipin antibody assay. Predictably, these tests do not identify unique groups of antibodies. In fact, the majority of anticardiolipin antibodies appear to be lupus anticoagulants, but the two groups are not equivalent. It seems all three tests may have some value in identifying patients with the antiphospholipid syndrome.

None of these antiphospholipid antibodies had recognized clinical significance until the early 1980s. Mueh[12] studied a group of patients with the lupus anticoagulant and found a surprising incidence of thrombotic events rather than bleeding. To date, despite considerable effort, a clear explanation for this thrombotic tendency is lacking. It is tempting to speculate that antibody adherence to platelet surface phospholipid produces abnormal coagulation factor activity and promotes thrombosis.[13] Other mechanisms involving vascular endothelium and prostacyclin have been proposed, but a coherent explanation remains elusive.

Another thread of evidence is the high rate of fetal loss found among SLE mothers with lupus anticoagulant or anticardiolipin antibody.[14,15] When studies of placentas suggested that thrombotic events were at least partially responsible,[16] the two lines of evidence began to merge. In short, some antiphospholipid antibodies have been associated with a hypercoagulable state that has multiple clinical manifestations.

Clinical Features. The antiphospholipid syndrome is defined by the presence of an antiphospholipid antibody and local or systemic thrombotic or thromboembolic disease. Recurrent episodes of deep venous thrombosis, fetal loss, or pulmonary emboli,[7,17] all suggest the diagnosis. Widespread arterial and venous disease has been described,[8,18] as well as superior vena cava syndrome,[19] aortic occlusion,[20] ocular vascular occlusion,[21] Budd-Chiari syndrome,[18,22] and thrombotic renal disease.[23]

Some patients appear to have a systemic disease with neurologic and cardiopulmonary disease. The neurologic manifestations include embolic strokes with multi-infarct dementia,[6,24,25] transient ischemic attacks,[26,27] and chorea.[28] Libman-Sacks endocarditis with large vegetations and valvular dysfunction is described,[26,27,29,30] as is intracavitary thrombus,[31,32] cardiomyopathy,[31] and myocardial infarction in young patients without risk factors.[25] Pulmonary manifestations of this syndrome extend beyond embolic disease to include pulmonary hypertension,[7] and hemorrhage with infarction.[33]

Hematologic abnormalities reported include thrombocytopenic purpura and hemolytic anemia,[34] and pure red cell aplasia.[35] Other serologic findings include a positive Coombs' test (with or without evidence of hemolysis) and hypocomplementemia.[36] Finally, livedo reticularis has been correlated with this disorder.[37]

An appropriately skeptical question is whether this disease represents primary vasculitis with secondary thrombosis or a primary thrombotic disorder. Pathologic studies tend to support the latter view, having found little if any vessel inflammation at the site of thrombosis.[2,39] Furthermore, the outcome for these patients has been poor in spite of aggressive antiinflammatory therapy.

Thus, a distinct systemic immune-mediated disease has emerged from the shadow of SLe. Antibodies directed against normal cellular constituents are present and seem to play some role in pathogenesis,[40] but the pathology of the disorder is thromboembolic rather than inflammatory or vasculitic.

Therapy. This leads to the question of therapy. It is not difficult to choose full-dose and chronic anticoagulation for the patient who has suffered a major thromboembolic event. The question of duration of therapy is open, but preliminary data suggest that the risk of thrombosis persists as long as antiphospholipid antibody levels remain high.[41] The more difficult problem is how (if at all) to treat the young person with a minor or questionable thrombotic event, or how intensively to anticoagulate the patient with other complicating medical problems. While simple antiplatelet therapy may be sufficient, there are no data to that effect. On the other hand, there are no data to suggest that chronic coumarin or heparin is superior to aspirin and dipyridamole. At this point in time there are few if any guidelines beyond one's clinical judgement.

Several caveats are in order. First, only a minority of patients with antiphospholipid antibodies are hypercoagulable, especially those with only a biologic false-positive test for syphilis.[42] Second, among women with idiopathic habitual abortion the frequency of antiphospholipid syndrome is very low, so screening this population will not yield many cases.[43] Third, there are no controlled data on treatment during pregnancy that support the use of chronic steroids, making it difficult to justify the risks of such therapy.[15] While the description of this syndrome and its natural history proceeds, it seems wise to make the diagnosis only in the most obvious cases and to treat in a conservative manner.

The Case in Context

This patient presented with a systemic disease that defied our best diagnostic efforts. While his elevated sedimentation rate, thrombocytopenia, renal disease, alopecia, serositis, and positive RPR all suggested SLE, that diagnosis was ultimately only partially correct and obscured the pathophysiology that caused his death. Thus, this case represents the antiphospholipid syndrome with ANA-negative lupus-like disease. As discussed earlier, this process has also been described as both primary and secondary to SLE. It seems appropriate that our concept of ANA- negative lupus be expanded to include this disorder. Recognition of the antiphospholipid syndrome also forces an extension of our concept of autoimmune pathophysiology to include thromboembolism. While the mechanism of hyper-coagulability remains speculative, the association with antiphospholipid antibodies is clear and a direct antibody effect seems likely. More importantly, the existence of a primary antiphospholipid syndrome suggests that a whole new family of autoantibodies associated with a separate set of clinical findings remains to be studied. The associations with LibmanSacks endocardial lesions and chorea are particularly intriguing.[44] In retrospect, the choice of therapy was both under-standable and belatedly instructive, emphasizing that immunosuppression is not an effective way to deal with this hypercoagulable state.[45] While it is possible that steroids helped suppress part of this patient's disease process, four months of aggressive steroid therapy did not prevent further thromboembolic complications.

Summary

Finally, this patient had a multisystem disease that was primarily thrombotic and thromboembolic associated with an antiphospholipid antibody. This disorder had many features of SLE but was persistently ANA-negative. Awareness of this syndrome can only help us further characterize, understand, and successfully treat this form of auto-immune disease.

References

1. Maddison PJ, Provost TT, Reichlin M: Serological findings in patients with "ANA-negative" systemic lupus erythematosus. Medicine. 1981;60:87-94.
2. Alarcon-Segovia D, Sanchez-Guerrero J: Primary antiphospholipid syndrome. J Rheumatol. 1989;16:482-488.
3. Hughes GR V, Asherson RR, Khamashta MA: Antiphospholipid syndrome: Linking many specialties. Ann Rheum Dis. 1989;48:355-356.
4. Colaco CB, Elkon KB: The lupus anticoagulant. Arthritis Rheuma. 1985;28:67-74.
5. Meyer O, et al: Antiphospholipid antibodies: A disease marker in 25 patients with antinuclear antibody negative systemic lupus erythematosus (SLE). Comparison with a group of 91 patients with antinuclear antibody positive SLE. J Rheumatol. 1987;14:502-506.
6. Asherson RA, et al: Cerebrovascular disease and antiphospholipid antibodies in systemic lupus erythematosus, lupus-like disease, and the primary antiphospholipid syndrome. Am J Med. 1989;86:391-396.
7. Anderson NE, Ali MR: The lupus anticoagulant, pulmonary thromboembolism, and fatal pulmonary hypertension. Ann Rheu Dis 1984;43:760-763.
8. Asherson RA, et al: Multiple venous and arterial thromboses associated with the lupus anticoagulant and antibodies to cardiolipin in the absence of SLE. Rheumatol Int 1985;5:91-93.

9. Mackworth-Young CG, Loizou S, Walport MJ: Primary antiphospholipid syndrome: Features of patients with raised anticardiolipin antibodies and no other disorder. Ann Rheum Dis. 1989;48:362-367.

10. Weidmann CE, et al: Studies of IgG, IgM and IgA antiphospholipid antibody isotypes in systemic lupus erythematosus. J Rheumatol. 1988;15:74-79.

11. Gharavi AE, et al: Anticardiolipin antibodies: Isotype distribution and phospholipid specificity. Ann Rheum Dis. 1987;46:1-6.

12. Mueh JR, Herbst KD, Rapaport SI: Thrombosis in patients with the lupus anticoagulant. Ann Intern Med. 1980;92:156-159.

13. Khamashta MA, et al: Immune mediated mechanism for thrombosis: Antiphospholipid antibody binding to platelet membranes. Ann Rheum Dis. 1988;47:849-854.

14. Lockshin MD, et al: Antibody to cardiolipin as a predictor of fetal distress or death in pregnant patients with systemic lupus erythematosus. N Engl J Med. 1985;313:152-156.

15. Lockshin MD: Editorial: Anticardiolipin antibody. Arthritis Rheum. 1987;30:471-472.

16. Hanly JG, et al: Lupus pregnancy: A prospective study of placental changes. Arthritis Rheum. 1988;31:358-366.

17. Asherson RA, Zulman J, Hughes GRV: Pulmonary thromboembolism associated with procainamide induced lupus syndrome and anticardiolipin antibodies. Ann Rheum Dis. 1989;48:232-235.

18. Asherson RA, et al: Budd Chiari syndrome, visceral arterial occlusions, recurrent fetal loss and the "lupus anticoagulant" in systemic lupus erythematosus. J Rheumatol. 1989; 16:219-224.

19. Steen VD, Ramsey-Goldman R: Phenothiazine-induced systemic lupus erythematosus with superior vena cava syndrome: Case report and review of the literature. Arthritis Rheum. 1988;31:923-926.

20. Drew P, et al: Aortic occlusion in systemic lupus erythematosus associated with antiphospholipid antibodies. Ann Rheum Dis. 1987;46:612-616.

21. Asherson RA, et al: Antiphospholipid antibodies: A risk factor for occlusive ocular vascular disease in systemic lupus erythematosus and the 'primary' antiphospholipid syndrome. Ann Rheum Dis. 1989;48:358-361.

22. Averbuch M, Levo Y: Budd-Chiari syndrome as the major thrombotic complication of systemic lupus erythematosus with the lupus anticoagulant. Ann Rheum Dis. 1986; 45:435-437.

23. Kincaid-Smith P, Fairley KF, Kloss M: Lupus anticoagulant associated with renal thrombotic microangiopathy and pregnancy-related renal failure. Q J Med. 1988;69:795-814.

24. Asherson RA, et al: Recurrent stroke and multi-infarct dementia in systemic lupus erythematosus: Association with antiphospholipid antibodies. Ann Rheum Dis. 1987;46:605-611.

25. Maaravi Y, et al: Cerebrovascular accident and myocardial infarction associated with anticardiolipin antibodies in a young woman with systemic lupus erythematosus. Ann Rheum Dis. 1989;48:853-855.

26. Asherson RA, et al Diagnostic and therapeutic problems in two patients with antiphospholipid antibodies, heart valve lesions, and transient ischemic attacks. Ann Rheum Dis. 1988;47:947-953.

27. Giansiracusa DF, Stafford-Brady F: A 35-year-old woman with recurrent strokes, an intracardiac lesion, anemia and thrombocytopenia. N Engl J Med. 1988;319:699-712.

28. Khamashta MA, et al: Chorea in systemic lupus erythematosus: Association with antiphospholipid antibodies. Ann Rheum Dis. 1988;47:681-683.

29. Chartash EK, et al: Aortic insufficiency and mitral regurgitation in patients with systemic lupus erythematosus and the antiphospholipid syndrome. Am J Med. 1989;86:407-412.

30. Ford PM, Ford SE, Lillicrap DP: Association of lupus anticoagulant with severe valvular heart disease in systemic lupus erythematosus. J Rheumatol. 1988;15:597-600.
31. Gur H, et al: Severe congestive lupus cardiomyopathy complicated by an intracavitary thrombus: A clinical and echocardiographic followup. J Rheumatol. 1988;15:1278-1280.
32. Leventhal LJ, et al: Antiphospholipid antibody syndrome with right atrial thrombosis mimicking an atrial myxoma. Am J Med. 1989;87:111-113.
33. Howe HS, et al: Pulmonary hemorrhage, pulmonary infarction, and the lupus anticoagulant. Ann Rheum Dis. 1988;47:869-872.
34. Deleze MC, Oria C, Alarcon-Segovia D: Occurence of both hemolytic anemia and thrombocytopenic purpura (Evan's syndrome) in systemic lupus erythematosus: relationship to antiphospholipid antibodies. J Rheumatol. 1988;15:611-615
35. Agudelo CA, Wise CM, Lyles MF: Pure red cell aplasia in procainamide induced systemic lupus erythematosus: Report and review of the literature. J Rheumatol. 1988;15:1431-1432.
36. Hazeltine M, et al: Antiphospholipid antibodies in systemic lupus erythematosus: Evidence of an association with positive Coombs' and hypocomplementemia. J Rheumatol. 1988;15:80-86.
37. Englert HJ, et al: Clinical and immunologic features of livido reticularis in lupus: A case-control study. Am J Med. 1989;87:408-410.
38. Alarcon-Segovia D, Cardiel MH, Reyes E: Antiphopholipid arterial vasculopathy. J Rheumatol. 1989;16:762-767.
39. Lie JT, Vasculopathy in the antiphospholipid syndrome: thrombosis or vasculitis, or both? J Rheumatol. 1989;16:713-715.
40. Alarcon-Segovia D: Pathogenic potential of antiphospholipid antibodies. J Rheumatol. 1988;15:890-893.
41. Asherson RA, et al: Anticardiolipin antibody, recurrent thrombosis, and warfarin withdrawal. Ann Rheum Dis. 1985;44:823-825.
42. Koskela P, et al: Significance of false positive syphilis reactions and anticardiolipin antibodies in a nationwide series of pregnant women. J Rheumatol. 1988;15:70-73.
43. Petri M, et al: Antinuclear antibody, lupus anticoagulant, and anticardiolipin antibody in women with idiopathic habitual abortion: A controlled, prospective study of forty-four women. Arthritis Rheum. 1987;30:601-606.
44. Asherson RA, Lubbe WF: Cerebral and valve lesions in sle: association with antiphospholipid antibodies. J Rheumatol. 1988;15:539-543.
45. Sturfelt G, et al: Anticardiolipin antibodies in patients with systemic lupus erythematosus. Arthritis and Rheum. 1987;30:382-388.

Case 21

Somatostatin in the Treatment of Acromegaly

Daryl A. Cottrell, MD, Samuel Cataland, MD, and Thomas O'Dorisio, MD

Case History

A 43-year-old white male with a history of hypertension, diabetes mellitus, coronary artery disease, and acromegaly presented to our hospital for treatment of diabetic ketoacidosis. The patient was diagnosed with acromegaly and insulin-dependent diabetes mellitus 20 years prior to admission. At that time, he had an increase in hand size, foot size, changes in facial features, sweating, and weakness. Two attempts at surgical resection 13 and 16 years prior to admission using transfrontal and transsphenoidal approaches were unsuccessful since the tumor could not technically be reached. The patient was not compliant over subsequent years and although counseled, refused therapy for his pituitary tumor, specifically, radiation or pharmacologic agents.

Over the past 5 years, the patient's ring size increased from 14 to 18 and his shoe size from 12E to 13EEE. The patient had multiple hospital admissions for hyperglycemia with serum glucoses in the 500 mg/dl range and insulin requirements exceeding 500 units daily to achieve only moderate to poor control.

He was brought to our hospital for the first time 9 months prior to the current admission with complaints of chest pain. Coronary artery catheterization demonstrated triple vessel coronary artery disease with diastolic dysfunction, mild pulmonary hypertension, left ventricular ejection fraction of 53%, severe apical hypokinesis, and segmental contraction abnormalities consistent with a myopathic process. Computerized tomography of the head revealed a large, 3 x 2.5-cm intrasellar mass with suprasellar extension and infiltration into the lower portions of the frontal lobes bilaterally. Serum growth hormone was markedly elevated at 51.6 ng/ml (normal < 5 ng/ml). Prolactin was also elevated at 35.2 ng/ml (normal < 15 ng/ml). Somatomedin C or insulin-like growth factor-1 (IGF-1) was 440 ng/ml (normal 83-378 ng/ml). Serum cortisol was 16.9 mg/dl and glycosylated hemoglobin 18.3% (normal 4.4-8.0%).

His acromegaly was treated with the somatostatin congener octreotide (Sandostatin®) at 150 μg s.c. daily and, with administration of an aggressive antianginal regimen, was associated with a significant decrease in insulin requirements from 420 to 95 units/day and resolution of his angina. The patient had two subsequent admissions for hyperglycemia, the last being one month prior to admission when he ran out of Sandostatin.

The patient presented on this occasion with nausea, vomiting, lethargy, lightheadedness, and 10 lb weight loss.

Family history was unknown for the father and unremarkable for the mother, siblings, and children of the siblings; specifically, no history of multiple endocrine neoplasia I.

Physical examination was significant for frontal bossing, protruding jaw, widely spaced teeth, acanthosis nigricans of the axillae, large hands and feet, large plantar foot pads, absence of deep tendon reflexes in the lower extremities, and absence of sensation to pain, vibration or light touch in the lower extremities bilaterally and in the ulnar aspect of the hands.

Laboratory. Electrolytes included a sodium of 134 mEq/liter, a normal potassium of 4.4 mEq/liter, chloride of 95 mEq/liter, bicarbonate of 22 mEq/liter, BUN of 20 mg/dl, and creatinine of 2.0 mg/dl. Anion gap was 17. His glucose on admission was 625 mg/dl and his glycosylated hemoglobin was 14.6% (normal < 8.0%). His hematocrit was 41.1 and his WBC was 8500. Arterial blood gases obtained at room air were: pH 7.28, pO_2 of 76, pCO_2 of 44, bicarbonate of 21, and an O_2 saturation of 94%.

Repeat head CT showed no changes from the previous scan obtained 8 months prior to admission.

Hospital Course. The patient was aggressively treated for ketoacidosis with intravenous fluids, insulin, and subcutaneous Sandostatin. The hyperglycemia was difficult to control until Sandostatin was increased to 300 μg s.c. daily, after which time the insulin requirements dropped from 200 to 66 units/day. The patient's initial response to Sandostatin was previously studied when the patient was medically stable, and is illustrated in Figure 1. Insulin requirements at that time decreased from 420 to 95 units/day. Serum glucoses improved dramatically from 200-600 mg/dl prestudy, to 60-200 mg/dl with lower insulin doses following Sandostatin therapy. Growth hormone fell from 81.6 to 7.8-12 ng/ml within 24 hr.

Discussion

This patient demonstrates many of the classic and a few atypical clinical findings and complications of acromegaly as well as the therapeutic value of treatment with the somatostatin analogue, Sandostatin, which has become the drug of choice in the treatment of end stage unresectable growth hormone-secreting tumors of the pituitary.

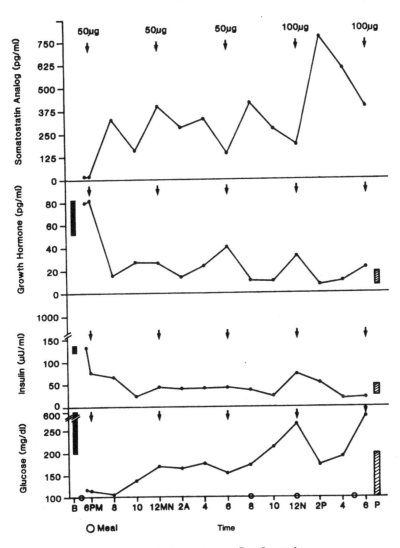

Figure 1. Response to Sandostatin

*Suppression of growth hormone and decrease in insulin requirement following sub-
cutaneous administration of somatostatin analogue over 24 hr. Arrows indicate times
of octreotide administration. The patient received continuous intravenous infusion of
insulin at 5-7 U/hr throughout the study. Bars represent ranges of GH, insulin, and
glucose concentrations obtained prior to the study (B, solid bars) and following
chronic octreotide therapy (P, hatched bars). Meals are denoted by open circles. See
text for discussion.*

Pathogenesis. Acromegaly is a disorder which results from the overproduction of growth hormone (GH) and growth hormone-dependent tissue growth factors such as insulin-like growth factor-1 (IGF-1 or somatomedin C). The etiologies of GH excess include GH-producing pituitary tumors; hypersecretion of GH-releasing hormone (GHRH) by hypothalamic or pituitary gangliocytomas[1]; ectopic GHRH production by tumors such as bronchial or intestinal carcinoids, pheochromocytomas, or pancreatic islet cell carcinomas[3,4]; GH-producing ectopic pharyngeal pituitary adenomas[2]; and ectopic production of GH by tumors of the breast, stomach, and lung.[5] Overproduction of tissue growth factors with normal GH production has also been described, resulting in the development of the physical characteristics of acromegaly without GH excess — termed "acromegaloidism."[6] Of the selected etiologies the most common cause of acromegaly is the GH-producing pituitary tumor, which accounts for over 99% of the reported cases.[5] Our patient is a classic example. Some pituitary adenomas may produce a variety of hormones in addition to GH, such as prolactin as seen in our patient, ACTH, or TSH. Malignant GH-producing carcinomas are extremely rare, and are associated with rapid growth and metastasis.[5]

GH secretion is normally regulated through the interaction of GHRH, somatostatin, and IGF-1. GHRH release by the hypothalamus stimulates the growth of and synthesis and release of GH from pituitary somatotrophs. Somatostatin inhibits GH release, and antagonizes the growth-promoting effect of GHRH in vitro, but apparently does not decrease GH synthesis.[7] IGF-1 may provide negative feedback inhibition of GH secretion and stimulate hypothalamic somatostatin release.[8] The neuromodulation of GH secretion involves complex interactions with many substances, including opioid peptides, thyrotropin-releasing hormone (TRH), VIP, glucagon, galanin, α-MSH, bombesin, secretin, calcitonin, CCK, CRF, various growth factors, acetylcholine, glucose, free fatty acids, gonadal hormones, and glucocorticoids.[9,10] The mechanisms involved have not been fully elucidated. There is some evidence that, rather than being a primary pituitary disorder, acromegaly may actually be the result of increased hypothalamic GHRH production.[11]

Clinical Characteristics. Acromegaly is typically insidious, with a delay between onset and diagnosis of 5-15 years.[5] The manifestations of GH and IGF-1 excess are multiple. Physical changes include enlargement of the sinuses, resulting in frontal bossing, protrusion of the jaw, increased spacing between teeth, tongue enlargement, coarsening of facial features, oily thick skin, increased perspiration, acanthosis nigricans, hirsutism, enlargement of the hands and feet, and kyphosis. Nearly all of these physical features were demonstrated by our patient. Patients may develop a noninflammatory arthropathy similar to osteoarthritis with involvement of the knees, hips, shoulders, elbows, and lumbosacral spine.[12] The arthropathy can be quite severe and one of the more clinically devastating problems of unstaged, untreated acromegaly. Muscle weakness can occur, as well as peripheral neuropathy or radiculopathy secondary to nerve compression. Our patient developed both peripheral neuropathy and nerve compression. Because the pituitary tumor is often large at the time of diagnosis,[13] compression of adjacent structures can result in deficits of cranial nerves II through V and VI, visual field defects, temporal lobe seizures, or CSF rhinorrhea.[5] Because of insulin resistance, as in our patient, glucose intolerance is common; however, frank diabetes is unusual because of compensatory hyperinsulinemia, and insulin-dependent diabetes is even more unusual. However, as noted in our patient, diabetic ketoacidosis may be a presenting symptom and, in the proper clinical setting, acromegaly should be suspected when diabetic ketoacidosis presents for the first time in a patient over the age of 40. Hypertension may be present as well. Cardiomyopathy or its complications of congestive heart failure and arrhythmias can be fatal.

Biochemical Diagnosis. GH levels are helpful when markedly elevated (< 50 to 100 ng/ml) or when very low (< 1 ng/ml), but levels within the normal range **do not** exclude the diagnosis of acromegaly because GH fluctuates markedly through the day. Renal failure, uncontrolled diabetes, malnutrition, physical exercise, and stress can also raise GH levels.[5]

Plasma IGF-1 levels correlate with mean 24-hr GH levels and provide a reliable diagnosis.[14] IGF-1 is very accurate for determining whether or not acromegaly is present.[15]

Other tests such as suppression of GH by oral glucose, TRH stimulation, suppression of GH by bromocriptine, or insulin-induced hypoglycemia may be helpful. GHRH measurement will distinguish GH-producing from GHRH-producing tumors.[4,5]

Therapy. Treatment modalities currently available include surgery, radiation, dopamine agonists, and octreotide (Sandostatin).

Surgery is most effective for small, noninvasive pituitary tumors and results in true normalization of GH levels in approximately 30% of patients.[5,16] Hypopituitarism requiring hormonal replacement may develop. With larger tumors, complete resection is difficult, and adjuvant radiation or medical therapy is required. This would have applied to our patient, whose tumor was too extensive for total resection.

Pituitary irradiation will effectively reduce GH secretion; however, the full effects may not be achieved until after 5-10 years. Because of this, radiation is not good as primary therapy except in cases where more effective therapy is contraindicated. In our patient, compliance was a major contraindication.

Bromocriptine and other dopamine agonists under investigation are used in conjunction with surgery or radiation to suppress GH secretion. This type of drug may also be effective if prolactin is co-released with GH-secreting tumors. Therefore, bromocriptine could have benefited our patient, who did have hyperprolactinemia, but was not compliant. Used alone, bromocriptine produces some symptomatic improvement and improved glucose tolerance, but suppression of GH is not as effective. Further, bromocriptine does not reliably reduce tumor size.

Octreotide (Sandostatin) is an octapeptide analogue of native somatostatin, which is effective in the treatment of acromegaly and other diseases. Octreotide can significantly and rapidly improve symptoms.[17,21] Suppression of GH and IGF-1 can be long term with continued therapy, but tumor shrinkage is variable.[13,17-21] A review of a number of long-term studies examining the efficacy of octreotide in the treatment of acromegaly showed normalization of somatomedin C in about 50% of patients, and tumor shrinkage in 30-50%.[32] Clinical improvement is rapid, occurring during the first few weeks of therapy. Combination therapy with Sandostatin and bromocriptine can produce an additive effect with further reductions of GH and IGF-1, since the two drugs appear to work by different mechanisms.[20,22] The response to octreotide appears to be related to the density and affinity of somatostatin receptors on the tumor surface.[23] Preoperative treatment with octreotide may or may not reduce tumor size, but does improve GH levels.[24,25] Even patients with acromegaly resistant to other therapeutic modalities have responded to somatostatin analogue, although sometimes requiring doses as high as 1500-3000 μg/day.[26,27] Octreotide will also suppress GH in acromegaly secondary to ectopic GHRH secretion, and has been reported to also suppress GHRH to a lesser degree.[28,29] In addition, it has been useful in the treatment of malignant pancreatic islet cell carcinomas (gastrinoma, insulinoma, VIP-producing tumors, glucagonoma), carcinoid tumors, and as adjunctive therapy for secretory diarrhea and acute variceal hemorrhage.[18,29-31]

Because absorption following oral intake of octreotide is poor, the drug must be delivered either intravenously or subcutaneously. The half-life of octreotide following subcutaneous injection is approximately 113 min, requiring a dosing interval of approximately 6 to 8 hr to achieve sufficient GH suppression.[18,31] For acromegaly, a starting regimen of 200-300 μg/day divided into three doses is recommended, although resistant tumors may require up to 1500 μg/day.[31] Gradual loss of sensitivity to the drug may develop, necessitating increased doses to control clinical disease.[31]

Common adverse reactions include pain at the site of injection. This can be lessened if the syringe is warmed by rubbing prior to injection and if a smaller volume with a higher concentration of Sandostatin is used. Other adverse reactions include crampy abdominal pain, diarrhea, abdominal bloating, flatulence, and steatorrhea. These gastrointestinal effects are transient, usually resolving within several weeks. They occur due in large part to the hypomotility effects of Sandostatin on the smooth muscle of the intestinal tract. Through a similar mechanism in addition to fat malabsorption, cholelithiasis may also occur.[32] Although native somatostatin will significantly inhibit insulin release, octreotide has less of an inhibitory effect on the ß cell.[5] Patients with acromegaly taking octreotide often demonstrate improved glucose tolerance and diminished hyperinsulinemia because of lower GH levels.[31] Our patient provides an excellent example of this improvement of severe insulin resistance and hyperglycemia following control of GH secretion with Sandostatin. Patients who develop non-insulin-dependent diabetes mellitus after prolonged therapy respond to oral sulfonylurea drugs.[31] No long-term adverse effects of octreotide therapy have, to date, been found.

Octreotide is a powerful and versatile agent which provides effective treatment in conjunction with other conventional therapies, or when other therapies have failed. It provides an important option in controlling the disabling and fatal disease of acromegaly.

References

1. Asa SL, Scheithauer B, Bilbao J: A case for hypothalamic acromegaly: A clinicopathological study of six patients with hypothalamic gangliocytomas producing GHRF. J Clin Endocrinol Metab. 58:796-803, 1984.
2. Warner B, Santen R, Page R: Growth hormone and prolactin secretion by a tumor of the pharyngeal pituitary. Arch Intern Med. 96:56-68, 1982.
3. Melmed S, Ezrin C, Kovacs K: Acromegaly due to secretion of growth hormone by an ectopic pancreatic islet-cell tumor. Engl J Med. 312:9-17, 1985.
4. Melmed S, Ziel F, Braunstein G: Medical management of acromegaly due to ectopic production of GHRH by a carcinoid tumor. J Clin Endocrinol Metab. 67:395-399, 1988.
5. Barkan A: Acromegaly:Diagnosis and therapy. Endocrinol Metab Clin North Am. 18(2):277-310, 1989.
6. Ashcraft M, Hartzband P, Van Herle A: A unique growth factor in patients with acromegaloidism. J Clin Endocrinol Metab. 57:272-276, 1983.
7. Billestrup N, Swanson LW, Vale WW: Growth hormone-releasing factor stimulates proliferation of somatotrophs in vitro. Proc Natl Acad Sci USA. 83:6854-6857, 1986.
8. Berelowitz M, Szabo M, Frohman L: Somatomedin C mediates growth hormone negative feedback by effects on both the hypothalamus and the pituitary. Science. 212:1279-1281, 1981.
9. Dieguez C, Page M, Scanlon M: Growth hormone neuroregulation and its alterations in disease states. Clin Endocrinol 28:109-143, 1988.
10. Dieguez C, Page M, Peters J, et al: Growth hormone and its modulation. J R Coll Physicians London. 22(2):84-91, 1988.
11. Barkan A, Stred S, Reno K, et al: Increased growth hormone pulse frequency in acromegaly. J Clin Endocrinol Metab. 69:1225-1233, 1989.
12. Layton M, Fudman E, Barkan A, et al: Acromegalic arthropathy: Characteristics and response to therapy. Arthritis Rheum. 31(8):1022-1027, 1988.
13. Bloom S: Acromegaly. Am J Med. 82(suppl 5B):88-91, 1987.
14. Barkan A, Beitins I, Kelch R: Plasma insulin-like growth factor-I/somatomedin-C in acromegaly: Correlation with the degree of growth hormone hypersecretion. J Clin Endocrinol Metab. 67:69-73, 1988.
15. Lamberts S, Uitterlinden P, Schuijff P, et al: Therapy of acromegaly with Sandostatin: The predictive value of an acute test, the value of serum SmC measurements in dose adjustment and the definition of a biochemical "cure." Clin Endocrinol. 29:411-420, 1988.
16. Oyen W, Pieters G, Meijer E: Which factors predict the result of pituitary surgery in acromegaly? Acta Endocrinol. 117:491-496, 1988.
17. Lamberts S, Uitterlinden P, del Pozo E: SMS 201-995 induces a continuous decline in circulating growth hormone and somatomedin-C levels during therapy of acromegalic patients for over two years. J Clin Endocrinol Metab. 65:703-710, 1987.

18. Gorden P, Comi R, Maton P, Go V: NIH Conference: Somatostatin and somatostatin analogue (SMS 201-995) in treatment of hormone-secreting tumors of the pituitary and gastrointestinal tract and non-neoplastic diseases of the gut. Ann Intern Med. 110:35-50, 1989.
19. Barkan A, Kelch R, Hopwood N, et al: Treatment of acromegaly with the long-acting somatostatin analog SMS 201-995. J Clin Endocrinol Metab. 66:16-23, 1988.
20. Chiodini P, Cozzi R, Dallabonzana D, et al: Medical treatment of acromegaly with SMS 201-995, a somatostatin analog: A comparison with bromocriptine. J Clin Endocrinol Metab. 64:447-453, 1987.
21. Sandler L, Burrin J, Williams G, et al: Effective long-term treatment of acromegaly with a long-acting somatostatin analogue (SMS 201-995). Clin Endocrinol. 26:85-95, 1987.
22. Lamberts S, Verleun T, Hofland L, et al: A comparison between the effects of SMS 201-995, bromocriptine, and a combination of both drugs on hormone release by the cultured pituitary tumor cells of acromegalic patients. Clin Endocrinol. 27:11-23, 1987.
23. Reubi J, Landolt A: The growth hormone responses to octreotide in acromegaly correlate with adenoma somatostatin receptor status. J Clin Endocrinol Metab. 68:844-850, 1989.
24. Barkan A, Lloyd R, Chandler W, et al: Preoperative treatment of acromegaly with long-acting somatostatin analog SMS 201-995 shrinkage of invasive pituitary macroadenomas and improved surgical remission rate. J Clin Endocrinol Metab. 67:1040-1048, 1988.
25. Spinas G, Zapf J, Landolt A, et al: Preoperative treatment of 5 acromegalics with a somatostatin analogue: Endocrine and clinical observations. Acta Endocrinol. 114:249-256, 1987.
26 Barnard L, Grantham W, Lamberton P, et al: Treatment of resistant acromegaly with long-acting somatostatin analogue (SMS 201-995). Ann Intern Med. 105:856-861, 1986.
27. Sandler L, Burrin J, Joplin G, et al: Effect of high dose somatostatin analogue on growth hormone concentrations in acromegaly. Br Med J. 296:751-752, 1988.
28. Moller D, Moses A, Jones K, et al: Octreotide suppresses both growth hormone (GH) and GH-releasing hormone (GHRH) in acromegaly due to ectopic GHRH secretion. J Clin Endocrinol Metab. 68:499-504, 1989.
29. Melmed S, Ziel F, Braunstein G, et al: Medical management of acromegaly due to ectopic production of growth hormone-releasing hormone by a carcinoid tumor. J Clin Endocrinol Metab. 67:395-399, 1988.
30. Kvols L, Buck M, Moertel C, et al: Treatment of metastatic islet cell carcinoma with a somatostatin analogue (SMS 201-995). Ann Intern Med. 107:162-168, 1987.
31. Lamberts S: A guide to the clinical use of the somatostatin analogue SMS 201-995 (Sandostatin). Acta Endocrinol Suppl. 286:54-66, 1987.
32. Battershill P, Clissold S: Octreotide: A review of its pharmacodynamic and pharmacokinetic properties, and therapeutic potential in conditions associated with excessive peptide secretion. Drugs. 38(5):658-702, 1989.

Index

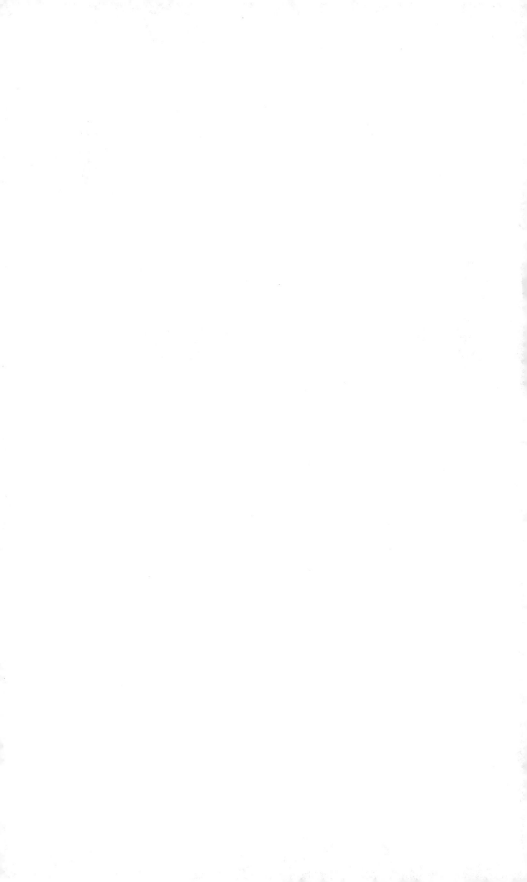

CPSIA information can be obtained
at www.ICGtesting.com
Printed in the USA
LVHW051255080622
720765LV00004B/94

9 780306 436840